clean
cuisine

clean
cuisine

an 8-week
anti-inflammatory
nutrition program that
will change the way you
age, look & feel

ivy ingram larson and
andrew larson, md, facs, fasmbs

BERKLEY BOOKS, NEW YORK

THE BERKLEY PUBLISHING GROUP
Published by the Penguin Group
Penguin Group (USA) Inc.
375 Hudson Street, New York, New York 10014, USA
Penguin Group (Canada), 90 Eglinton Avenue East, Suite 700, Toronto, Ontario M4P 2Y3, Canada
(a division of Pearson Penguin Canada Inc.) • Penguin Books Ltd., 80 Strand, London WC2R 0RL,
England • Penguin Ireland, 25 St. Stephen's Green, Dublin 2, Ireland (a division of Penguin
Books Ltd.) • Penguin Group (Australia), 707 Collins Street, Melbourne, Victoria 3008, Australia
(a division of Pearson Australia Group Pty. Ltd.) • Penguin Books India Pvt. Ltd., 11 Community
Centre, Panchsheel Park, New Delhi—110 017, India • Penguin Group (NZ), 67 Apollo Drive,
Rosedale, Auckland 0632, New Zealand (a division of Pearson New Zealand Ltd.) • Penguin Books,
Rosebank Office Park, 181 Jan Smuts Avenue, Parktown North 2193, South Africa • Penguin China, B7
Jiaming Center, 27 East Third Ring Road North, Chaoyang District, Beijing 100020, China

Penguin Books Ltd., Registered Offices: 80 Strand, London WC2R 0RL, England

This book is an original publication of The Berkley Publishing Group.

While the author has made every effort to provide accurate telephone numbers and Internet addresses at the time of publication, neither the author nor the publisher is responsible for errors, or for changes that occur after publication. Further, the publisher does not have any control over and does not assume any responsibility for author or third-party websites or their content.

Every effort has been made to ensure that the information contained in this book is complete and accurate. However, neither the publisher nor the author is engaged in rendering professional advice or services to the individual reader. The ideas, procedures, and suggestions contained in this book are not intended as a substitute for consulting with your physician. All matters regarding your health require medical supervision. Neither the author nor the publisher shall be liable or responsible for any loss or damage allegedly arising from any information or suggestion in this book.

The recipes contained in this book are to be followed exactly as written. The publisher is not responsible for your specific health or allergy needs that may require medical supervision. The publisher is not responsible for any adverse reactions to the recipes contained in this book.

The opinions expressed in this book represent the personal views of the authors and not of the publisher.

CLEAN CUISINE

Copyright © 2013 by Ivy Larson and Andrew Larson, MD, FACS
Jacket design by Judith Lagerman
Jacket photograph © Maks Narodenko / Shutterstock
Book design by Pauline Neuwirth

Clean Cuisine® is a registered trademark of Flourishing Health, Inc.

FIRST EDITION: February 2013

ISBN: 978-0-425-25285-7

An application to register this book for cataloging has been submitted to the Library of Congress.

PRINTED IN THE UNITED STATES OF AMERICA

10 9 8 7 6 5 4 3 2 1

To our dear son, Blake.
We are so very proud of the young man you are turning out to be.
We love you.
Mom and Dad

CONTENTS

FOREWORD

by natalie morales

I'm an enormous believer in the principles behind Clean Cuisine. Providing my body with the best and most nutritious options without having to sacrifice flavor is important to me. We are all aware of the news lately, how the nation as a whole has packed on the pounds and how we have one of the highest childhood obesity rates because we are feeding ourselves and our kids more and more processed foods that fill us with empty calories and excess sugar, nitrates, saturated fats, and sodium. It's enough to literally make you sick to your stomach!

As a television news anchor I have spoken with a lot of people about many different subjects. One of the focal topics of these conversations is health. I know people today are actively looking for a sustainable way of eating that does not require extreme dieting or deprivation. People want to learn how to change their bodies. They want to look and feel better, both inside and out.

As a working mom and athlete with a grueling schedule, what I eat is critical to help me have enough energy to power me through the day. I also want to share with my family and friends the healthiest choices that will appeal to even my youngest kids' difficult tastes. What Clean Cuisine is—it's a lifestyle that will make you feel and look better in just days. This book offers you a good start to get you and your family on the path to a healthier way of living and being.

Natalie Morales
News anchor of NBC News' *Today*
Cohost of *The Third Hour*

INTRODUCTION
A Tale of Life, Love, Food, and Lasting Good Health

Ivy

I know when people look at me today it is hard for them to imagine I have ever had a worry in the world. And for the first two decades of my life I truly was happy, healthy, and carefree. But, as you will read in just a bit, my life has not always been picture perfect. But let's start with the good old days . . . and food.

I was born in 1976 to a loving family with a stay-at-home mom who cooked a "square meal" every night of the week. My parents were health conscious for their time; Dad was an avid exerciser and Mom never brought processed foods into our house. In fact I still remember Mom sending me to preschool with a box of raisins as a substitute for the Oreo cookie snack the teacher gave the rest of the kids. My parents were far ahead of the game because at least they made a sincere effort to care about nutrition. In retrospect I know we could have done even better; they just weren't exposed to the best information.

My parents believed a healthy balanced meal meant eating from the four food groups, which meant a serving of meat, a starch, and a vegetable (iceberg lettuce counted) with every meal. Milk was also encouraged (it was believed to build strong bones), and dessert would typically be ice cream or some sort of fruit crisp concoction. Although dieting was never done in our house, occasionally my parents would hear about a trendy health fad and might even hop on the bandwagon. One of their doctors was a marathon runner, and I remember him getting my parents on a big pasta energy kick. I also still remember my mom and dad arguing about whether it was healthier to eat butter or margarine; Mom was convinced anything artificial like margarine couldn't possibly be healthy, but Dad had high cholesterol and was firmly convinced margarine was the superior substitute for artery-clogging butter. I now know they were both wrong, but Mom was less wrong than Dad!

Certainly the homespun meals and the foods I ate were better from a nutritional standpoint than the fast-food pizza and snack-food dinners many of my friends ate, but I now know and my parents now realize the food I ate growing up and the foods my parents thought were healthy could have been even better. Still, despite not eating the absolute best diet in my childhood and teens I was relatively healthy. I was also extremely active, athletic, lean, and fit. And, admittedly, when I was out of Mom's sight I pretty much ate what I wanted. Sweets were, and still are, my vice so I can assure you I had my fair share of sweet treats when I was out of the house.

Not only did I not have an understanding of nutrition, I actually believed the only people who needed to watch their diets were people who were overweight, had heart disease, or had diabetes. If you didn't have these old-person medical conditions, which I didn't, I figured you were home free and could pretty much eat what you want . . . as long as you exercised. And exercise I did! I thought exercise was the ultimate elixir for good health. My motto was Exercise and You Can Eat Whatever You Want!

Andy

I grew up in a wonderful family environment where hard work was encouraged and rewarded. We were thrifty, and because of this we were ultimately able to live quite well. I don't remember eating at a restaurant until I was nearly twelve, save for the very occasional fast food and, perhaps, a get-together for the extended family. Consequently, the food I did eat was also relatively healthful, though as I now know certainly not perfect. Ivy chides me now for having eaten Cheerios for breakfast every morning, but at least I ate them without milk!

As I started driving and got further into high school my diet declined . . .

much more fast food, much more fried food, fewer balanced meals, foot-long white bread subs. I gained over twenty pounds by the time I graduated high school. It took a concerted effort to lose the weight my freshman year of college. I mostly kept it off the next few years by cutting down on the fast food and exercising portion control, but this seemed to be more challenging with each passing year. I wondered if there might be an easier way to stay healthy; perhaps they would teach me in medical school. By late 1998, I was close to graduating but I never gained more than a passing knowledge of nutrition, mostly specialized stuff, such as learning how to feed burn patients intravenously and things like that. As you will see, to my great and lasting benefit, my high school friend (really, my sweetheart) gave me the motivation to learn the secret to healthful living for myself and ultimately for the benefit of tens of thousands of readers, patients, clients, and friends.

Ivy

My entire view on food and the trajectory of my life changed in the summer of 1998. I was twenty-two years old, had just acquired my American College of Sports Medicine fitness instructor certification and was excited to be working in a hospital wellness center as an exercise specialist. I was working with clients who had fibromyalgia, arthritis, heart disease, osteoporosis, and many other degenerative conditions. While trying to develop an exercise prescription for these patients I distinctly remember thinking to myself that if these people had just exercised more in the first place they could have avoided their health issues. I actually believed this.

It wasn't long before I began to feel sick myself. It started with embarrassing episodes of incontinence and extreme bladder urgency. I was waking up in the middle of the night six or seven times to go to the bathroom. I felt the urge to go every fifteen minutes in the middle of the day and soon was literally planning my days around access to a toilet. I was having overwhelming exhaustion, a fog overwhelmed my thoughts, and numbness crept down my right leg. My right thigh muscle would spasm so severely I could see the muscles twitch for hours on end. I developed a weakness in my right leg that made it difficult for me to use my hip flexors to raise my knee. My right foot would suddenly give out as I was walking, and I'd stumble for no reason. I visited three doctors but none had a clue what was wrong. I then had a very scary medical emergency, an episode of urinary retention where I couldn't go to the bathroom at all. I ended up in the ER and left wearing a catheter. This doctor correctly informed me something was seriously wrong, and he urged me to go to the University of Miami to obtain a diagnosis.

At the University of Miami I was first seen by a urologist and then by a neurologist. After an extensive and exhausting series of bladder tests and MRIs of my brain and cervical spine the neurologist, Dr. William Sheremata, sat me down, with my parents in the room, to tell me the most terrifying thing I had ever been told. He said I was in the early stages of multiple sclerosis (MS). At this point my thoughts went into a complete tailspin. I was certain a diagnosis of MS meant I would end up in a wheelchair. I wouldn't be able to walk; I'd never get married or have children. I was convinced my life was over. Dr. Sheremata calmly explained what MS was and what I could expect. In one visit I learned more about MS than I cared to learn. I learned MS changes your brain in a way that can cause depression, anxiety, impaired memory, and loss of mental clarity; in addition, there are physical symptoms, including impaired vision, paralysis, inability to swallow, and loss of bladder or bowel control.

My neurologist said I had the option of going on one of a few disease-modifying medications available to treat MS at the time, I could enter a trial to test a new drug, or I could try changing my diet. I was told about Dr. Roy Swank's research and his book, *The Multiple Sclerosis Diet Book,* and I was told that MS is a disease that is made worse by inflammation but can often be made better by adopting a nutrient-dense, anti-inflammation diet. The way I understood it, the diet wouldn't cure the disease but neither would the medication. The medications were contra-indicated during pregnancy—so I knew they had to be some heavy-duty drugs—and also came with very serious side effects, including suicidal ideation. I was already struggling with episodes of depression, and I can tell you right now, I did *not* want to take medication. I was so confused, and I was so scared.

To say that period of time was a low point in my life would be a drastic understatement. As I struggled to accept the fact that I had been given a life-changing diagnosis, I managed to remain hopeful that somehow, someway I would have as normal a life as possible. But I also knew I couldn't just ignore the diagnosis. I had to do *something.* Of the options I had been given, the change in diet appealed to me the most. The biggest obstacle at first, to be honest, was I just couldn't imagine how a change in diet could really be powerful enough to improve *my health* considering I wasn't overweight, I didn't have diabetes, I didn't have heart disease, and I was exercising all the time.

I trusted my neurologist and eventually learned he was considered among the top in his field, but I still felt I needed a second opinion. It was within days of my diagnosis that I called Andy to ask whether he thought changing my diet would be the best first step. I didn't have any close family doctor friends to call, and Andy was the only person I knew who was in medical school at that time. He wasn't at just any medical school; he was at the University of Pennsylvania, one of the top three medical schools in the country. Besides, I trusted Andy and I knew he was incredibly smart. I just prayed he knew, or at least had the training and patience necessary to research, whether a change in diet could in fact help me.

Andy

I was shocked and saddened to hear about Ivy's diagnosis, but perhaps even more shocked to hear her neurologist would suggest dietary modi-fication as a means of treatment. I was vaguely aware that some people could lower their cholesterol level with diet and I knew you needed extra nutrition if you were in the burn unit, but I had never been exposed to treating something like MS with food. Ivy seemed strongly encouraged and intrigued by that approach so I spent an entire weekend researching MS and diet belowground at the university's medical library; I still wasn't quite up to speed with the Internet! Later, I flew down to Miami to meet with Dr. Sheremata, who I came to realize was one of the world's foremost authorities on MS; he was a full professor and had authored more than sixty scientific papers at that time.

I concluded Ivy should absolutely change her diet because the research was clear, crystal clear. I remember the research on diet being too over-whelming to ignore. I remember feeling cheated that I had to learn the facts about the correlation between diet and disease on my own. As a result of Ivy's phone call and that one weekend at the library, I remember being excited and motivated to read abstract after abstract and article after article proving the benefit of diet for the treatment of a constellation of conditions, ranging from MS to cancer to heart disease to chronic fatigue syndrome.

The more we learn about MS and other chronic diseases the more we learn that the brain, and body, is constantly remodeling itself. For example, in MS patients, the brain has a significant reserve capacity that it can use to repair itself. Activities that exercise your brain and body (such as our fitness program in Chapter 8) appear to be critical to the development of the cognitive reserve needed to work around the areas of damage caused by MS. In fact, an important emerging theory is that disease progression in MS happens because the brain is no longer able to repair itself. On average, you renew about 1 percent of the cells in your body daily, and those new cells come in either stronger and younger or weaker and older; your overall lifestyle plays a tremendous role in cell regeneration—for better or worse. Exercising regularly and giving your body the right nutrients, eating anti-inflammatory and antioxidant foods, and eating the right types of fats (especially the omega-3 fats) all work to keep your brain flexible and fluid, giving it the edge it needs to manage MS. And of course MS isn't the only disease that can benefit tremendously from lifestyle choices!

Ivy embraced what she called *nutritional therapy* wholeheartedly; she promptly changed the way she ate. She also used her fitness background to develop a workout program to keep her strong. Her diagnosis brought the two of us together; no longer just good friends, we were married a year and a half later. Our son, Blake, was born one year after that. By this time Ivy had radically changed her diet and regained her health. Knowing what I now know, and having Ivy's help to make the great meals, I too dramatically changed my diet. I was no longer eating hospital food but instead was eating "Ivy food." I lost the extra weight for good and have not had to exercise painful portion control since. I'm prone to high blood pressure and have kept this in check as well. By the time our son was born Ivy and I were both 100 percent committed to her diet. Blake has known only healthful eating. He is now eleven and has taken antibiotics just once in his life. Last year he was one of only six kids in his one-hundred-person grade to earn the Presidential Physical Fitness Award.

Ivy

I am now in my mid-thirties and remain in wonderful health. As you will read more in Chapter 8, by far my greatest health problem has actually *not* been MS but instead a congenital hip disorder called *femoral retroversion* in which my femoral head was angled twenty-two degrees off normal. The hip issue was misdiagnosed for years, and resulted in significant pain for over a decade. I had two major surgeries, including a femoral derotational osteotomy during which my thigh bone was broken in half and the shaft was rotated to put my femoral head in the normal position; then I went through extensive rehabilitation for more than a year. People always hear about my MS and think that the diagnosis sounds so terrible and so scary, but for me, the hip ordeal has been much, *much* worse. I tried every non-invasive, nonsurgical alternative therapy under the sun for my hip. You name it, I tried it. And nothing worked. It was very depressing because until I got the proper diagnosis I really didn't have control over the issue—or the pain. The type of workouts I outline in Chapter 8 helped me stay strong and lean for years without putting strain on my hip or other joints, but they still didn't fix the underlying orthopedic abnormality of my femur (or the pain.) But compared to the hip ordeal, I have always felt much more in control of the MS diagnosis because I really did see a significant change in how I felt simply by changing my diet and my lifestyle. I know there is no surgery that can be done to cure MS, and I know the medications on the market today are suboptimal, but at least I feel like the lifestyle choices I make have an impact. And for me, this is comforting and reassuring.

With the MS in remission and my hip issues behind me, I now have the luxury to start worrying just a little bit about those things the stereotypical metro-Miami thirty-something starts to fret about. Aging, for one. Gladly, I can say without a doubt that the dietary habits I have adopted over the last fourteen years and the nonimpact strength training programs I did to help compensate for my hip problems have made a tremendous difference in the way I age. And, of course, the way I age absolutely affects the way I look. I have exercised consistently and have been conscious of what I eat for over a decade, and I am a firm believer the lifestyle you lead and the food you eat are the most powerful factors in optimizing health, boosting energy, slowing the aging process, and improving appearance.

The older we get the more our lifestyle choices are most blatantly apparent in our appearance. There is no greater beauty truth than the old saying that at age twenty you get the face you were born with but at age fifty you get the face you deserve. It's pretty darn hard to look good at age fifty if you aren't leading a healthy lifestyle. If you've ever noticed the sallow, wrinkled skin of a smoker or the complexion of a junkaholic, you've seen for yourself the signs of premature aging, and that's just on the outside!

Andy

Dietary phytonutrients, beneficial substances found only in plant-based foods, and antioxidants help us age slower and feel and look better. Nutrition scientists now know how specific molecules affect precise functions of certain cells in our body, and we know for a fact that eating a nutrient-dense, anti-inflammation diet based on unrefined whole foods with a hearty emphasis on plant foods is healthy for everyone. The science to back this up is just irrefutable.

Two diets strongly associated with longevity and decreased disease burden, the traditional Japanese diet and the Mediterranean diet, are similar in that they are both notable for their favorable omega-3 to omega-6 fat balance (at least in part as a result of their both including moderate amounts of fish), their emphasis on vegetables, their near total exclusion of refined and processed foods made with omega-6-rich vegetable oils such as corn oil and cottonseed oil, and their relatively minimal reliance on milk and meat. Those of you who are familiar with these diets will notice Clean Cuisine is similar, yet places even more emphasis on eating a fruit- and vegetable-forward, plant-strong plate and on obtaining all carbohydrates from *unrefined* sources (for example, insisting on brown rice and whole grain pasta instead of white rice and traditional pasta).

Our work is based on human studies and human epidemiology, the study of cause and effect as it relates to human health and disease, and is sourced back in numerous locations throughout this book to the primary scientific literature. If something makes a rat live longer but hasn't been tested on people, then you won't find that recommendation in *Clean Cuisine*. The concept of nutrient density—getting more nutrition per calorie eaten—is heavily emphasized. Given the realities of industrial agriculture and mass-produced meat, we place special emphasis on organic foods when necessary. We fervently believe genes are not your destiny. The science that studies how the food we eat affects the way our genes express themselves is called nutrigenomics. Based on this philosophy, the food you eat provides the building blocks for your body: You actually do become what you eat. Certain foods create a youthful, energetic, lean, and disease-proof body whereas other foods do the exact opposite. The foods you eat can actually communicate with your cells, and your cells behave the way the food you eat tells them to. Nutrigenomics puts the power in your own hands to change the way you age, look, and feel. Regardless of your current state of health, without regard to your genetic makeup, you can make the choice to eat foods that nourish your body, reduce inflammation, slow aging, and protect against disease.

Clean Cuisine can greatly minimize some of the biochemical mechanisms, including free-radical-induced cellular damage, that lead to disease and premature aging. The study of nutrition is rapidly evolving, and many progressive mainstream medical doctors are starting to take notice. Although nutrition is still not emphasized in medical school, nutritional epidemiology is taking hold as an entire discipline devoted to the study of connections among nutrition, disease, and health. Thousands of studies and evidence-based medicine link poor nutrition to disease and accelerated aging. The medical community is no longer ignoring the proof.

The lifestyle you lead and the foods you eat greatly affect the health of your very own lifelines, your blood vessels. Your blood vessels supply nourishment to your skin, and if your blood vessels are in poor health you can rest assured you will look, and feel, older than your years. A few factors that keep your blood vessels young and the many organs that depend on blood flow healthy are reducing blood pressure, reducing inflammation, reducing certain species of cholesterol in your blood, and reducing the propensity of the fats in your blood to oxidize. Our Clean Cuisine lifestyle accomplishes all of these goals.

The problem for many of us in the medical community is we don't have a pill to prescribe that changes the way you age, look, and feel so patients must take their health into their own hands. Unfortunately, the reality is that the way medicine is set up today does not allow physicians the time to educate their patients on how to optimize their health. The other reality is that taking care of yourself by eating clean, exercising, and living healthfully requires a commitment, but it's a commitment to yourself that pays big dividends. Although it is never too late to start the Clean Cuisine lifestyle, an ounce of prevention is worth a pound of cure. In many ways, Ivy's MS diagnosis was one of the best things that happened to her; it happened at a relatively young age, and I believe the dietary changes she made in her early twenties are the reason she is aging so beautifully now.

Ivy

Adopting our Clean Cuisine lifestyle works on many levels to reduce inflammation, improve the clarity of your skin, boost your energy level, lift your mood, and as Andy can explain, even change your blood work. Antioxidant- and phytonutrient-rich Clean Cuisine foods even act as a form of edible sunscreen, helping prevent premature environmental- and sun-induced skin aging.

Clean Cuisine will also help you lose weight because the side benefit of improving health is attaining a healthy weight, without hunger I might add! If you are overweight, reaching a healthy weight is one of the greatest makeovers you can possibly treat yourself to. In fact, losing weight and ridding your body of excess fat are two of the most effective ways of removing toxins from your body; after all, toxins are stored in fat cells, so a toxin-free body is going to look a heck of a lot better than a toxin-laden body!

It doesn't matter who you are or how genetically blessed you are, food and staying fit matter on every level for all of us. Nobody is so genetically blessed that he or she can get away with eating poorly without negative consequences at some point. Nobody is so genetically blessed that he or she can get away without exercising either. I had a grandfather who lived well into his nineties and was skinny as a rail his whole life, but because he didn't exercise he had a hard time getting out of his chair. He died from the consequence of a fall that broke his hip. The thing is, it doesn't matter who you are, you have to eat healthy, and you have to exercise or there will be negative consequences. I know this sounds doom and gloom but it's the truth. I wish I had started eating clean in childhood. I'm glad I had the exercise habit early on because I know it's a hard habit to get into the older you get. However, it is never too late (or too early!) to eat healthy and exercise.

We've been personally following the prescription outlined in *Clean Cuisine* for years now, and as new research is published we add more healthy recommendations. When I learned about the health and cleansing power of green smoothies and started making them for Andy a couple years back, he joked that blending kale, frozen fruits, and powdered greens in a Vitamix might be going a bit too far. He worried I might be teetering toward fringe recommendations. But now, not only does Andy drink his greens but he *craves* them. Me too! And we are not the only ones either. Everybody who starts drinking greens regularly gets hooked. Once you start making certain diet changes you just feel too good to not continue.

It is true some of the recommendations you'll read in this book might not yet be mainstream, but that doesn't mean they are difficult or not enjoyable. One thing we have held firm to over the years is the fundamental belief that healthy living can and should be a joyful life. Andy and I believe restricting your diet and lifestyle too much is unhealthy. We have never nor will we ever encourage you to micromanage your diet; to measure or count your carbs, calories, and fat; to deny your hunger; or to ask you to calculate the ratio of macronutrients that provide the greatest weight loss. This sort of obsessive preoccupation with food and dieting is not the prescription for good health or a healthy mind.

As a certified food lover I can tell you eating good-tasting food is a top priority for me. I love everything about food—from writing about it to cooking it, shopping for it, and most important, eating it. I also love cooking for my husband and son, entertaining friends and family, and enjoying a glass of wine with dinner. The last thing I want to do is deprive myself or live a life of dietary austerity all in the name of health and life extension. My desire to live an enjoyable life, dine on great food, and enjoy wine with dinner while also trying to be as healthy as possible have led to the development of a new way of cooking and eating we call Clean Cuisine. I firmly believe food can be powerful medicine, but I also believe a good portion of the power of food comes from the enjoyment it provides. And I assure you eating healthful, nourishing food can be extremely pleasurable.

Andy

The only way a lifestyle program is going to be effective is if people actually do it. Both of us, Ivy in particular, are very motivated people when it comes to healthy eating but even we would be unable to follow an unnecessarily austere program. We feel firmly a lifestyle program cannot be overly strict or people just won't do it, and therefore it won't work. What we have done with the Clean Cuisine lifestyle is taken all of the available research and put together a program that is enjoyable and effective. Could you adopt a more extreme way of living? Sure thing! Will doing so substantially improve your health, energy, or appearance? Based on all the available science, that's highly doubtful. Our primary goal is life-enhancement; we want to enjoy our life maximally in every way possible. The Clean Cuisine lifestyle is strict when and where it counts most and lenient where it doesn't matter so much. It's a balanced lifestyle that will not decrease the pleasure in your life.

As a doctor, as a surgeon who specializes in treating severely overweight persons with a host of chronic conditions, I feel confident in promising that if you change your diet, you will change your health. The Clean Cuisine diet we recommend combats inflammation and eliminates malnutrition, twin pariahs that create disease, accelerate aging, and worsen preexisting conditions. Ivy and I have held numerous Health and Body Makeover Programs over the years, and I can tell you from the results we have had that if you adopt the Clean Cuisine diet you will truly be able to see measurable improvements in medical markers that are a proxy for good health: lower triglycerides, decreased blood pressure, reductions in CRP levels, and diminished body fat in as little as four or five weeks. If you have an inflammation-mediated condition such as asthma, fibromyalgia, or arthritis, you will also feel better and enjoy symptomatic improvement in as little as four to five weeks. These overlapping and far-reaching results trump what is offered by medications, without the negative side effects.

Clean Cuisine works to improve the way you age, look, and feel for all the reasons other popular diet plans don't. We offer sound science, no gimmicks. There is no deprivation, and you'll not leave the table feeling hungry. Clean Cuisine doesn't make you count calories or measure your food portions in little cups. It doesn't require the mathematical skills of an engineer. It makes food your ally, not your enemy. It meets your body's need for energy and nutrients and minimizes the risk of chronic disease. And, thanks to Ivy's creative recipe development, Clean Cuisine tastes incredible. Her exercise interest also pays off because her Full Fitness Fusion workout programs really are super time-efficient, tremendously effective, and absolutely not boring.

Although some physicians might argue it is neither practical nor convenient to advise patients to totally change their diet and lifestyle, I would argue it is neither practical nor convenient to consider the alternative. There is a relationship between poor nutrition and disease. If you ignore nutrition then the odds are stacked against you that you will get sick. And as Ivy can tell you, sickness is the ultimate inconvenience. It is absolutely not convenient to be obese and undergo weight-loss surgery, or to have coronary artery disease that requires bypass surgery. It is not convenient to need to take insulin injections on a daily basis to control diabetes, and it certainly is not convenient to suffer from a debilitating stroke or undergo chemotherapy for cancer. It is far more convenient, and more enjoyable I might add, to eat Clean Cuisine. Changing your diet and adopting the Clean Cuisine lifestyle requires a lasting change, but this is a change that will improve the way you age, look, and feel and will truly change your life.

From Both of Us

Clean Cuisine, the book, is an offshoot of our cleancuisine.com website, a site we started in September 2010. On the site we strive to provide a snapshot of our daily lives but we also realize sometimes a guide is more helpful than a snapshot. With this book we have done our best to simplify the science behind our recommendations as well as to lay out an eight-week roadmap that will help you clean up your diet and your lifestyle, without feeling overwhelmed or deprived. Think of Clean Cuisine as an eight-step, eight-week recipe for preserving youth, staying healthy, and enjoying delicious food. The Clean Cuisine lifestyle is not a quick fix, but it does work and it is doable.

Of course after the eight weeks we don't expect you will go back to your old ways, the idea is that you will continue eating and living clean. We also hope you will connect with us on our website so we can share more tips, recipes, and healthy product suggestions.

Keep in mind, we did not change our diets overnight, and we don't expect you to either. Think of adopting the Clean Cuisine lifestyle as a journey; it's something new, but it is also something exciting and life changing.

Wishing you and your family good health and happiness always.

Bon Appetit!

Ivy & Andy

Ivy Larson and Andy Larson, MD

PART 1

The Spirit of Clean Cuisine

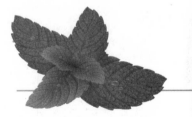

LAYING THE FOUNDATION
Whole Foods Nutrition

It is a wise man who knows what he is eating nowadays.
—HENRY T. FINCK (1913)

In no period of history have people been so preoccupied with the subject of nutrition as they are today. Yet, ironically, never before have we been so overweight and suffering such an alarming number of early-onset degenerative and inflammatory diseases. Modern medicine might keep us alive, but are we really *living*? Obesity, hypertension, multiple sclerosis, diabetes, gallstones, rheumatoid arthritis, asthma, osteoporosis, vascular dementia, and cancer are but a few of the diseases related to poor nutrition and inflammation. As a population do we *thrive* with good health? If you head to the closest airport, mall, or amusement park and take a picture of the people around you, you are not going to see a vibrant healthy-looking community. Instead, people simply look and feel much older than their years. Many of us are fat and sick. And the worst part is so many people think that being fat and sick is normal. It's not! Being fat and sick and looking and feeling older than your years doesn't need to be the norm. It is entirely possible to eat in a way that can slow aging and dramatically improve how you age, look, and feel. Best of all, we have a program that can help you look and feel like a million bucks *without feeling deprived.*

While it is true people are living longer thanks to modern medicine, the advancements we've made in medicine run parallel to the giant step

3

backward we've taken with our diets. Even our children are being affected. Just 100 years ago the obese child was an anomaly. Today, according to the Centers for Disease Control and Prevention (CDC), approximately 17 percent (or 12.5 million) of children and adolescents aged 2 to 19 years are obese. Since 1980, obesity prevalence among children and adolescents has almost tripled.[1] Human genes have not changed; what has changed is our diet. We do not eat real whole food anymore.

Our current diet patterns are a far cry from clean, and they certainly are not healthy. The average person eating the modern-day diet consumes way too many animal foods, too many calories, too much refined oil, too many refined carbohydrates in the form of sugar and refined flour, an abundance of processed junk foods, far too few vegetables, too little fiber, too few *true* whole grains (we're not talking crackers here), too few fat-soluble vitamins, too few essential fats, and far too few plant-based, disease-fighting phytonutrients. It's amazing anyone is healthy eating this way!

The animal-food-rich, processed-junk-food-rich standard American diet (SAD) most of us around the world eat today is making us fat and sick. A drastic dietary overhaul is in order. What is more, to meet the needs of a growing and increasingly busy world population, there is a need for a sustainable way of eating that doesn't require extreme measures, lengthy prep time, or gustatory deprivation and that can still change our bodies, both inside and out. It's time to clean our plates. Clean Cuisine is the long-term answer to eating for optimal health, disease prevention, weight loss, vitality, longevity, and good taste. Clean Cuisine will help change your life, and your body, one delicious bite at a time.

Clean Cuisine Is Based on *Real* Whole Foods

What is *real food*? Real food is nutrient-dense whole food found in its most natural and unrefined state.

Real food is also traditional, meaning it is produced and prepared more or less as it once was, long before factories and big companies started manufacturing inferior cheaply processed versions. Industrial food delivers pasteurized orange juice, enriched flour, and high fructose corn syrup—foods that are rich in calories and poor in overall nutrition. Eating industrial foods is the fastest way to expedite the aging process and get sick and fat simultaneously. In comparison, eating nutrient-dense, fresh, whole food is the simplest solution to staying young, healthy, slim, and disease free.

The whole foods our family eats and the whole foods that form the foundation of Clean Cuisine are as nutrient dense and close to their natural state as possible. We choose steel-cut oats over instant oatmeal. We eat apples (with the skin!) instead of commercially packaged applesauce. We drink whole orange juice made from whole orange segments including the fiber-rich and flavonoid-rich pulp, instead of commercial pasteurized orange juice. We eat corn on the cob instead of cornflakes. We choose sprouted whole grain bread made with a blend of unrefined whole grains, beans, and legumes instead of bread made with enriched and refined flour. The eggs we eat come from healthy pastured chickens, not chickens that were fed a diet that deviates from the natural diet chickens are supposed to eat. The small amount of beef we eat is from healthy pastured cows that live and eat the way nature intended. The two big ideas here are that first, the closer to nature your food, the more nutrient dense and the more healthful it will be and second, you can't separate the health of the animal from your own health.

Unlike the vast majority of highly processed foods filling today's supermarket shelves, whole foods are brimming with nutrients in a natural and bioavailable form that your body can actually recognize and use. *Real* nutrients from real whole foods will help keep your body younger and healthier. Because a nutrient deficiency can cause food cravings and interfere with your body's ability to burn fat, real nutrients from whole foods can also help you manage your weight. Some real nutrients, such as certain antioxidants, phytonutrients, and essential fats, are highly anti-inflammatory and can therefore help you control symptoms of inflammatory conditions such as multiple sclerosis, asthma, allergies, and fibromyalgia.

In contrast, your body can't necessarily assimilate or recognize the synthetic nutrients found in enriched, processed foods. The word *enriched* is actually a keyword telling you the food has been processed and refined. Start reading food labels, and you'll notice many manufacturers of breads, cereals, pastas, and so on actually promote the fact that their foods are enriched, as if it were a good thing! Keep in mind whole foods don't need to be enriched with synthetic vitamins and minerals because whole foods already contain these nutrients intact and in a bioavailable (usable) form!

Besides, *real* whole foods taste delicious and look beautiful *naturally,* so they don't need to be pumped with artificial flavors or food coloring either.

6

The *Cleanest* Cuisine Emphasizes More Plants, Less Meat

While whole foods are the foundation of Clean Cuisine, unrefined plant-based foods are lower on the food chain and can truly be considered the cleanest whole foods on earth. In addition to being whole-foods based, Clean Cuisine is also exceptionally plant forward. We aren't saying you need to be a vegan or even a vegetarian; as far as we know there are no traditional vegan cultures, and we certainly aren't vegans. We also know the vegan lifestyle can be extremely difficult to follow, especially if you want to eat a *nutrient-dense* and *anti-inflammatory* vegan diet (vegan cupcakes are not nutrient dense and aren't exactly going to boost anybody's health!). Instead, Clean Cuisine bridges the gaps among what we should eat, what tastes good, what is scientifically proven to be best for our bodies, and what is actually *doable* in the real world. Clean Cuisine aims to shrink America's carnivorous obsession via a reduced-animal-food diet that is nutrient dense, anti-inflammatory, and based on unrefined whole foods with an emphasis on unrefined plant-based nutrition. It is a medically sound way of eating that has the power to reverse diabetes, improve cholesterol and blood pressure, and ease the symptoms of other inflammatory diseases, such as fibromyalgia, asthma, allergies, and arthritis. Hunger-free weight loss is an inevitable side benefit of eating a plant-forward Clean Cuisine diet. Clean Cuisine unrefined plant foods are bulky and take up a lot of space in your stomach, so they work mechanically to help you stay full. Plant foods also are high-volume foods that stimulate your digestive system's distention nerves (stretch receptors) and send the memo to your brain to stop eating. By eating a whole foods diet filled to the brim with plenty of unrefined plant foods, you will give your body the nutrients it needs to fight fat, aging, and disease. It's just about that simple.

Certain plant foods in particular contain exceptionally few calories, yet they take time to eat and they take up quite a bit of room in your stomach. These foods have a low energy density. Vegetables are your best source of low energy density foods, and fruits are the second best source. Eating more vegetables and more fruits is fundamental to following Clean

Cuisine. This one dietary change alone is perhaps the safest, best way to achieve a healthy body weight without hunger and without creating a nutrient deficit while simultaneously optimizing health and protecting against disease. You absolutely do not need to eat smaller portions on Clean Cuisine; in fact, you should be eating *bigger* portions! If you eat big portions of fruits and vegetables, these low energy density foods will naturally and painlessly displace nutrient-poor calorie-rich foods like pretzels, ice cream, and hamburgers. On Clean Cuisine you will eat more, weigh less, and be exceptionally well nourished too.

Quenching Food Cravings

Having a full stomach is not the only factor that contributes to hunger-free weight loss. Extinguishing food cravings is every bit as important. Time and again we hear from Andy's patients that one of the main reasons they can't lose weight and can't stick to a healthy diet is because they are constantly experiencing food cravings. The bulk of the plant-forward Clean Cuisine diet comes from low energy density whole foods that are brimming with all sorts of nutrients that quench food cravings. We can't emphasize enough that keeping hunger and food cravings under control is a crucial factor in facilitating weight loss and improving health. Keep in mind, the malnourished body is hungrier than it needs to be, and it experiences unnecessary food cravings; if you are constantly hungry and your body is always fighting food cravings, you are at a high risk for gaining weight and acquiring degenerative disease. A body that is lacking in nutrients will also age faster. Even though many diets seem to focus more on the things you shouldn't eat, they really should be teaching you how to ramp up the nutrient intake of your food choices. Getting more nutrients into your diet is another fundamental concept central to Clean Cuisine. Eating more unrefined plants, less animal foods, and less processed foods is a simple and surefire way to maximize nutrition to lose weight and gain health!

Inflamed, Overfed, and Undernourished

It's hard to believe anyone could be malnourished living in the land of plenty. But the reality is that people who eat a modern diet of cheap, highly processed convenience foods are not getting the nutrients they need to thrive. Sure they might be getting calories, and too many at that, but they are not getting the nutrients needed to fight cancer, support a healthy metabolism, and look and feel their very best.

Malnutrition refers to "improper nutrition," not necessarily inadequate calorie intake. Even though plenty of people get more than enough calories to eat, they are getting the vast majority of their calories from packaged convenience items—fake foods that have actually had nutrients and even antioxidants destroyed during the refinement process. If you were to visit any modern family's home and peek inside the refrigerator or pantry, we bet you a hundred dollars to a nickel the vast majority of the foods you would find would not be whole foods, but rather processed and refined foods wrapped in brightly colored packages. Orange juice is a good example. Pasteurized pulp-free orange juice is not nearly as nutritious and contains less than 10 percent of the antioxidant vitamin C as is found in fresh whole orange juice, which can easily be made in a blender with whole orange segments and includes the flavonoid and fiber-rich pulp. Pasteurizing juice is done for safety reasons to keep bacteria from growing and to keep orange juice shelf stable for upward of a year. The problem is pasteurized orange juice is not only a concentrated source of fiber-free calories but is also devoid of enzymes and lower in flavonoids, antioxidants, and carotenoids compared to the fresh and raw whole juice alternative.[2] In the body, flavonoids and vitamin C work together, supporting health through their interaction. When the pulpy white part of the orange is removed in the processing of orange juice, flavonoids are lost too. This loss of flavonoids is one of the many reasons eating oranges in their whole food form or making completely whole orange juice is considerably healthier than just drinking the pasteurized orange juice you buy from the grocery store. In just about every scenario, anytime a food is manufactured for the purposes of extending shelf life, its nutrition deteriorates. As we'll discuss later, there are a few exceptions. Some traditionally fermented foods such as kimchee, natto, and sauerkraut actually contain more nutrients than the original product. These traditionally fermented foods are important exceptions.

As mentioned earlier, a body that is not properly nourished is going to be hungrier than it needs to be and is going to experience excessive food cravings. A false sense of hunger leads to overeating, and if the foods that are overeaten are nutrient poor and calorie dense, then weight gain is inevitable. It is probable that one of the reasons many women today find themselves gaining an excessive 60, 70, or more pounds during pregnancy is because they are not eating a nutrient-dense diet. Pregnancy is a time when a woman's body demands nutrients, and if nutritional needs are not met she will experience intense food cravings. Keep in mind, pregnancy does *not* drastically increase calorie needs, yet many women eating a modern-day diet of processed foods find it almost impossible to feel satisfied without overeating calories. It is not healthy for mom or baby to gain 60 plus pounds during pregnancy, but if mom is not getting the nutrition she needs from her food, she will ultimately overeat calories and gain too much weight in an effort to meet those needs. Whether you are pregnant or not, the best way to control your weight is by eating a nutrient-dense diet.

9

Inflammation is another problem intimately related to eating a highly processed, low-nutrient diet. Eating too many animal foods and too much animal-based saturated fat also increases inflammation. It is important to understand that inflammation per se is not intrinsically bad because it is actually part of the body's natural defense system against infection, toxins, and foreign molecules. Although a properly functioning immune system needs to be able to activate an inflammatory response, chronic, constant inflammation is not desirable. Chronic inflammation leads to pain, illness, and accelerated aging. It is the *chronic* inflammation that Clean Cuisine is designed to extinguish. Approximately half the people Andy sees in his medical practice are in a state of chronic inflammation. It is no surprise that so many of the degenerative diseases people suffer from in our modern world have chronic inflammation as the common thread. Seemingly unrelated conditions that affect millions of people, including Crohn's disease, heart disease, asthma, rheumatoid arthritis, ulcerative colitis, psoriasis, and multiple sclerosis, all have one common denominator: inflammation.

C-reactive protein (CRP) is a marker of inflammation that can be measured with lab testing. Physicians measure CRP to evaluate silent and nonsilent systemic inflammation. Silent inflammation may have no symptoms, but it still accelerates the aging process and contributes to disease. Nonsilent inflammation produces symptoms that can be seen by answering the questionnaire "Are You Inflamed, Overfed, and Malnourished?" on page 12. Another inflammation test is the high sensitivity C-reactive protein (hs-CRP), which can be used to measure cardiac inflammation and is widely used by cardiologists to help prevent and treat cardiovascular disease. These tests are valuable for physicians to better treat their patients, and we encourage you to proactively ask your healthcare provider to search for inflammation.

Although a lab measurement is most accurate, it is possible to gauge how much nonsilent inflammation is present in the body just by looking in the mirror. Visible symptoms of inflammation include puffy eyes, acne, enlarged pores, android (big belly, smaller thighs) fat distribution, and edema. Research also links obesity to inflammation. Because fat cells are metabolically active contributors to the inflammatory process, being overweight promotes inflammation. In a circular manner inflammation itself promotes the tendency toward weight gain in a dreadful vicious circle.

Inflammatory conditions have reached epidemic proportion, and they are a big boon for the pharmaceutical industry. Current mainstream medical treatments for blocking inflammation include steroid drugs and aspirin, ibuprofen, and other nonsteroidal anti-inflammatory drugs (NSAIDs). But in many cases these medications, especially steroids, are like taking a sledgehammer to your foot just to kill a red ant; the smashed foot is more likely to end up being a bigger problem than the red ant bite. The point is, all anti-inflammatory prescription medications have very serious side effects, and sometimes the side effects can be worse than the initial problem.

The good news is you can modify your body's inflammatory response and reduce the chronic low-grade inflammation that exacerbates inflammatory conditions simply by changing the foods you eat. This is because some foods are pro-inflammatory and other foods are anti-inflammatory. For example, omega-3 fish oil happens to have extraordinary anti-inflammatory properties. In fact, omega-3s can lower your level of interleukin 1 (IL-1), a marker of inflammation, by as much as 50 percent, a degree of suppression similar to that caused by some powerful drugs.[3] Even just increasing fiber intake by eating more plant foods lowers inflammation and C-reactive protein levels.[4] Food, as we have learned, is very powerful medicine.

By adopting the whole foods–based and plant-forward Clean Cuisine lifestyle and choosing anti-inflammatory foods over pro-inflammatory foods you can directly control the amount of inflammation in your body and simultaneously slow the process of aging. As a general rule, any food that causes inflammation is going to increase your risk of disease, promote obesity, and accelerate aging. Any food that is anti-inflammatory is going to do the exact opposite.

The Clean Cuisine Food Pyramid
An Easy Anti-Inflammatory Diet Guideline

Vegan Dark Chocolate
(60% cocoa)

Sweets, Flour,
Organic Pastured
Cheese

Wine

Extra Virgin Coconut Oil

Green or White Tea

Organic Pastured Beef, Lamb & Chicken

Garlic, Herbs, Ginger, Spices & Unsweetened Cocoa Powder

Organic "Whole" Soy
Edamame Beans, Tofu, Tempeh, Miso, etc.

Organic Pastured Eggs

Omega-3 Oils: Flax Oil, Walnut Oil, Hemp Oil
or
Monounsaturated Oils:
Extra Virgin Olive Oil, Avocado Oil, Macadamia Nut Oil

"Whole" Fats:
Raw Nuts, Raw Seeds, Hemp Seeds, Raw Nut Butters & Avocados

Wild Sea Omega 3:
Wild Fish and Shellfish

Vegan Omega 3:
Chia Seeds or Flaxseeds

Non-Flour "Whole" Grains & Sprouted "Whole" Grains
Brown & Black Rice, Barley, Quinoa, Millet, Oatmeal, etc.

Beans & Legumes

Starchy Vegetables
Sweet Potatoes, Potatoes, Corn, Butternut Squash, Peas, Parsnips

Large Raw Salad:
Dark Leafy Greens & Raw Veggies

Dark Leafy Greens (Cooked)

All Fruits
Bananas, Apples, Oranges, Acai, Blueberries, etc.

Non-starchy Vegetables (Lightly Cooked)
Rainbow of Colors— Peppers, Eggplant, Broccoli, etc.

ARE YOU INFLAMED, OVERFED, AND MALNOURISHED?

ANSWER YES or NO to the following questions. See the score sheet that follows for an interpretation.

- Do you have intense food cravings? ___N___
- Do you have acne, psoriasis, or eczema? ___N___
- Is your waist circumference more than 34 inches/91 cm (women) or more than 38 inches/102 cm (men)? _____
- Do you have frequent constipation, Irritable Bowel Syndrome, or Crohn's disease? ___N___
- Do you have puffy eyes? ___N___
- Do you have any autoimmune disease such as multiple sclerosis or rheumatoid arthritis? ___N___
- If so, do you have active symptoms? ___N___
- Do you have heart disease or have you ever had a heart attack? ___N___
- Do you have osteoarthritis? ___N___
- Do you have either fibromyalgia or chronic pain? ___N___
- Do you have diabetes? ___N___
- Do you have allergies? ___N___
- Do you have asthma? ___N___
- Do you eat fewer than 5 servings of fresh fruits and vegetables each day? ___N___
- Do you eat more than 2 servings of packaged, processed foods each day? ___N___
- Do you eat more than 2 servings of animal food other than fish (dairy, meat, eggs, chicken, etc.) each day? ___N___
- Do you ever eat packaged foods containing added vegetable oil other than olive oil (vegetable oil, cottonseed oil, soybean oil, canola oil, etc.)? ___N___
- Do you find it difficult to lose weight or to maintain your current weight? ___Y___
- Are you often fatigued? ___N___
- Have you ever been told you need to take cholesterol-lowering medication? ___N___

- Has your CRP level ever been abnormally high (other than when you had an active infection)? ___*N*___
- Do you require more than one medication to keep your blood pressure normal? ___*N*___

13

- Do you routinely suffer from more than one cold per year?

_____

- Have you ever been diagnosed with any kind of cancer?

___*N*___

- Do you have a disease that causes you to routinely take drugs called corticosteroids, such as prednisone? ___~___

SCORE SHEET

COUNT UP HOW many times you answered yes.

- 0–3 = probably not inflamed
- 4–7 = borderline inflamed
- 8–11 = moderately inflamed
- 12–16 = overinflamed
- 17–25 = severely inflamed

Excess Intake of Nutrient-Poor Calories Accelerates Aging

Clean Cuisine is rich in antioxidants and phytonutrients, substances that play a key role in disposing of free radicals. Most people who read about health and nutrition recognize free radicals are bad. The thing is they are much worse than you might realize, and minimizing them can do wonders to help you look and feel younger than your years. Free radicals cause oxidative damage to tissues, proteins, fat, and even your DNA. In fact, tissue damage by free radicals is thought to underlie the entire process of aging. The production of free radicals occurs during the natural process of metabolism in turning the calories from the food you eat and the oxygen from the air you breathe into usable energy by your body. The oxidative damage that occurs from free-radical production accelerates the aging process of every part of your body, including the visible parts like your skin and the behind-the-scenes organs and internal tissues. When free radicals are left to run amok they cause the oxidative damage that accelerates biological aging. Free-radical damage can also promote inflammation and has been associated with weight gain, a decreased sensitivity to insulin, diabetes, and heart disease. The single most important controllable factor in minimizing free-radical damage and oxidative stress is better attention to the foods you eat.

Antioxidants and certain phytonutrients (these are plant-based substances that have antioxidant properties) are some of your best anti-aging allies. They quench the oxidative fire by gobbling up free radicals. This means if you are eating a colorful whole foods diet rich in antioxidants and phytonutrients (think red berries, green leafy vegetables, yellow corn, purple grapes, and the like), the amount of free-radical production that occurs every time you eat is greatly minimized. If, on the other hand, you are eating a diet containing nutrient-poor empty calories (white bread, pretzels, and processed foods, for example) and eating too many animal foods, which are completely devoid of phytonutrients, you aren't giving your body the substances it needs to keep free-radical production in check. Free-radical production is made even worse by an excessive calorie load, which is almost impossible to avoid if you are eating anything other than a nutrient-rich whole foods diet. The more calories you eat, the more oxidative stress occurs simply because the process of metabolism itself generates free radicals. For this reason, increased calorie intake can in many cases cause you to age faster. As a side note, when you eat more whole foods, especially from plants, you feel full faster and naturally begin to eat fewer calories, reduce oxidative stress, and, yes, lose weight, too. Another problem with eating nutrient-poor foods is that certain vitamins and minerals found naturally in whole foods are necessary for your body to manufacture its own antioxidants. If you aren't getting a broad spectrum of nutrients from whole foods, you'll be shortchanging your body's natural ability to quench the free-radical fire.

In summary, the spirit of Clean Cuisine is to choose tasty, nourishing foods that enhance your health on many levels. In the next six chapters we are going to give you an in-depth education on exactly what real food is before we outline the 8-week Clean Cuisine program. We don't want to simply give you a program without providing an explanation for our recommendations because we feel motivation stems from education and an understanding of the why. We'll share the science behind why eating a plant-strong diet is one of your best anti-aging weapons. We'll explain in detail how to identify nutrient-dense and anti-inflammatory foods. We'll empower you to choose antioxidant-rich foods that will fight free radicals. In short, we'll show you how to use food to change the way you age, look, and feel. And we'll make sure you won't feel deprived at any step!

2

ALL CALORIES ARE NOT CREATED EQUAL
The Case for Micronutrients

Everything should be made as simple as possible, but no simpler.
—ALBERT EINSTEIN

To understand the concept of nutrient density we alluded to in the last chapter, it is important to understand the difference between macronutrients and micronutrients. *Macronutrients* are the calorie-containing substances that give us energy: carbohydrates, fats, and protein. The nutrition facts labels you see on food products can make it appear as though all carbohydrates, all fats, and all proteins were equal. This is not the case. There are good, healthful unrefined sources of carbohydrates, fats, and protein and then there are bad, unhealthful, and highly processed sources too. Whole grains, fruits, and vegetables are excellent sources of carbs; high fructose corn syrup, enriched or all-purpose flour, and white rice are poor sources of carbs. Raw nuts, flaxseeds, and avocados are good sources of fat; vegetable oil, butter, and shortening are bad sources. Fish, nuts, beans, seeds, and whole soy products (such as tofu and tempeh) are good sources of protein; isolated soy protein, hot dogs, milk, and cheese are not. The best sources of macronutrients are unrefined whole foods, primarily plant-based.

16   The *micronutrients* in food do not contain calories and do not directly provide energy, but they do play a tremendous role in optimizing health and even appearance. Micronutrients consist of vitamins, minerals,

antioxidants, and phytonutrients. Modern diets are highly deficient in micronutrients. Although it is true highly processed modern foods such as enriched flour and most breakfast cereals are often fortified with vitamins and minerals, such synthetic versions are not recognized or used by your body in the same way as naturally occurring vitamins and minerals. Synthetic nutrients are not nearly as bioavailable, or absorbable, as the real deal. For example, in nature, foods rich in vitamin E, such as avocados, spinach, sunflower seeds, wheat germ, nuts, and whole grains, contain vitamin E in the form of at least eight separate chemical compounds including a variety of mixed "tocopherols" and "tocotrienols." In its natural form, vitamin E is more than just one chemical; it is a mixture of beneficial chemicals. However, when foods are fortified with extra vitamin E the norm is to use a single-chemical synthetic form of vitamin E called DL-alpha-tocopherol. This form is also often found in cheap multivitamins and cheap vitamin E supplements. Studies show synthetic vitamin E in the form of DL-alpha-tocopherol is not handled by your body in the same way as is the natural vitamin E found in whole foods. There are many studies showing differential effects of each individual form of vitamin E in the body. In general it is known that gamma-tocopherol, a vitamin E found in many plant foods and plant seeds, inhibits inflammation, whereas alpha-tocopherol alone, the vitamin E most commonly included in supplements, does not. As a matter of fact, high doses of supplemental vitamin E in the alpha-tocopherol form can deplete your body of the naturally occurring gamma-tocopherol subtype of vitamin E and may have the net result of increasing inflammation and increasing the risk of chronic disease.

In addition, although processed foods may be fortified with a few vitamins, they are not fortified with all the other good things, such as antioxidants and phytonutrients, present in natural, whole foods. These good things are destroyed during food processing and are not added back. In fact, you can obtain phytonutrients, powerful anti-aging and anti-inflammatory substances, only from plant foods; they are not found in animal foods and only rarely can be obtained from supplements. Even if a food is fortified with an isolated phytonutrient or antioxidant, such as with a lycopene-fortified beverage, your body does not recognize or use the isolated substance in the same manner as it would if the nutrient had been ingested as part of a whole food. Without a doubt, food-sourced vitamins and minerals are superior to their laboratory-created counterparts.

Although vitamins, minerals, antioxidants, and phytonutrients are all lumped together under one category as micronutrients, there are several distinct differences. Vitamins and minerals are absolutely essential for life, whereas antioxidants and phytonutrients are not. While it is true you could probably survive for a while eating nothing but vitamin and mineral-fortified processed breakfast cereal or bread made with enriched flour, you certainly wouldn't *thrive* on such a diet! To thrive and enjoy vibrant health and a vibrant appearance you need a rich and steady supply of antioxidants and phytonutrients. And when it comes to *naturally occurring* antioxidants and phytonutrients, more is better. (It's important to note that with vitamins and minerals, especially when they are obtained from synthetic supplements or artificially fortified foods, more is often *not* better. In fact, if you get too many of certain vitamins or minerals, the effect can actually be dangerously toxic. However, toxicity resulting from an overconsumption of vitamins and minerals is next to impossible when whole foods are the source; the bulk and fiber in whole foods prevent overconsumption.)

A NOTE FROM DR. LARSON

WE ARE NOT saying we don't advocate or believe in any nutritional supplementation, because we do. We believe that even if you eat a nutrient-dense Clean Cuisine diet you can still benefit from select nutritional adjuncts. But you do need to be careful because not all supplements are helpful or even safe. We'll show you how to safely supplement your diet for maximum health benefits in Chapter 9 when we outline the 8-week Clean Cuisine program.

All Calories Are *Not* Created Equal

These are words you never thought you'd hear from the president of a $2.7 billion weight-loss empire. "Calorie counting has become unhelpful," David Kirchhoff stated on the Weight Watchers International website. "When we have a 100-calorie apple in one hand and a 100-calorie pack of cookies in the other, and we view them as being 'the same' because the calories are the same, it says everything that needs to be said about the limitations of just using calories in guiding food choices." We couldn't have said it better ourselves.

When calories are burned in a laboratory, they are indeed created equal, and the same amount of energy is released. In the lab, there is no difference between 500 calories of carrots and 500 calories of carrot cake. But don't be fooled; *your body* handles the calories from carrots and carrot cake very, very differently. Carrots and carrot cake are absorbed at completely different rates and have totally different amounts of nutrients, fiber, antioxidants, carbohydrates, fat, and protein, all of which affect health, weight, oxidative stress, hunger, and metabolic rate at the cellular level. The more nutrients per calorie you eat, in this case by choosing carrots over carrot cake, the better protection you'll have against disease and the slower you'll age. You'll also weigh less and be less hungry.

19

It's important to realize foods are so much more than just a source of energy. Try eating 1,000 calories of French fries and see how energetic you feel! The secret to having tremendous energy, what Ivy calls "zip, pep, and go!" is consuming the vast majority of your calories from unrefined, nutrient-dense plant foods. Plant foods flood your body with a plethora of anti-aging micronutrients. In addition, the nutrients in plant foods are more bioavailable (absorbable) than the nutrients in processed foods or animal foods. The quicker nutrients are extracted from your food, the sooner the food can be eliminated, and this is a key factor in optimizing health as well as eliminating the fatigue, bloating, and other unpleasant symptoms of poor digestion. A diet with lots of easily digested and easily absorbable micronutrient-rich plant foods will speed digestion and thus help reduce toxins from settling in your colon and infiltrating your body. Raw and low-temperature cooked plant foods are especially beneficial because their high enzyme content helps your body use the energy and nutrients in the food best. While you certainly don't need to eat all of your foods raw, it is a great idea for energy and health purposes to consciously increase your consumption of raw fruits and vegetables as well as raw nuts and seeds.

What is of utmost importance is getting enough nutrients. Contrary to what you might think, your brain—not your gut—plays the biggest role in your appetite, and your brain craves nutrients. If you starve your brain of nutrition you will experience a constant, nagging hunger that can lead you to over consume calories. And, as we see daily, even those patients and clients who have eaten thousands of extra empty calories and consequently weigh in excess of 100 pounds more than their ideal body weights are often still always hungry because the calories they eat are nonnutritive calories. When it comes to health and weight management, there's just no way around the fact that nutrients matter. Counting calories is a waste of time; you have to make your food count nutritionally if you want to look and feel your best and age slower.

We aren't the only ones who dispel the conventional wisdom to simply eat everything in moderation and just reduce total calories without paying attention to what those calories are made of. A federally funded analysis of data collected over 20 years from more than 120,000 U.S. men and women in their 30s, 40s, and 50s found striking differences in how various foods and drinks—as well as exercise, sleep patterns, and other lifestyle choices—affect whether people gradually gain weight or not.[1] This 2011 Harvard study was published in the prestigious *New England Journal of Medicine* and, although the study was not perfect by any means, it was a prospective investigation based on a large number of people followed over multiple 4-year periods and should absolutely make proponents of the Calories In, Calories Out mantra rethink their tune. After adjusting for age, baseline body mass index, and lifestyle factors such as exercise and sleep duration, the authors found that the foods most associated with adding pounds over a 4-year period were French fries, potato chips, sugary drinks, meats, sweets, and refined grains. The foods most associated with weight loss were yogurt, nuts, whole grains, fruits, and vegetables. The study showed some foods clearly cause people to put on more weight than others. The foods that cause the most *weight gain* are the ones that have the most calories with the fewest nutrients. It should be no surprise that the foods that cause the most *weight loss* are the ones with the most nutrients per calorie.

There are many factors involved in why all calories are not burned the same in our bodies as they are in machines that measures calorie content. It may be that calories packaged with nutrients, including antioxidants and phytonutrients, are just biochemically different from empty calories so our bodies process them differently. And when it comes to promoting health and slowing aging, slurping 100 calories of soda pop as opposed to 100 calories of the truly whole orange juice we talked about in Chapter 1 does offer a profound difference. We couldn't agree more with Dr. Mozaffarian from the Harvard School of Public Health who led the study: "All foods are not equal, and just eating in moderation is not enough."

Don't Count Your Food, Make Your Food Count!

We don't support counting calories nor are we supporters of "counting your food" in the form of measuring macronutrient content. We don't count carbs, fat grams, or proteins. As mentioned, even Weight Watchers, the largest diet company in the world, has finally acknowledged calorie counting does not work. Low-fat, low-carb, no-fat, and no-calorie foods are not the solution *but the problem*. Instead of asking you to try to precisely gauge how many carbohydrates are in your pasta or how many fat grams are found in a handful of nuts, we want to encourage you to first and foremost consume foods in their natural, whole form. Eating whole foods is the first step to eating clean; eating substantially more unrefined plant foods is the second step. Eating these unrefined plant foods gives you the most nutritional bang for your calorie buck.

As you'll learn throughout this book, plant foods are the richest source of micronutrients. Plant foods are also the *only source* of phytonutrients. Plant foods are the lowest on the food chain (meaning they have the fewest toxins) and contain the cleanest sources of macronutrients. You don't need to fear eating bananas because they have too much sugar; besides, as you'll learn later, bananas are one of the very best sources of healthful resistant starch. And regardless of what those of you familiar with the glycemic index fad might have been told, carrots are absolutely healthful and should certainly be a part of your Clean Cuisine diet. There is no reason to not eat brown rice and potatoes because they have too many carbs either. Raw nuts, raw seeds, and raw nut butters should not be feared for their fat grams. The point is, if the foods you eat are unrefined whole foods mostly from plant sources, you do not have to worry about counting your food. Once you get into the mind-set of trying to make every bite count from a nutritional standpoint, you can look beyond the carbohydrates, fat grams, and protein and focus instead on the quantity of healthful micronutrients delivered relative to the energy calories the food supplies.

Faulty Nutrition Facts Labels

We are a society obsessed with counting our food: We count our calories, carbs, fat grams, sodium, and so forth. And the existence of the Nutrition Facts on food labels helps perpetuate this obsession. One of the biggest mistakes people make when trying to eat healthfully or lose weight is they often turn to the Nutrition Facts for reference. In the United States the Food and Drug Administration (FDA) requires all packaged foods to include the Nutrition Facts on the food labels. *Note that fresh foods, like apples and oranges, do not need to include Nutrition Facts on the label.* Ironically the Nutrition Facts tell you absolutely nothing about the intrinsic health and nutrition properties of the food. A perfect example is the Lean Cuisine Baja-Style Chicken Quesadilla frozen entrée. If you were someone who liked to count your food in the form of calories, carbs, fat grams, fiber, and so forth and you were to rely totally on the Nutrition Facts then you might think this would be a good choice for a meal, with just 280 calories, only 7 grams of fat, and less than 6 percent of your daily allotment of cholesterol. But the reality is you're kidding yourself if you think eating this meal is going to reduce inflammation or help change the way you age, look, and feel for the better. We can assure you it won't help you full feel and it won't help you achieve lasting weight loss either.

Before we go further, take a look at exactly what is in the Lean Cuisine Baja-Style Chicken Quesadilla frozen entrée.

Ingredients in Lean Cuisine Baja-Style Chicken Quesadilla

Tortilla (Bleached Enriched Flour (Bleached Wheat Flour, Niacin, Reduced Iron, Thiamine Mononitrate, Riboflavin, Folic Acid), Water, Soybean Oil, Salt, Sugar, Sodium Bicarbonate, Sodium Aluminum Phosphate, Potassium Sorbate (A Preservative), Mono And Diglycerides, Calcium Propionate (A Preservative), Fumaric Acid, Sodium Metabisulfite (Dough Conditioner)), Corn And Black Bean Blend (Corn, Black Beans (Black Beans, Water), Poblano Chilies, Red Bell Peppers, Extra Virgin Olive Oil), Reduced Fat Mozzarella Cheese (Cultured Milk And Non-Fat Milk, Modified Corn Starch*, Salt, Vitamin A Palmitate, Enzyme. (*Ingredient Not In Regular Mozzarella Cheese)), Light Pasteurized Process Monterey Jack Cheese (Cultured Milk, Water, Potassium Citrate, Salt, Sodium Citrate, Whey*, Sorbic Acid, Cream, Enzymes, Sodium Phosphate, Lactic Acid (*Ingredient Not In Regular Pasteurized Process Monterey Jack Cheese)), Cooked White Meat Chicken (White Meat Chicken, Water, Seasoning (Salt, Flavorings, Maltodextrin, Modified Food Starch, Sugar, Autolyzed Yeast Extract, Flavor (Maltodextrin, Smoke Flavor), Spices, Caramel Color, And Citric Acid), Isolated Soy Protein, Modified Rice Starch, Chicken Flavor (Dehydrated Chicken Broth, Chicken Powder, Flavor, Salt), Sodium Phosphates), Light Pasteurized Process Cheddar Cheese (Cultured Milk, Water, Potassium Citrate, Salt, Sodium Citrate, Whey*, Sorbic Acid, Cream, Apo Carotenal And Beta Carotene Color, Enzymes, Sodium Phosphate, Lactic Acid (*Ingredient Not In Regular Pasteurized Process Cheddar Cheese)), Tomato Puree, Water, 2% Or Less Of Tomato Paste, Soybean Oil, Seasoning (Flavor (Autolyzed Yeast Extract, Chicken Powder, Maltodextrin, Flavoring (Contains Canola Oil), Grill (Contains Sunflower Oil)), Salt, Spices, Onion And Garlic, Lime Juice Powder (Corn Syrup Solids, Lime Juice Solids, Natural Flavor), And Jalapeño Powder), Corn Starch

This Lean Cuisine entrée is clearly not a clean and nutrient-dense choice when you see it has ingredients like modified corn starch, isolated soy protein, cream, soybean oil, and all sorts of preservatives. The problem is if you rely on the Nutrition Facts for guidance you could easily be fooled into thinking this is in fact a good choice. Not true.

The Nutrition Facts label is actually so difficult to interpret, the FDA publishes a 10-page-long, color-coded, and awfully complex guide that is supposed to help the public make smart choices. It's not working. The truth is, the Nutrition Facts label does not echo superior nutrition; rather, it is a reflection of what various government entities have agreed to say to keep the big food companies happy. Keep in mind it is highly profitable for food companies to include cheap, nutrient-poor, and highly processed ingredients such as corn syrup solids in their foods. If corn syrup is fat free and cholesterol free, it makes a good selling point on the Nutrition Facts label. If a food happens to have less than 0.5 gram of trans-fat, then a food manufacturer can claim it is trans-fat free on the Nutrition Facts label, another good selling point. These selling points are great for moving products off the shelves, but they aren't doing a thing to help people make the food choices that will improve their health or reduce the inflammation epidemic. In the case of trans-fats, even a teeny tiny bit matters, and if you eat a lot of packaged foods or you dare eat more than a single serving (does a normal person really eat only ¾ cup of cereal?) then the trans-fat can add up quick. Studies show a teeny-tiny increase of less than 3 grams of trans-fat a day is enough to result in an astounding 50 percent increase in heart attacks and deaths.[2] Bottom line, the Nutrition Facts label is influenced by forces other than science and tells you nothing about whether the food is nutrient dense.

THE MOST NUTRIENT-DENSE FOODS USUALLY DO NOT HAVE NUTRITION FACTS LABELS

AS MENTIONED IN this chapter, whole foods like apples and oranges don't have Nutrition Facts labels. Neither do carrots, kale, beets, radishes, corn on the cob, raspberries, blueberries, watermelon, tomatoes, spinach, onions, bananas, and red peppers. *All* fresh fruit and vegetables are among the most nutrient-dense foods in the world, and unless you buy them frozen or packaged—still healthful by the way—these nutritional all-star superfoods will not have the

Nutrition Facts label. Throughout this book you will learn all about which foods are in fact nutrient-dense and healthful and which ones are not. Then, instead of relying on the misleading Nutrition Facts you can read the ingredient list, find out exactly what is in your food, and make an informed and educated choice.

Ingredient Lists, on the Other Hand, Do Not Lie

Once you know how to distinguish between nutrient-dense whole foods and nutrient-poor refined foods, you will soon realize an astounding number of packaged foods are not healthful. But some are. Ezekiel 4:9 Sprouted 100% Whole Grain Bread made by Food for Life is a perfect example. This is a packaged food containing the following ingredients:

Ingredients in Food for Life Ezekiel 4:9 Sprouted 100% Whole Grain Bread

Organic Sprouted Whole Wheat, Filtered Water, Organic Malted Barley, Organic Sprouted Whole Millet, Organic Sprouted Whole Barley, Organic Sprouted Whole Lentils, Organic Sprouted Whole Soybeans, Organic Sprouted Whole Spelt, Fresh Yeast, Organic Wheat Gluten, Sea Salt.

Every single ingredient on the label is healthful and nutrient dense.

If you do buy packaged foods, the ingredients list is, without a doubt, the most important bit of information on the entire package. This means the ingredients list is more important than the total calories, total carbs, fat grams, fiber, sodium content, and cholesterol listed on the Nutrition Facts. As we move on to Part Two of this book, you'll gain a solid understanding of how to identify truly healthful ingredients.

Eat More (Plants), Weigh Less!

The China-Cornell-Oxford Project is considered a landmark study. In fact, the *New York Times* called it the "Grand Prix of all epidemiological studies" and "the most comprehensive large study ever undertaken on the relationship between diet and the risk of developing disease."[3] The study is analyzed in the bestselling book *The China Study*[4] and provides compelling evidence that a vegan diet causes an increased calorie burn after meals, meaning plant-based foods generate increased levels of cellular metabolism, as opposed to being stored passively as fat. In other words one can eat more calories worth of food yet weigh less by eating plant foods. The study showed that people living in rural China, even those who worked sedentary jobs, consumed significantly more calories per pound of body weight than did Americans with similarly sedentary lifestyles. But despite eating more calories, those Chinese who consumed a plant-based diet actually weighed less. The difference in body weight was not attributed to activity because the comparison was between average (not very active) Americans and the least active Chinese (office workers). Instead, the difference has primarily been attributed to thermogenesis, which is the generation or production of heat. The more heat generated, the more calories burned.

25

Research in the *American Journal of Clinical Nutrition* shows vegetarians by weight have a slightly higher rate of metabolism during rest, meaning they burn slightly more of the calories ingested as body heat rather than depositing them as body fat.[5] In the case of the China Study, the average calorie intake per kilogram of body weight was 30 percent higher among the least active Chinese than among the average American, yet body weight was 20 percent lower in the Chinese. We cannot say with certainty why such a difference exists in body weight between the rural Chinese and Americans. What we do know is that vegetarian populations tend to be slimmer than those that are heavy meat eaters, and they also experience lower rates of heart disease, diabetes, high blood pressure, and other life-threatening conditions linked to overweight and obesity.

In addition to the findings from the China Study, a study of more than 55,000 Swedish women showed meat eaters are more likely to be overweight than are vegetarians or vegans.[6] The results are similar in the United States. The type of vegetarian you are also seems to matter. A study population made up of 22,434 men and 38,469 women in the Adventist Health Study 2 showed that the mean body mass index (BMI), a measure of weight that also factors in height, was lowest in vegans and incrementally higher in lacto-ovo vegetarians, pesco-vegetarians, semi-vegetarians, and nonvegetarians.[7] The difference in this study was substantial enough for its authors to conclude that a vegan or vegetarian diet can protect against obesity (see the figure on the following page).

Body Mass Index (BMI) in kg/m² as it Relates to Adherence to Vegetarian Lifestyle in the Adventist Health Study-2

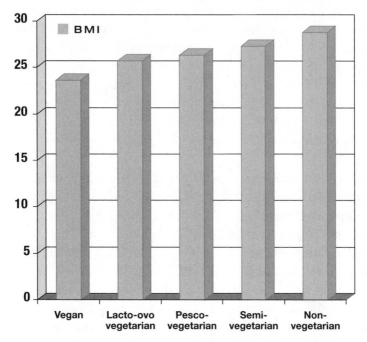

Mean BMI was lowest in vegans (23.6 kg/m²) and incrementally higher in lacto-ovo vegetarians (25.7 kg/m²), pesco-vegetarians (26.3 kg/m²), semivegetarians (27.3 kg/m²), and nonvegetarians (28.8 kg/m²).

It could very well be the calories in unrefined plant foods are more likely to be burned off through increased cellular thermogenesis and less likely to be stored as body fat. It could also be that unrefined plant foods are simply less toxic and therefore maximize movement, activity, and metabolism encouraging a leaner more healthy state. Insulin sensitivity could also be a key factor because insulin sensitivity is improved by a whole foods, plant-based diet, thus allowing nutrients to enter the cells of the body more rapidly to be converted into heat energy rather than stored as fat. We can see the meat-loving readers getting nervous. Don't worry, as we mentioned in Chapter 1, you don't need to give up animal foods and convert to veganism to follow the Clean Cuisine program. In Part Two we will show you how to incorporate the healthiest and cleanest animal foods into your diet along with simple tricks for keeping your overall animal food consumption low without feeling deprived. On Clean Cuisine you can reap the health and weight-loss benefits of a vegan diet without actually becoming a vegan. We will go a step further and say that on Clean Cuisine you will actually be healthier than if you became a vegan.

Nature's Detox

Although *detox* is primarily thought of as a treatment for alcohol or drug dependence, the term is also used to refer to diets, herbs, and other methods of removing environmental toxins from your body for general health. Body cleansing is a method of helping your body eliminate toxic waste stored in its tissues. Cleansing, or detoxifying, is a process that occurs naturally and regularly in your body. The Clean Cuisine lifestyle and micronutrients in the foods we recommend provide support for your body's natural cleansing functions.

We do not support drastic detox methods such as colonics and prolonged fasts because they can be dangerous and because they aren't really necessary. Nature provides all the nutrients your body needs for gentle yet effective detoxification. You simply need to feed your body a steady supply of detoxifying foods and adopt the lifestyle habits we recommend. The problem is, if you eat a highly processed, animal-foods-rich diet you are not only introducing toxins such as hormones, antibiotics, and preservatives into your diet you are also displacing the unrefined plant foods that are the richest source of the micronutrients and substances your body needs to naturally cleanse itself. If you eat too many toxin-promoting foods and not enough detoxifying foods, you get sick, tired, and fat. You end up looking and feeling older than your years. It is not surprising that the most nutrient-dense, plant-based foods— fruits, raw nuts, raw seeds, unrefined whole grains, beans, legumes, whole soy, and so forth—are also the most detoxifying of foods.

Ridding your body of accumulated toxins and boosting your natural detoxification system will improve energy, support a healthy immune system, and optimize health. Your skin will become clearer. You'll decrease inflammation and improve symptoms of inflammatory conditions. You'll lose toxic body fat without hunger. You'll also improve digestion and will even have an improved clarity of thought. The Clean Cuisine plant-forward way of eating will help your body gently and safely get rid of toxins through several different mechanisms:

- Cleanse the colon through improved bowel regularity and improved bile flow
- Assist the liver in filtering toxins from the body and in breaking down excessive fats
- Decrease the propensity your body has to store fat (body fat tends to concentrate toxins within its mass)
- Increase hydration status through water naturally found in fruits and vegetables
- Improve circulation of the blood and lymph system
- Flood the body with detoxifying essential nutrients

Stored Toxins Affect Your Body Weight and Fat Loss

Your body stores most toxins in fat tissue. (Better there than in your bloodstream!) Because of this you can also assume the more body fat you have, the more stored toxins you have. Bummer, we know. The problem is once you accumulate toxins in your fat cells, your body doesn't want to let go of them for the simple reason it doesn't want them getting loose and running wild throughout your body. When the toxins do get loose they can slow your metabolism down. A study published in *Obesity Reviews*[8] concluded that during weight loss, pesticides (organochlorines) and polychlorinated biphenyls (PCBs) from industrial pollution are released from fat tissue where they are typically stored. These toxins can interfere with your metabolism and make additional weight loss challenging. Another study found that individuals who released the most pesticides from their fat stores during weight loss had the slowest metabolisms after weight loss.[9] Yet more studies suggest toxin release during weight loss can interfere with thyroid function and inhibit mitochondrial metabolism, which can reduce your ability to burn fat and calories.

The good news is, if you have excess fat to lose you can take steps to detoxify and provide your body with the essential nutrients it needs to assist in the natural toxin elimination process and therefore prevent the metabolic dysfunction associated with toxin release. Nature provides all the nutrients your body needs to detoxify; you simply need to get those nutrients into your body. We will show you how.

In conclusion, it should be empowering to know that you have the option to choose micronutrient-dense, anti-inflammatory, antioxidant-rich, and naturally detoxifying foods that can truly make a difference in the way you age, look, and feel. By using the information in this book, you can learn to make educated decisions based on the nutritional value of a food. If you have struggled with food cravings and have never been able to lose weight permanently due to an ongoing battle with hunger, you should feel elated that there is, in fact, a way to eat that doesn't require starvation or deprivation, that tastes good, and that can help you maintain your weight effortlessly. You should feel delighted that simply by choosing nutrient-dense foods you can slow the aging process, both internally and externally. You should feel excited that to a large degree you do have control over your body. While it's true you can't alter your genes, you *can* alter your food choices and you *can* make a big dent in your overall health and appearance. Once you appreciate the power of plant foods and the anti-aging miracle of phytonutrients you will be even more excited and even more motivated to eat Clean Cuisine. Let's press on.

3

PLANT POWER
The Antiaging and
Anti-Inflammatory Miracle
of Phytonutrients

While nutritionists have been recommending we eat more fruits and vegetables for years, recent research points to the astounding health and antiaging benefits of many other plant-based foods including beans, nuts, seeds, whole soy, and a wide variety of unrefined whole grains. All plant foods contain a vast array of vitamins, minerals, essential fats, and fiber that are vital for health. But plant foods are also the *only* source of phytonutrients. Phytonutrients are the substances that protect the plant and fortify it against illness, but they also offer invaluable disease protection and anti-inflammatory benefits to *you*, the plant eater. The power-packed phytonutrients that keep plants healthy and give fruits and vegetables their many vibrant colors are also one of Mother Nature's very best antiaging substances.

Phytonutrients act in myriad health promoting ways. Many phytonutrients are sources of natural antiaging antioxidants. The antioxidants in phytonutrients help protect fruits and vegetables from free-radical attack; they do the same thing in humans by protecting your cells from damage. Other phytonutrients act as anti-inflammatory substances and help reduce pain and decrease the chronic inflammation associated with many diseases. Some phytonutrients modulate and enhance immune function, maintaining the body's healing system. Phytonutrients are also known to stimulate enzymes that detoxify cancer-causing carcinogens. Some phytonutrients lower cholesterol levels, whereas others offer hormonal benefits, easing menopausal symptoms and protecting against osteoporosis. The point is phytonutrients do a whole lot of good for your body. With phytonutrients, more is better.

More Plant Foods = More Phytonutrients

Phytonutrients are *not* found in processed foods and they are not found in animal foods such as eggs, chicken, beef, milk, and cheese. The phytonutrients found in plants are a major contributing factor to why plant foods play such an important role in Clean Cuisine. And, for whatever it's worth, most people who eat the standard modern-day diet are in less than optimal health, so it's not surprising that their diets are exceptionally low in the phytonutrient-rich foods that form the foundation for Clean Cuisine.

We are not the only ones who are praising the powers of phytonutrient-rich plant foods either. The American Heart Association Nutrition Committee, the American Cancer Society, the American Academy of Pediatrics, the American Dietetic Association, the Division of Nutrition Research Coordination of the National Institutes of Health, and the American Society for Clinical Nutrition all agree that we should eat more phytonutrient-rich unrefined plant foods and less foods from animals.

> NOTE: *We didn't say no animal food, we said less animal food; there's a big ditfference!*

Phytonutrients offer tremendous health, anti-inflammatory, and anti-aging benefits independent of their nutritional value. These plant-based superstar antiagers help cells repair themselves by stimulating the release of protective enzymes. In other words, flooding your system with phytonutrients can help you stay looking and feeling younger by providing your body with the raw materials it needs to repair damaged cells. Your body's ability to repair damaged cells on a regular basis is a key factor in staying youthful. Without a sufficient supply of phytonutrients, your cells age more rapidly, and they lose their ability to remove and detoxify waste products, increasing the risk for disease.

A phytonutrient-rich diet is also an essential component of preventing the development of degenerative diseases. Research shows populations with low death rates from such diseases and populations with low obesity rates consume upward of 75 percent of their calories from unrefined phytonutrient-rich plant foods. Scientific evidence supports the idea that phytonutrients play an important role in preventing and even treating some of the most deadly diseases, including heart disease and cancer.[1] It is believed phytonutrients inhibit cancer-producing cells. Cancer starts out as a cell growing out of control. It is now believed some cancer cells are probably formed in every person every day. If you have a strong immune system, your body recognizes these cancer invaders and attacks. Almost always the healthy body with a healthy immune system wins this combat so cancer cells either never have a chance to develop or are destroyed before they have a chance to spread or cause damage. The body can fight and even cure cancer, in some cases even when rather advanced. Phytonutrients from a wide variety of plant-based foods help fight cancer on many levels and help keep your cells healthy and strong. A review of 206 human population studies shows raw vegetable consumption to offer the strongest protective effect against cancer among the phytochemical-rich fruits and vegetables.[2]

WHAT IF YOU *HATE* VEGGIES?

LIKE MANY SMALL children, certain adults don't want to eat their veggies. This can be a real problem if you are trying to follow the Clean Cuisine lifestyle because eating lots of veggies is a principal component of our nutrition recommendations. But if veggies just are not your thing yet (we say *yet* because the more you eat them, the more you will like them. We promise!), you can take advantage of the findings from researchers at Pennsylvania State University. They discovered that adding puréed vegetables to the favorite foods of preschool children boosted their veggie consumption by 50 percent and helped them consume 11 percent fewer calories.* Although decreasing the calorie intake of a child's diet might not sound politically correct, when you consider childhood obesity rates are on the rise from eating nutrient-poor, empty-calorie diets we don't see a decrease in calories accompanied by a 50 percent veggie boost as being a bad thing. Not a bad thing at all! Similar results have been found for adults.†

Another idea, which is incredibly simple, is to roast your veggies.

Roasting naturally caramelizes and sweetens veggies. Even kids who will barely touch a vegetable will almost always eat them roasted.

33

* M. K. Spill, L. L. Birch, L. S. Rose, and B. J. Rolls, "Hiding Vegetables to Reduce Energy Density: An Effective Strategy to Increase Children's Vegetable Intake and Reduce Energy Intake," *American Journal of Clinical Nutrition* 94, no. 3 (2011): 735–41.

† A. D. Blatt, L. S. Roe, and B. J. Rolls, "Hidden Vegetables: An Effective Strategy to Reduce Energy Intake and Increase Vegetable Intake in Adults," *American Journal of Clinical Nutrition* 93, no. 4 (2011): 756–63.

It's the Mix That Matters

For optimal health, you need lots and lots of phytonutrients from a mix of all sorts of different plant foods. There are scores of plant foods to eat and each plant food has its own unique phytonutrient makeup. In fact, scientists have identified over 10,000 different phytonutrients to date. It's important to remember there is no such thing as a magic bullet, single best phytonutrient because these powerful substances work synergistically as team players. Just like *our* favorite football team, the Miami Dolphins, couldn't have enjoyed the only unbeaten, untied record in modern sports history through the isolated efforts of one star player, one single phytonutrient can't get the job done either. You need to have the whole team.

Although each phytonutrient plays a special role in promoting health and slowing the aging process, some are more well known and more thoroughly studied than others. Some of the best known phytonutrients are the carotenoids, flavonoids, and isoflavones. Carotenoids include yellow, orange, and red pigments in fruits and vegetables. Dark green, leafy vegetables are also rich in carotenoids such as beta-carotene, but their usual yellow color is masked by chlorophyll, the green pigment in these vegetables. Flavonoids are reddish pigments found in red grape skins and in citrus fruits, and isoflavones can be found in peanuts, lentils, soy, and other legumes. In general, the more colorful a food is, the more phytonutrients it contains, which is why you want to expose your body to a rainbow of colors. Although there is nothing wrong with foods like whole grain brown rice and potatoes, black rice and purple potatoes are the more healthful choices simply because they contain more phytonutrients. Here are some examples of just a few of the thousands of phytonutrients that exist, the foods they are found in, and what they can do for you.

- **Chlorophyll:** This is the green pigment abundant in green vegetables. Chlorophyll carries oxygen to our red blood cells, helping fight off disease. In cancer studies, it reduced carcinogens binding to DNA and diminished metastasis. It also has critical antioxidant and anti-inflammatory properties.

- **Carotenoids:** These are naturally occurring colorful compounds with potent antiaging properties. There are hundreds of different carotenoids but some of the more familiar ones are alpha-carotene, beta-carotene, lycopene, lutein, zeaxanthin, and cryptoxanthin. Carotenoids are found in a wide variety of fruits and vegetables, including those colored orange (carrots, apricots, squash, and sweet potatoes), green (spinach, kale, and collards) and pink-red (tomatoes, guava, and grapefruit).

- **Capsaicin:** This is the active compound in chili peppers. Capsaicin has been widely studied for its pain-reducing effects and cardiovascular benefits. It has also been show to assist with weight loss by increasing thermogenesis, the rate at which your body burns calories at the cellular level, and decreasing appetite.

- **Flavonoids:** This group of phytonutrients has potent antioxidant properties, helps prevent blood clotting, and offers protection against heart disease. They are also believed to protect veins and help prevent cataracts and even boost mood. Foods particularly rich in flavonoids are green tea, wine, apples, chocolate, and pomegranates.

- **Glucosinolates:** These phytonutrients help activate enzymes that detoxify the liver. Glucosinolates are found in broccoli, Brussels sprouts, cabbage, and cauliflower.

- **Isoflavones:** These plant compounds are considered to be natural selective estrogen receptor modulators (SERMs) that partially inhibit the activity of excess human estrogens. Isoflavones are believed to play a role in protecting against hormone-sensitive cancers, such as breast cancer and prostate cancer, and also offer protection from osteoporosis. Isoflavones can be found in soy beans, peanuts, chickpeas, fava beans, alfalfa, and all members of the legume family.

- **Lignans:** These are potent antioxidants that fight free-radical damage and offer protection against hormone-sensitive cancers, such as breast, ovarian, uterine, prostate, and colon cancer. Flax-seeds are by far the richest source of lignans, but these phytonu-trients can also be found in sunflower seeds, cashews, sesame seeds, and peanuts.

Supplements Are Not a Supplement

First, we are not against nutritional supplementation in general—as you'll read in Chapter 9 we do suggest considering certain phytonutrient supple-ments (including whole food–based phytonutrient supplements such as Juice Plus+, Barlean's Greens, and Green Vibrance), but we are against supplementation with *isolated* phytonutrients and with certain synthetic vitamins and antioxidants. Lycopene is a good example: As a phytonutri-ent, it has been a media darling now for some time. Although research shows lycopene from food sources seems to reduce the risk of certain types of cancer and even heart disease, scientists cannot determine if it is *only* the lycopene that provides the benefit. It might be that lycopene is found in the same foods as some other, undiscovered superstar food substance. And this undiscovered food substance might be the *real* reason foods containing lycopene are so healthful. The thing is, food is really ultracom-plex. Foods contain thousands and thousands of phytonutrients along with other antioxidants and nutrients that can't possibly be isolated, pack-aged and bottled into a pill. You really need to get the *whole food* to reap the benefits of the phytonutrients found within the food. Each one of the hundreds, perhaps thousands, of yet-undiscovered phytonutrients helps the others biochemically in the food and in your body. For example, eating tomato sauce is far better than eating a food boosted with lycopene that has been isolated from the tomato. This is because a tomato contains more than 10,000 different phytonutrients; lycopene is not the only player on the team! For phytonutrients to be effective they need to be eaten as part of the whole food the way nature designed.

While we know that phytonutrient-rich diets do conclusively offer pro-tection against disease and slow the aging process, it is certainly not proven that taking isolated phytonutrients is in any way helpful. Worse, isolating phytonutrients can even be harmful. Beta-carotene is a good example of isolation gone wrong. For years scientists noted that diets high in beta-carotene from *plant-based whole foods* (not supplements) reduced the risk of many types of cancer, including lung cancer in smokers. But when researchers tested isolated beta-carotene supplements in people who smoke, they noticed an increased cancer risk.[3]

36   Beta-carotene supplements also increased the risk of other cancers, heart attack, and stroke. In comparison, plant-based whole foods such as carrots that contain beta-carotene are consistently associated with a decrease risk of cancer. It really is the same logic with lycopene. What is known is that *foods* (not supplements) containing lycopene, beta-carotene, and other phytonutrients are associated with decreased risk of cancer, better health, and better aging. So when it comes to phytonutrients, don't isolate them and don't try to take short cuts; you need to get them from plant-based whole foods.

EAT VEGGIES WITH FAT FOR MORE BIOAVAILABILITY AND MORE FLAVOR!

AS LONG AS vegetables are properly prepared, most grown-up palates are pleasantly surprised how delicious they truly are. By preparing vegetables and salads with a little bit of healthy fat (think chopped raw nuts and seeds, olives, extra-virgin olive oil, flax oil, walnut oil, avocado, and so forth), you'll greatly enhance their flavor, increase your satiety, and even boost the absorption of many nutrients, including certain phytonutrients. Keep in mind fat is one of the best natural substances known to convey the flavor of food most effectively, which is one reason why diet-style steamed asparagus tastes so bland and blah compared to asparagus roasted with just a little bit of extra-virgin olive oil. And besides, the assimilation of fat-soluble vitamins such as A, D, E, and K as well as certain phytonutrients such as lycopene actually requires the presence of a little bit of dietary fat.

A fascinating study published by the *American Journal of Clinical Nutrition* showed people who consumed salads topped with fat-free salad dressing absorbed far less of the helpful phytonutrients and vitamins from spinach, lettuce, tomatoes, and carrots than those who consumed salad with a dressing containing some fat.[*] This is certainly good news for your taste buds! On top of this, dietary fat actually activates a satiety hormone called cholecystokinin, which acts like an appetite suppressant, sending the message to your brain that you are full. Bottom line, eat your vegetables, but be sure to eat them with a little bit of healthy fat for optimal taste, health, and satisfaction.

37

* M. J. Brown, M. G. Ferruzzi, M. L. Nguyen, et al., "Carotenoid Bioavailability Is Higher from Salads Ingested with Full-Fat Than with Fat-Reduced Salad Dressings as Measured with Electrochemical Detection," *American Journal of Clinical Nutrition* 80, no. 2 (2004): 396–403.

Pass the Fruit and Veggie Platter

One of the most consistent findings in the epidemiological and nutritional literature is that as fruit and vegetable consumption increases in the diet, chronic disease and premature deaths decline. The CDC, the National Cancer Institute, the American Heart Association, and the U.S. Department of Agriculture all recommend adults eat 7 to 13 servings of fruits and vegetables every day for better health. One of the reasons fruits and vegetables are so important to eat in abundance is because they offer such incredible nutrient and phytonutrient bang for such a teeny-tiny calorie buck.

Vegetables in particular offer big nutrient package for basically zero calories. It is just impossible to overeat vegetables. For example, eating 1 cup of raw spinach delivers hefty amounts of fiber, vitamins, minerals, and phytonutrients for a paltry 10 calories. Yet, while spinach is great, you can't eat only spinach for optimal health. You need to eat lots of different colored vegetables and fruits, and the more variety in color you get, the broader the protection. This is because each fruit and vegetable contains its own unique set of phytonutrients. Red fruits and red vegetables have different phytonutrients from green fruits and green vegetables. Even red strawberries have a different phytonutrient profile from red tomatoes.

Are Raw Veggies Best?

Raw is not always best. While we are big advocates of eating plenty of raw vegetables (raw fruits, too!) this certainly doesn't mean we are against cooked vegetables. In fact, some of the nutrients in vegetables, including certain phytonutrients, are actually better absorbed after the vegetables have been cooked. For example, the carotenoids in carrots are made more bioavailable by eating cooked carrots. The lutein found in tomatoes and corn is made much more absorbable after the tomatoes and corn have been exposed to heat and are even more absorbable when eaten with a little fat too. Although not technically vegetables, mushrooms contain toxic compounds that are broken down and eliminated by cooking. When it comes to members of the allium family, such as onions and garlic, heat actually increases the variety of health-promoting, sulfur-containing substances found in these foods. The point is, heat is not always bad.

However, it is true that heating vegetables (as well as other foods) above around 110°F or so destroys enzymes that raw food advocates believe are essential to human health. The fact that raw food is rich in enzymes is a big feather in the raw food advocate's cap. Yet we can't give full credit to the enzymes as the main reason why raw foods are healthful because as soon as those enzyme-rich foods hit the acidic environment of your stomach, they start to unravel. Instead, we believe the unrefined phytonutrient and plant-rich foods and the kaleidoscope of vegetables raw food advocates enjoy in abundance have far more to do with the health-promoting benefits of their diet than the enzymes. On the other hand, if you overheat your vegetables (or any food) with char-grilling techniques or you cook vegetables in oils that are not heat stable (more on these in Chapter 5) you can generate carcinogens that can absolutely be harmful. And of course if you overcook your vegetables in big batches of water that you toss out once the vegetables are cooked you could also lose important vitamins and minerals right along with the discarded water. So, while you don't necessarily need to go raw with your vegetables or any other foods, you do want to take care when preparing all foods to preserve nutrients and reduce your exposure to carcinogens.

The other thing to keep in mind is that raw vegetables are not always easy to digest, and how well you digest your food makes a *big* difference in the bioavailability of the nutrients from that food. If you eat a food but don't absorb its nutrients you're sort of wasting time. When you eat raw instead of cooked vegetables, your body depends much more heavily on chewing in order for the food to be properly digested. Cooking a vegetable, even for as little as 1 minute, can be a way of enhancing its digestibility. As a side note, blending raw vegetables into a smoothie or cold soup, like a gazpacho, can also increase the bioavailability of the nutrients in the vegetables, which is one reason we love our daily SuperGreen smoothie (more details in later chapters).

One more thing to keep in mind: Although it is true most animals thrive on diets consisting almost exclusively of raw, uncooked food, we are unaware of modern human cultures that have thrived exclusively on a raw foods diet. Eating your vegetables raw is not an either/or decision. For optimal health, not to mention taste and variety in food choices, you should eat both raw *and* cooked vegetables. And because most people don't even come close to eating the amount of vegetables they should, adding the one huge raw salad we recommend to your daily diet should have great benefits because even small increases in the percentage of raw foods eaten (especially fruits and vegetables) have been shown to have significant benefits in lowering blood pressure and cholesterol naturally. And, while there is no scientific study on this, Ivy swears a daily salad makes your skin glow! But again, you absolutely do not need to go overboard eating an exclusively raw foods diet. We don't recommend that.

39

Sunny News!

Did you know phytonutrients can even help protect your skin from the damaging and aging effects of the sun? We made this connection a few years back after Andy noticed his skin take on a little bit more color than usual when Ivy started giving him green smoothies and more vegetables in general. In particular, he was eating more carrots (two or three raw carrots almost every day with lunch), more tomatoes (a sliced tomato salad with balsamic vinaigrette) most days for dinner, a green smoothie either at breakfast or before dinner, plus a green salad nightly. It is interesting that, after increasing his vegetable consumption Andy also noticed he tended to sunburn less and tan better. Perhaps the tan color mixed with the carotenoid hue in a pleasing way, and he could spend more time outside without having to put on his shirt or apply sunscreen.

The question then arose, Was Andy imagining this benefit or was there real research to support nutritional approaches to sun protection? As we began to dig into the medical literature we discovered natural foods, especially those rich in phytonutrients, *do* in fact provide sun protection. Of the phytonutrients, flavonoids and carotenoids were shown to be particularly helpful. Omega-3 fats, tocopherols, and tocotrienols were nonphytonutrient substances shown to also provide internal natural sun protection. One study showed the flavonols in high-quality chocolate—not conventional mass-market chocolate—and cocoa beans more than doubled the length of time necessary to develop sunburn. Ivy, who *loves* chocolate, was especially pleased to hear about this study! Yet another study showed that tomato extract provided about a 40 percent increase in the length of time necessary to develop reddening of the skin. We're not saying you should trade in your sunscreen for a chocolate bar, but you should be encouraged to know that adding more phytonutrients to your diet can help thwart sun-induced skin damage.

40

EASY WAYS TO BOOST PHYTONUTRIENT INTAKE

- Eat fruits and vegetables in a rainbow of colors. The more color and the more variety, the more variety of phytonutrients you'll get.
- Eat a serving of isoflavone-rich whole soy foods such as tempeh, soy milk, edamame, and tofu once a day.
- Drink resveratrol-rich red wine (we drink it regularly!).
- Eat beans (see CleanCuisine.com for free bean recipes).
- Enjoy small amounts of polyphenol-rich dark chocolate with a minimum cocoa content of 70 percent or, better yet, vegan and sugar-free cocoa nibs or unsweetened cocoa powder.
- Drink more green and white tea.
- Go for flavor! The more flavor you can add to your food from garlic and from fresh and dried herbs (dill, basil, oregano, thyme) and spices (ginger, cardamom, turmeric, cumin, cinnamon), the more antioxidants and phytonutrients you'll get. Not to mention that your food will taste better too!

Detox

Another way phytonutrients keep you healthy, looking renewed, and feeling good is by helping you cleanse your body. While all phytonutrients support detoxification and boost your body's natural detoxifying abilities, certain phytonutrients are particularly effective. Phytonutrients that generate glutathione production at the cellular level play a key role in detoxification.

Glutathione is a critically important super-antioxidant and cell protectant that is naturally produced in the body. Glutathione directly quenches free radicals and plays a vital role in the cell's defense against inflammation-generating free radicals and oxidative stress as well as the breakdown of toxins and carcinogens. This super-antioxidant even has the ability to regenerate other antioxidants, including vitamins C and E and coenzyme Q10 (CoQ10).

41

Glutathione is your brain's most important antioxidant and is absolutely critical for proper brain function. It is interesting that what is good for the brain is also good for the skin. We made this connection a while back when researching a brain healthy diet for MS. Over and over we noted that just about every nutritional recommendation for brain health coincided with the same recommendations for healthy skin. This is because both the skin and the brain are derived from the same embryonic tissues. It is no surprise that any substance that boosts the health of your brain by quenching free radicals and reducing inflammation will do the same for your skin. This also helps explain why Ivy noticed a definite improvement in her own skin clarity and overall appearance shortly after changing her diet to the brain healthful MS diet in her early 20s.

The super-antioxidant glutathione is found in high concentrations in the liver, and when it encounters a toxin it attaches to it and makes it water soluble, thus allowing the toxin to be flushed out in the urine. The problem is glutathione levels decline with age, and oral glutathione supplements are poorly absorbed. The oral supplements alpha-lipoic acid and N-acetylcysteine are precursors to glutathione and can help boost glutathione levels.

> NOTE: *Intravenous glutathione therapy is recommended by integrative neurologists because it is effective at boosting glutathione levels, but we acknowledge this method can be rather inconvenient.*

The good news is that certain phytonutrient-rich foods activate pathways that generate glutathione production as well as anti-inflammatory chemicals. Studies show that these pathways may remain activated for as long as 24 hours after being stimulated by an appropriate phytonutrient. The phytonutrients that are currently thought to be most effective for boosting antioxidant capacity include the following:

- **Curcumin in turmeric:** Curcumin is the most active phytonutrient component of the spice turmeric and has powerful

42

antioxidant and anti-inflammatory properties. You can boost your intake of curcumin by cooking with turmeric (a delicious ingredient in many Indian dishes) or boosting your intake of good old American mustard. You can also supplement with turmeric by taking turmeric extract, but we do not recommend supplementation with isolated curcumin. Supplementation with turmeric extract is especially helpful for inflammatory disorders such as arthritis and autoimmune diseases. The downside is that compared to the actual spice, turmeric supplements are not well absorbed. However, research shows that by adding piperine (a compound found in black pepper) the absorption of turmeric is greatly enhanced. It's interesting that cultures that consume turmeric regularly also cook with pepper. One economical turmeric supplement we found containing piperine is Turmeric Extract with BioPerine (a standardized piperine extract obtained from black pepper). You can purchase Turmeric Extract with BioPerine online at VitaCost.com.

NOTE: *Ginger is also frequently paired with turmeric, and ginger is known to help boost its absorption.*

- **Catechins in green tea or white tea:** White tea is the least processed and therefore has the most catechins, but green tea is more widely available. The benefits associated with drinking antioxidant-rich green tea have been touted for centuries. The catechins in green tea are known to improve liver function. Catechins also promote weight loss by increasing the metabolism of fats by the liver, inhibiting fat absorption, and providing a feeling of satiety and fullness.[4] Adding bioflavonoid-rich citrus juice, such as a squirt of lemon, in your green tea significantly boosts the absorption of catechins. But don't add milk! The milk protein casein has been shown to bind to the catechins in tea, thus making them unavailable to the body. We both drink oodles of tea each day, Ivy in particular states 6 cups or more is perfectly acceptable, unless you are sensitive to the caffeine component.
- **Sulforaphane in cruciferous vegetables:** The sulforaphane in cruciferous vegetables like broccoli, cauliflower, kale, cabbage, and Brussels sprouts is one of the strongest and most widely studied activators of antioxidation pathways. Sulforaphane

has significant anticancer and anti-inflammatory benefits, and studies show it helps cells defend against oxidants that damage DNA. Epidemiological (population) data have shown that diets high in sulforaphane-containing cruciferous vegetables result in fewer instances of certain cancers, especially lung, colon, breast, ovarian, and bladder cancer.

43

- **Pterostilbene (pronounced tero-STILL-bean) in blueberries and grapes:** Pterostilbene, like its cousin resveratrol, is gaining worldwide attention for its rather dramatic ability to improve human health and slow aging. Pterostilbene enhances the production of key antioxidants, including glutathione, that are critical for protecting cells against free radicals. Studies also show when pterostilbene enters a cell, it easily binds to peroxisome proliferator-activated receptors (PPARs), thus enabling improved metabolism of triglycerides, cholesterol, and blood sugar.[5]

The Clean Cuisine Flavorful and Functional Approach to Boosting Phytonutrient Intake

Once upon a time the bland diet was a staple of clinical diet prescriptions. But these days experts in nutrition recognize a healing and health-promoting diet need not and should not be bland or boring. Just the opposite! Today nutritionists are viewing kitchen spice racks and fresh herb gardens with more interest than ever before. Chock-full of phytonutrients, herbs and spices are nature's apothecary. These culinary superstars offer tremendous healing, antiaging, and anti-inflammatory benefits with no negatives, only flavor-enhancing benefits.

Exploring a wide variety of traditional global cuisines reveals richly flavored meals that offer intrinsic health-promoting properties enhanced by the creative use of herbs and spices. In fact, many of the most flavor-forward meals in the world are among the most healthful, thanks in large part to herbs and spices. Herbs and spices are a natural and tasty source of preventive healthcare, and their isolated phytonutrients have been a great resource for discovering a large proportion of commercially available medications for the treatment of many different diseases. Throughout the world, botanists and chemists actively search the plant kingdom for new phytonutrients. In fact, over 40 percent of medicines now prescribed in the United States contain chemicals derived from plants. For example, aspirin was initially derived from extracts of willow bark, and the breast cancer drug Taxol was initially harvested from the Pacific yew tree. Phytonutrients isolated from plants have also been a great help for the treatment of a wide range of human diseases, including pulmonary diseases, cardiovascular diseases, diabetes, and cancers.

Study after study shows the benefits of different herbs and spices. One 2003 trial of 60 people with type 2 diabetes reported that consuming as little as 2 teaspoons of cinnamon daily for six weeks reduced blood glucose (sugar) levels significantly. It also improved blood cholesterol and triglyceride levels, perhaps because insulin plays a key role in regulating fats in the body.[6] Studies have shown cumin to significantly reduce allergy symptoms. The more you read, the more benefits associated with herbs and spices you discover.

SPOTLIGHT ON THREE SUPER HERBS

WE LOVE AND use a wide variety of culinary herbs in preparing Clean Cuisine but these are three we find ourselves using over and over:

- **Oregano:** Oregano contains numerous phytonutrients, including thymol and rosmarinic acid, that have also been shown to function as potent antiaging phytonutrients. According to a study in the *Journal of Agriculture and Food Chemistry,* oregano has 42 times more antioxidant activity than apples, 30 times more than potatoes, 12 times more than oranges and—most surprising of all—4 times more than blueberries!* The warm, aromatic flavor of oregano is particularly delicious for boosting flavors of Mexican and Mediterranean cuisine. We whisk minced oregano into vinaigrettes or mix with olive oil, lemon slices, olives, and capers to make a marinade for fish.
- **Parsley:** There are actually more than 30 varieties of parsley, but our favorite is the peppery Italian, or flat-leaf variety. Parsley is best known for its detoxification properties and it's the world's most popular herb. We routinely put a big handful of parsley in our daily green smoothies; it's delicious when blended with frozen pineapple, frozen mango, and coconut water. In addition to its detoxifying properties, parsley is also

rich in phytonutrients as well as vitamin K, calcium, and a mega amount of vitamin A. And did you know the ergosterols found in parsley are vitamin D precursors? So eating more parsley can actually help boost your vitamin D levels, something most of us could certainly use!

> **NOTE:** Try shredding parsley in your food processor then sprinkle it on top of salads, soups, and whole grain pilafs. Mmmm. . . .

■ **Rosemary:** Rosemary is chock-full of a wide variety of specific phytonutrients called flavonoids. It's also rich in antioxidants like vitamin E. Rosemary has particularly strong anti-inflammatory properties and has been shown to be helpful for people with inflammatory conditions like asthma and even heart disease. The phytonutrients in rosemary also aid in detoxification by enhancing the action of liver enzymes responsible for metabolizing and detoxifying chemicals. One of our family's favorite ways to eat rosemary is to dip sprouted whole grain bread in a mixture of chopped fresh rosemary, flaxseed oil, sea salt, and freshly ground pepper. It's also great for sprinkling on almost any vegetable just before roasting.

* B. Shan, Y. Z. Cai, M. Sun, and H. Corke, "Antioxidant Capacity of 26 Spice Extracts and Characterization of Their Phenolic Constituents," *Journal of Agricultural and Food Chemisty* 53, no. 20 (2005): 7749–59.

Variety Is the Spice of Life

Because Clean Cuisine is so rich in phytonutrients, not only from plant foods but also from herbs and spices, it is by default, also exceptionally flavor forward. But just as we encourage you to eat a variety of different phytonutrient-rich foods, you should also strive to eat a variety of phytonutrient-rich spices and herbs. This is because each spice and herb offers its own unique range of health-promoting properties. Every time you season a recipe with herbs and spices you substantially boost your intake of powerful disease-fighting phytonutrients and maximize nutrition for zero added calories. Every little bit you add counts too! If you look at the culinary history of ethnic cuisine, you'll notice traditional cultures such as Italian, Indian, Thai, and Japanese all incorporate herbs and spices into their food; therefore Clean Cuisine relies heavily on flavor combinations borrowed from a number of different cultures (one day we will have to do a Clean Cuisine around the world cookbook!).

Once you start putting phytonutrient-rich foods on your radar; start consciously to increase your consumption of a kaleidoscope of fruits and vegetables and other plant-rich phytonutrient-rich foods like nuts, seeds, beans, and whole grains; and start to season these natural and nourishing foods with all sorts of flavor-boosting herbs and spices, you'll be amazed at how incredibly tasty your meals will become. And you won't just be enjoying better-tasting food either. You'll start to look better and feel better too. You'll also start to wonder why on earth you haven't been eating like this all along.

PART 2

The Nutritional
Nuts and Bolts
of Clean Cuisine

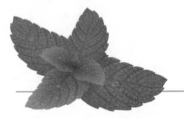

4

CLEAN CARBS
Maximum Nutritional Bang for Minimum Calorie Buck

We've talked about the spirit of Clean Cuisine, the concept of whole foods nutrition, and the amazing powers of plant foods to change the way you age, look, and feel. The next three chapters discuss our philosophy as it pertains to the three macronutrients: carbohydrates, fats, and proteins. All are necessary for lasting good health, but there are clean sources of these nutrients and there are less clean sources. We'll start with carbohydrates, probably the most unfairly maligned macronutrient of all.

The truth about carbohydrates has been trapped in a labyrinth of erroneous information for decades. The average person, even the average health- and nutrition-conscious person, is admittedly confused about carbohydrates on *some* level. In this era of food subtraction—low-calorie, low-fat, and low-carbohydrate dieting—the benefits associated with eating a whole foods diet that includes plenty of whole carbohydrates have been largely overlooked, despite the fact that the whole foods approach to eating has been shown to be superior to all other dietary lifestyles when it comes to preventing heart artery disease.[1] For example, the difference between a healthful whole foods diet that incorporates plenty of whole carbs and a conventional Western diet that is not based on eating whole foods and whole carbs when it comes to slowing the progression of heart artery disease can be greater than 70 percent, far greater than the benefits offered by medications such as aspirin, beta-blockers, cholesterol-lowering drugs, and any other pills on the market for that matter. Low-carb diets are not only unhealthful but can actually be dangerous; complications such as increased cancer risk, lipid abnormalities, impairment of physical activity, osteoporosis, kidney damage, and even sudden death can all be linked to long-term restriction of carbohydrates in the diet.

And, no, whole carbohydrates won't make you fat either, just the opposite. In fact, a multicenter study of 4,451 people published in the *Journal of the American Dietetic Association* found the slimmest people actually ate the most carbs, (from whole plant sources such as fruits, vegetables, and whole grains), and the heaviest people at the fewest carbs.[2] This research concluded your odds of getting and staying slim are best when carbs make up at least 64 percent of your daily calorie intake, obviously a far cry from the typical low-carb diet! The truth is, the quickest way to gain weight is to routinely avoid whole carbohydrates in favor of calorie-dense, proinflammatory, phytonutrient-poor foods like meat, cheese, oils, sugar, and flour. Swapping calorie-dense, yet not-so-filling meat, oil, dairy, flour, sugar, and refined packaged snack foods (chips and pretzels) for calorie-poor but nutrient-dense, whole food, clean carbs such as fruits, vegetables, unrefined whole grains, and beans is one of the easiest things you can do to lose weight without hunger and without food cravings. There is no doubt that whole carbs are your very best bet for maximizing nutrition for minimal calorie buck.

The Antiaging Superfoods!

Whole carbs work beyond keeping your heart healthy and waist trim; their supporting cast of antioxidants and phytonutrients fight aging and disease on many levels too. While oxygen is essential to life, some unstable oxygen molecules (free radicals), can attack cell membranes and even damage our genetic code (DNA), thus lighting the spark that can begin a deadly cancer cascade. Yet whole carbs contain a broad spectrum of antiaging antioxidants, such as vitamins A and C and lycopene, that can actually neutralize the damaging effects of free radicals and fight cancer and other diseases at the cellular level, before disease begins. The powerfully protective phytonutrients present in whole carbs (such as chlorophyll, flavonoids, and carotenoids) have additional antiaging, antioxidant properties that not only help plants in nature defend against bacteria, insects, and bad weather but also help *you*, the plant eater, fight inflammation, slow aging, and prevent disease. And so for all these reasons, plant-based unrefined whole carbs lay the foundation for Clean Cuisine. In other words, the bulk of the calories you eat should come from clean carbs.

Fiber Is a Nutrient Found Only in Whole Carbs

Fiber is another critical nutrient naturally present in all plant-based whole carbs. Although fiber is not digested and has basically no calories, it is still absolutely essential for optimal health and achieving a healthy body weight, and it is considered to be a nutrient. In general, the more fiber you eat from whole carbs, the healthier you will look and be. Simply adding more fiber-rich foods to your diet also appears to be associated with decreased inflammation and C-reactive protein levels.[3] It is not surprising that people who eat the most fiber from whole carbs have smaller waists, lower insulin levels, and a reduced risk of type 2 diabetes and many other diseases. As a general and bariatric surgeon, Andy frequently sees the negative complications associated with a low-fiber diet, including obesity, colon cancer, and intestinal diseases.

Fiber that is eaten the way nature packages it, in whole food form and *not* as fiber from isolated supplements, has been proven to provide tremendous health benefits. It is important to note that the scientific literature does *not* support fiber supplements for promoting health or weight loss. This means you cannot spike your Lucky Charms with a sprinkling of Metamucil and expect to reap the same benefits you would get from eating a breakfast of unrefined whole carbs, such as steel-cut oats. Fiber from real whole and unprocessed foods provides many benefits:

- Fiber-rich "whole carbs" are particularly detoxifying and help remove nondigestible and potentially carcinogenic toxins from your body.
- Fiber-rich whole carbs slow down the digestion of all the foods you eat, thus helping control both blood sugar levels and appetite.
- Fiber-rich whole carbs help lower cholesterol and improve your cholesterol profile.[4]

- Fiber-rich whole carbs offer significant protection against cancer, including reducing colon and rectal cancer by as much as 50 percent. Almost every week, Andy treats a patient with colon cancer and he would love to have half of those weeks off! Researchers have concluded that if Americans simply ate an additional 13 grams of fiber a day from whole carbs then about a third of colorectal cancers in the United States could be avoided.[5]

- Fiber-rich whole carbs prevent diverticulitis and diverticulosis, potentially lethal diseases of the colon that Andy deals with in his surgical practice on a weekly basis. In countries where high-fiber diets are eaten, diverticulosis and diverticulitis are very rare. Studies suggest that about half of all symptomatic cases of these diseases could be prevented by eating a fiber-rich diet.

- Fiber-rich whole carbs create a sense of fullness, satisfy hunger, and minimize the overconsumption of calories.

The Ultimate Clean Fuel

Our brain and muscle cells are designed to operate on carbohydrates. In fact, glucose, a carbohydrate, is the primary fuel for your brain and muscles, and your body does just about everything it can to make sure you have enough glucose available at all times. Carbohydrates are also nature's cleanest-burning fuel source for your body. Carbohydrates burn clean because they turn into only glucose, water, and carbon dioxide (CO_2) when metabolized. If your body doesn't get enough carbs, it senses starvation and sends "Feed Me" signals pretty loud and clear.

It is absolutely true that if you restrict carbs, your body will turn to fat reserves for fuel—but it also uses protein in muscle for fuel too. The problem is stored fat and protein do *not* burn clean. Toxic by-products of protein and fat metabolism called ketones and aldehydes will make you miserable and sick. These toxic by-products make your skin smell, cause bad breath, cloud your thinking, and do nothing to promote health. Your body turns to protein and fat as a mechanism of survival all in an effort to get the clean carb fuel in the form of glucose it needs. Yes, you might lose weight temporarily on a carb-restricted diet, but only a portion of the weight is actually from fat. The rest of the weight loss is from water (low-carb diets are dehydrating) and metabolically active lean muscle mass.

Because of the bariatric surgery Andy does, he talks with thousands of patients a year about weight loss. By the time the patients get to Andy, their situation is often dire. Many of Andy's patients are morbidly obese, weighing in excess of 300 pounds with numerous health issues. It's sad that they often feel weight-loss surgery is their only hope. Even sadder is when Andy inquires about their diet history and nutritional knowledge, he learns 99 percent of them have made some serious efforts to lose weight, but they are also victims of seriously bad nutrition advice. It's the same story over and over, with slight variations, but it goes something like this: Jane was either a normal weight (or slightly overweight) teenager. She started to put on pounds (or decided to go on a diet) in her mid-20s. She reduced her calories and used willpower to overcome her hunger. She lost weight at first, but then hunger ultimately derailed her best dieting intentions. She began to eat normally again and slowly but surely she regained the weight and then some. And then she dieted again. Rinse and repeat. As she became more "educated" about nutrition Jane eventually went on a low-carb diet. Weight loss was rapid and quick, but so was the rebound weight gain. Eventually Jane ended up weighing almost double what she did in her early 20s.

The point is, diets don't work and carb deprivation doesn't either. As soon as you eat carbs again your carb-starved body quickly replaces lost reserves and you often gain more weight, including fat and water weight, than you had before. Your metabolism naturally slows with age because you lose metabolically active muscle, unless you combat this process with regular resistance exercise (see Chapter 8 for how to combat muscle atrophy), but low-carb dieting actually speeds up the muscle loss normally associated with aging. Ugggh. Low-carb diets are not a healthful, sustainable, or clean way of eating. Period. In fact, the best diet for weight loss *and optimal health* is a diet rich in whole carbs.

Satiety and the Science of Appetite

Satiety is one the most important factors in developing a nutrition program designed to help you achieve a healthy body weight and improve the way you age, look, and feel. Satiety is a position of being and feeling full to the point at which no more food is required for your body to be satisfied. When you feed your body enough of the right foods, your stomach sends signals your brain to stop eating. If you do not eat in a way that creates satiety, your nutrition program will ultimately fail. Why? Because hunger will override willpower in the long run. Hunger is proven to derail the very best diet intentions even among individuals who are exceptionally motivated and educated about the dangers of being obese. Controlling hunger with nutrient-dense foods is one of the most important components to the Clean Cuisine program. If hunger is not satiated, and you end up eating an excess amount of the wrong types of food, you not only will gain weight but will also accelerate the aging process, increase your risk of many different diseases, and increase inflammation, thus making you feel miserable. You absolutely must learn to eat in a way that allows you to feel satiated after your meals.

Because of his bariatric patient population, Andy has spent a great deal of time researching the science of appetite. And the literature is fascinating. Research shows infants are born with an instinct that sends a Stop Eating, I'm Full! signal to the part of their brain (the hypothalamus) that controls appetite. This instinct is referred to as *appestat,* and it has the potential to be of help to you for a lifetime. In a perfect world, this instinct would last a lifetime and work for almost everyone. Sure, some of us would eat a bit more than others and be a bit larger (just like some folks are five foot six and others are five foot ten), but clearly the variability when it comes to weight is much greater. Is this because some of us have wildly dysfunctional appestats? Do we have no control over satiety? How do we explain skyrocketing rates of obesity over the last hundred years? Has psychology changed, has genetics changed? Of course not. There is only one reasonable explanation for the apparent complete dysfunction of the appestat in the modern world. Let's press on.

Scientists and surgeons trying to help morbidly obese patients lose weight and gain health have spent tremendous time trying to understand the science of appetite and how some people can eat so much that they end up weighing in excess of 300, 400, and even 500 pounds. The latest Gallup-Healthways Well-Being Index shows 62.6 percent of adults in the United States were either overweight or obese in April 2012.[6] This is more than half the country. Other countries are catching up fast. Most alarming, obesity is on the rise among many cultures in which it was once rare. There are multiple theories to explain this phenomenon, but a wholesale change in population genetics cannot possibly be the main reason. On an individual level there are always some people who are born lucky, with an appestat that works well no matter what they eat. There are also others who are unlucky, whose appestats have been damaged or even destroyed by factors beyond their control. For example, although many psychologists attribute obesity to psychological issues, including those that stem from childhood trauma and sexual abuse, and although this is certainly true for some patients, we do not believe half the population have psychological problems that causes them to overeat. The primary problem in our experience is *excessive hunger*. This excessive hunger is *not* because the modern appestat is different from that of our ancestors', but rather the modern appestat is not able to function properly because we are now exposed to nutrient-poor foods we as humans have not evolved to handle.

We believe certain people have a genetic predisposition to overeat because they don't feel full on the foods they are eating. And although genetics does play a role in how well your appestat functions, genetic predisposition need not be your destiny! Clean Cuisine foods are the best possible foods available to maximize the function of your appestat. You can't change your genes, but you *can* change the foods you eat. Because the foods you choose to eat play a tremendous role in regulating your appetite, you *can* gain control of your weight and your appetite simply by eating different foods.

Weight-loss surgery would not exist if people weren't excessively hungry. While any weight-loss surgeon can give you plenty of scientific mumbo jumbo about the intricacies of bariatric surgery, when you get down to the nitty-gritty he or she will tell you the surgery primarily works because it curbs hunger. This is why hunger control should be at the core of any weight-loss program. When patients are not hungry they don't overeat. And they lose weight. Lots of it.

The mechanism by which weight-loss surgery works is very complicated, and the powerful influence the surgery has on complex appetite-controlling hormones is still not fully understood. However, what is understood is that when the stomach is surgically made smaller the patient feels full with less food and the brain receives Stop Eating, I'm Full! signals. The good news is you don't need to resort to weight-loss surgery to feel full. You can simply choose to eat different foods. And the absolute very best foods for appetite control and filling up your stomach mechanically are whole carbs.

Whole carbs activate stretch receptors in your stomach, signaling satiety. This is because whole carbs are bulky and take up a lot of space or volume in your stomach. By eating plenty of whole carbs, you can eat a tremendous volume of food for very little calories. In addition to volume, you also get massive amounts of vitamins, minerals, phytonutrients, antioxidants, and fiber, substances that all work synergistically to curb food cravings and appetite even further. If you don't get enough nutrients, you will feel hungrier than you should feel.

Choosing voluminous whole carbs as your foundation to a healthy diet is one of the very best ways to make your food count nutritionally. The absolute best whole carbs for providing lots of volume for barely any calories are raw, dark leafy greens (kale, spinach, mache, arugula, watercress, and such) followed by other raw vegetables and cooked vegetables—in that order. To maximize nutrition while simultaneously filling your stomach with voluminous foods you need to eat considerably more vegetables than you think. We are talking *mega*-size servings here. Eating *huge* salads (in excess of 2 cups) and *very large* portions of cooked vegetables (such as ¾- to 1-cup servings) daily is essential to feeling full and satisfied while simultaneously supplying a tremendous amount of nutrition from antioxidants, phytonutrients, fiber, vitamins, minerals, and more. Raw fruits, beans, legumes, whole grains, and even potatoes are also excellent sources of slimming whole carbs. While we recommend you don't eat *massive* amounts of these foods, you can still eat large servings of these foods— enough so that you feel satisfied—without gaining weight.

One of the most important tenets of Clean Cuisine is to make sure you eat enough of the good whole carb foods every day so that you feel full and satisfied and don't have room for—or cravings for—unhealthful foods. It's not that you can't still enjoy foods like beef, eggs, cheese, and a little sugar as part of a treat, it's just that you shouldn't be eating excessive amounts of these foods, which is what most people eating a modern-day diet are doing. The bottom line here is that for satiety and long-term success, the bulk of your diet needs to come from unrefined whole carbs (especially the *super whole carbs* we discuss later in the chapter). This is a concept few people really get, but it's a concept that will substantially reduce inflammation and make a world of difference in how you age, look, and feel. If you shortchange yourself on eating whole carbs, *especially* vegetables and fruits, you will age faster. End of story.

Go for the *Whole* Shebang!

Here's the deal: Eating a diet rich in carbs is going to do absolutely *zilch* to reduce inflammation and optimize the way you age, look, and feel if the carbs you choose are not nutrient-dense, fiber-rich whole carbs. In fact, if the majority of carbs you eat are bad empty carbs you will accelerate aging, increase inflammation, and increase your risk of heart disease and type 2 diabetes. And you'll gain a lot of unwanted pounds too.

The bad empty carbs we are talking about are highly refined and stripped of all the good stuff we need to support a speedy metabolism and stay healthy. Refined empty carbohydrates are devoid of naturally occurring nutrients, they contain no fiber, and they are easily overeaten, contributing substantially to obesity and type 2 diabetes. If eaten in excess, refined carbohydrates can also be converted by your body into saturated fat, which increases inflammation, worsens the symptoms of numerous inflammatory conditions, and can even contribute to heart disease. Refined carbohydrate consumption can cause the proteins in your body to be less functional and, as a result, directly age your immune and arterial systems and even your joints.

Processed empty carbs contain almost no bioavailable antioxidants or phytonutrients or any of the other many substances found in whole carbs that are essential for cellular normalcy, prevention of disease, and slowed aging. For example, to make enriched wheat flour, whole wheat kernels are first stripped of their nutrient and antioxidant-rich germ and then their fiber-rich bran is removed, leaving behind nutrient-poor, fiber-free, calorie-rich starch that is then enriched with synthetic nutrients your body can't use in the same manner as the naturally occurring nutrients found within the original whole wheat kernel. Even worse, digestion of empty refined carbohydrates calls on your body's own store of vitamins, minerals, and enzymes for proper metabolism. Naturally occurring bioavailable B vitamins are absent in most refined carbohydrates, yet the breakdown and metabolism of carbohydrates cannot take place without B vitamins! If all this weren't bad enough, refined carbs enter our bloodstreams very quickly, igniting a nasty flood of insulin that then causes blood sugar levels to tailspin, stimulates hunger, and promotes fat storage. It's no wonder carbs have gotten such a bad rap because the majority of the ones most of us eat are from refined, fattening sources that include white rice, white pasta, high-fructose corn syrup, sugar, and baked goods made with enriched or bleached flour such as bagels, breads, crackers, snack foods, and muffins.

58   Plant-based whole carbs, on the other hand, are the ones found in their most natural and unrefined form, the form that comes naturally packaged with nutrients and bulk from calorie-free fiber. Whole carbs give us the *whole shebang*! They fuel us with maximum energy and mega nutrition for a minimal calorie buck. Examples of super healthy whole carbs are all fruits and vegetables, beans, legumes, potatoes, and whole grains (such as steel-cut oats, quinoa, millet, brown rice, and corn). When consumed in their whole, unprocessed form, these carbohydrates are nutrient dense, low in calories, loaded with fiber, full of disease-fighting phytonutrients, and chock-full of antiaging antioxidants.

Whole carbs enter your bloodstream slowly, raise blood sugar slowly, offer solid nutrition, and keep us healthy on many levels. These are the carbs that will help fight heart disease by lowering cholesterol and triglycerides, control blood sugar levels, curb food cravings, boost energy, preserve metabolism-boosting lean muscle mass, keep you feeling full for hours, and even improve your mood. Whole carbs are the carbs your body craves and needs most.

The reason we innately crave carbs is because we crave nutrition, and in nature, whole carbs are one of our best sources of nutrition. Whole carbs provide vitamins to support a healthy immune system; minerals to assist with proper cell function; antioxidants and phytonutrients to fend off disease, slow aging, and reduce inflammation; and fiber for detoxification and natural appetite control. Our bodies instinctively know whole carbs are healthful, which is one reason why food cravings can become unbearable on a low-carb diet. There's even a scientific explanation for why we crave sweets. Fruits, for example are a whole carbohydrate that also happen to naturally be one of the sweetest things on earth. Not incidentally, fruits are also jam-packed with a whole array of nutrients. If we didn't have our natural sweet tooth and we happened to live tens of thousands of years ago, we might be happy to hunt and eat nothing but animal foods like buffalo and deer. But luckily, nature saw to it we craved natural sweet foods that would make us healthy. If you don't get enough of the right whole carbohydrates, you will absolutely have food cravings and you won't be healthy.

The solution is not to eliminate carbs from our diets but to simply change the type we are eating. Go for the whole shebang! Choose whole carbs for whole body health.

Meet the Miracle Starch

You've probably heard of soluble fiber and insoluble fiber, but there is a third type of fiber known as resistant starch. Resistant starch is as close to a miracle starch as it gets. Considered a functional fiber, resistant starch actually resists digestion, meaning the calories in resistant starch are much less likely than the calories in other foods to be stored as fat. And because resistant starches such as those found in the foods listed on the following page are only partially digested yet are even more filling than simple starches like sugar and flour (which are completely digested), you end up with lower blood sugar levels, fewer insulin spikes, and a better ability to burn fat after a resistant starch–rich meal. In other words, you feel like you've eaten more due to the taste and volume satisfaction resistant starch brings, but your body treats these foods as if you've eaten less because only a small portion of the food is metabolized. If your body needs more energy than can be absorbed from the resistant starch it has no choice but to burn fat! Studies show a diet rich in resistant starch not only helps control blood sugar levels and reduce fat storage after meals but also helps you feel more full, so you eat less.[7] The resistant starch found in the plant-based whole carbs that make up the bulk of the rural Chinese diet might help explain the findings outlined in the Campbells' *China Study* book showing that per kilogram of body weight, the rural Chinese ate a generous 30 percent more calories than the average American yet weighed 20 percent less despite having comparable activity levels.[8] All of this is a perfect example of how not all calories are created equal. It is time to retire calorie counting for good from the weight-loss vernacular. Resistant starch is bulky, so it takes up space in your digestive system and you simply feel more satisfied after eating. By promoting a sensation of fullness or satiety, improving your body's sensitivity to insulin, and increasing the breakdown of fat, resistant starch from plant-based whole carbs is an essential component to losing weight without feeling hungry.

Not only will resistant starch help you shed pounds but it can improve your health in many additional ways. Resistant starch helps heart health by binding to dietary cholesterol and removing it from the body, thus lowering serum (blood) cholesterol levels. Diets rich in resistant starch also help remove toxins from your body and can lower the risk for colon cancer. And, finally, because resistant starch is a prebiotic fiber that promotes good bacteria and suppresses bad bacteria, it can help normalize bowel function and support a healthy digestive system in general. Having more good-for-you bacteria in your digestive system will also improve your immune function and make it easier for your body to fight disease.

CLEAN CUISINE–APPROVED PLANT-BASED WHOLE CARBS RICH IN RESISTANT STARCH

- Bananas
- Oatmeal
- Beans
- Lentils
- Whole wheat pasta (*sprouted* whole wheat is best)
- Potatoes
- Peas
- Barley
- Millet
- Polenta
- Corn
- Yams
- Brown rice

Does Eating Bananas and Potatoes Make You Fat?

We won't name names, but we are well aware numerous fad diets have been responsible for popularizing the myth that foods like carrots, potatoes, bananas, and beets are fattening. The reasoning, albeit false, is that these carbohydrate-containing foods increase insulin levels too much and therefore make you gain weight. Diet gurus who forbid foods like bananas and potatoes (both of which contain resistant starch by the way!) encourage dieters to be conscious of the glycemic index (GI) score of the carbohydrate-containing foods they eat. Low GI foods such as pizza, Snickers bars, and potato chips are considered good, whereas high GI foods, like carrots and beets, are considered bad.

So, what exactly is the glycemic index and how does it have anything to do with foods like bananas and potatoes anyway? The glycemic index is a numerical system of measuring how quickly a carbohydrate-containing food turns to glucose (blood sugar). Once glucose is absorbed from the intestine into the bloodstream, blood glucose levels go up and your pancreas starts secreting insulin to help get that sugar out of your bloodstream and into your brain and muscles where it is needed. On the GI index, the slower a carbohydrate-containing food is turned to sugar the better and the lower the GI score will be. Here's a very general scale:

- A GI of 70 or more is considered high
- A GI of 56 to 69 is considered medium
- A GI of 55 or less is considered low

The theory behind the glycemic index is simply to minimize insulin-related problems by identifying and avoiding foods that spike blood sugar levels. The problem is scientific evidence indicates that the GI rating of ingested foods is *not* a reliable predictor of the effect the food has on blood glucose levels, cholesterol, or insulin.[9] Additional research shows a diet revolving around unrefined whole carbs, such as bananas, carrots, whole potatoes, whole grains, and beans will not raise blood sugar or insulin levels. In fact, studies have shown that a diet based on such whole carbs can actually reduce fasting insulin levels by 30 to 40 percent in just three weeks.[10] The key is that the diet must be based on *unrefined* and fiber-rich whole carbs. Foods like pretzels, fat-free cookies, pizza dough, and white bread are not what we are talking about.

Another flaw with the GI rating system is that measuring the GI value of food does not take into consideration the normal portion size a person would eat. The GI value of a food is assessed by giving 10 or more volunteers a serving of a carbohydrate-containing food with 50 grams of digestible (this would not include fiber or the nondigestible portion of the resistant starch) carbohydrate. Scientists then take blood samples every 15 minutes to test how long it takes the 50 grams of carbohydrates to turn into blood sugar. The subject's response to the carbohydrate being tested is compared with the subject's sugar response to 50 grams of pure glucose. Because glucose is standard, it is the reference food, and the testing of glucose on the subject's blood sugar levels is done on a separate occasion. The average blood sugar response from 8 to 10 people will determine the GI value of that particular carbohydrate-containing food. Using this method, carrots rank high on the glycemic index. But—and this is where the GI scale is not very useful—a typical 3-ounce serving of carrots contains just 9 grams of carbohydrates and 2 grams of fiber (7 grams of digestible carbs). It's not accurate to say that carrots have a high GI because it's practically impossible to eat 21 ounces of carrots, the amount needed to obtain the 50 grams of net carbs used to measure the GI of a food. Bananas have a high GI rating too, but you would need to eat nearly three whole bananas in order to obtain 50 grams of net carbs.

When you choose to eat whole carbs you really don't need to worry about overeating or the GI value. Whole carbs are difficult to overeat because they stimulate the digestive system's distention nerves, which then send nerve impulses to your brain via your vagus nerve to calm your appetite, so you simply feel too full to overeat! Need proof? An Australian study showed that 240 calories of plain boiled potatoes (which are whole carbs and rather bulky) satisfied test subjects an astounding *seven times* as much as a very nonbulky (but low GI) 240-calorie croissant serving. The boiled potato versus croissant study clearly demonstrates one reason food volume and bulk is so important in weight management; the more space a food takes up in your stomach, the more full you feel and the fewer calories you eat.[11]

The intrinsic *portion distortion problem* with the glycemic index ultimately led scientists to come up with the idea of the glycemic load (GL). The GL considers the total amount of absorbable carbohydrate—starch or sugars—in a 100-gram serving portion of the food being measured as well as the GI of that food. Because the glycemic load factors in quantity (and therefore calories) it is a much better system than the GI. So low-density foods like potatoes, watermelons, and carrots that happen to have a high GI have a relatively low glycemic load. But regardless, we think both the glycemic index and the glycemic load are a ridiculously complex way to approach eating. Like the misleading Nutrition Facts label, the GI food-ranking system is just not the best way to plan your meals.

Good whole carbs are easy to identify. They are unrefined and packaged just the way nature intended, in their whole, beautiful, delicious natural form. For optimal health and effortless (hunger-free) weight management, you need to make the bulk of your daily calories come from whole carbs. If you follow our simple guidelines for making sure you eat enough whole carbs each and every day you will age less, both inside and outside.

Clean Cuisine *Super* Whole Carbs

While you absolutely want to eat a variety of whole carbs every day, you should be aware that certain whole carbs are jam packed with so much nutrition for so few calories that we consider them Clean Cuisine super whole carbs. Getting the minimum recommendation of super whole carbs into your daily diet is essential for maximizing health and offering the greatest protection from heart disease, cancer, stroke, and hypertension. If you have extra pounds to shed and you start eating as many super whole carbs as we recommend you will shed pounds pronto! Furthermore, eating plenty of super whole carbs will do wonders for improving your appearance too. These carbs are filled to the brim with antioxidants and antiaging phytonutrients that protect internal and external cells from free-radical damage. Less damage to internal organs and blood vessels means they wear out more slowly and stay young longer; less damage to collagen in your skin means fewer wrinkles and younger-looking skin. There is no way around it, eating tons of super whole carbs is essential for feeling and looking younger.

Super Whole Carb 1: Dark Leafy Greens

Romaine lettuce, kale, collards, spinach, Swiss chard, parsley, dandelion greens, beet greens, and all the other dark leafy greens are the first category of super whole carbs. Calorie for calorie, dark leafy greens provide more nutrients than just about any other food on earth. They are super rich in chlorophyll, which works to cleanse and oxygenate your body. They are also a good source of fiber and essential minerals, especially calcium and iron.

As you will learn when we get to the 8-week program in Chapter 9, we not only eat our greens but drink them too (as fresh whole smoothies), we take them as powdered greens like Green Vibrance and Barlean's Greens, and we supplement greens in the form of whole food capsules like Juice Plus+. You just can't get enough of the mind-blowing good stuff dark leafy greens have to offer.

Dark leafy greens are absolutely a case in which more really is better. Research shows that as vegetable portions per day increase, intravascular inflammation decreases and elasticity and endothelial function improves, thus reducing risk of heart attack and stroke.[12] The endothelium is a thin membrane that lines the inside of your heart and blood vessels; keeping your endothelial function and blood vessels in tip-top shape is a key factor affecting how you age, look, and feel. Your blood vessels supply nourishment to your skin, and if your blood vessels are in poor health you can rest assured you will look, and feel, older than your years. Eating more vegetables each day can help keep your blood vessels, and your body as a whole, younger longer. Dark leafy greens are rich in antioxidant plant pigments known as carotenoids, which enhance immune response, protect skin cells against UV radiation, and spare liver enzymes that neutralize carcinogens and other toxins. Their important antioxidant, anti-inflammatory effects reduce the risk of heart disease and block sunlight-induced inflammation in the skin that can lead to wrinkles and skin cancer.

Eating one huge salad made with mixed greens and a wide assortment of raw vegetables each day is an important part of the Clean Cuisine lifestyle. (If eating a huge salad every day doesn't sound particularly exciting be sure to see page 322 on how to build a four-star salad that tastes out of this world delicious!) Raw leafy greens and raw vegetables of all sorts contain important enzymes and vitamins that are heat sensitive and can be destroyed by standard cooking methods, so it's important to consume a good portion of these vegetables raw. Plus, if you are trying to lose excess pounds, getting in the habit of eating a huge salad each day will help you shed pounds and decrease your blood pressure with effortless ease.[13] In addition to your daily raw salad, you should also have one SuperGreen Smoothie—these are fruit and green veggie cleansing smoothies that we promise will boost energy and mental clarity like nothing else (see Part Four for recipes) *and* one additional serving of cooked dark leafy greens each day. For your cooked dark leafy greens we suggest just adding a side dish of greens such as garlic braised spinach or broccoli rabe to dinner each night (recipes in Part Four). To really bump your nutrient content even further we also suggest adding a scoop of freeze-dried concentrated powdered greens like Barlean's Greens to a glass of water each day. You could also take Juice Plus+ as a nutritional fruit and veggie booster in capsule form. Although we have incorporated the following recommendations into our 8-week program outlined in Part Three, here is an overview of what your goal for eating dark leafy greens should be each day.

DAILY GOAL FOR EATING DARK LEAFY GREENS

■ Consume 1 huge raw salad (with about 2 cups of assorted mixed dark green lettuce such as watercress, spinach, arugula, and romaine) plus 1 cup of raw chopped vegetables.

■ Consume 1 big serving (¾ to 1 cup) cooked dark leafy greens, preferably as a side dish with dinner.

> *NOTE: A time-saving strategy is to have tons of frozen dark leafy greens (chopped kale, chopped collards, chopped spinach) in the freezer at all times. In less than 5 minutes you can thaw the greens in the microwave and drizzle with a little olive oil, truffle oil, or a yummy sauce (Rao's marinara is one of our favorites, but we also have an entire sauce collection in Part Four). Another option is to quickly stir-fry frozen greens in a large skillet with crushed garlic and a bit of extra-virgin olive oil or coconut oil. Or, for a green veggie boost, try adding frozen chopped greens to soups—invariably a handful of greens blends in perfectly! We also chop fresh parsley and cilantro in a mini–food processor so we have herb "crumbs" to toss into all sorts of dishes for an ultra-easy and tasty greens booster. (See CleanCuisine.com for additional ideas.)*

■ Have one SuperGreen Smoothie made with greens and fruit each day. Believe it or not, a handful of raw leafy greens, particularly kale, cilantro, and parsley, can easily hide out pretty much undetectable tastewise in fruit smoothies; we didn't say the greens wouldn't color your smoothie green, we just said you can't necessarily *taste* them!

■ Add one scoop of a freeze-dried concentrated greens powder (such as Barlean's Greens or Green Vibrance) to a glass of water or to your fruity greens smoothie. If you find the powder to be inconvenient you can also try taking your greens in capsule form, such as Juice Plus+. Or do both! Just remember, you can't overdo greens!

WANT STRONG BONES? GET GREENS!

DARK LEAFY GREENS such as spinach, collards, turnip greens, and parsley are a fabulous source of bone-building nutrients, including calcium, magnesium, and vitamin K. As you will read on page 164 when we discuss dairy, people make the mistake of thinking dairy is the best source of calcium and the best food for building strong bones, but this just isn't true. Dairy is in fact a good source of calcium, but when it comes to keeping your bones strong, calcium alone is not enough. There are a number of other vital nutrients that help your body absorb and make use of the calcium you consume. The most important of these nutrients are magnesium, vitamin K, and vitamin D. The magnesium in dark leafy greens helps your body absorb and retain calcium and works like calcium's teammate to build and strengthen bones and prevent osteoporosis. Because your body is not good at storing magnesium, it is vital to make sure you get enough of it in your diet on a daily basis. The vitamin K in dark leafy greens helps activate certain proteins that are involved in the structuring of bone mass.

Dark leafy greens do not contain vitamin D, nor do dairy products in their natural form: Dairy is artificially enriched with vitamin D. To get a natural vitamin D fix, make sure to eat fatty fishes like salmon, eat egg yolks from pastured hens, and make it a point to get a bit of sunshine exposure.

If you want strong bones and a healthy disease-free, inflammation-resistant, younger-feeling body one of the best things you can do is to get in the habit of getting enough dark leafy greens on a daily basis, which is one of the reasons our 8-week program includes a SuperGreen Smoothie each day. Instead of asking whether you've Got Milk?, ask instead if you've Got Greens! Greens are the *true* super food (they just don't have a multibillion-dollar industry like the National Dairy Council behind them for marketing).

Super Whole Carb 2: Kaleidoscope of Nonstarchy Vegetables

Bok choy, eggplant, fennel, onions, tomatoes, rutabaga, radishes, bell peppers, broccoli, cauliflower, artichoke, asparagus, leeks, spaghetti squash, green beans, snow peas, zucchini, cucumber, Brussels sprouts, and the like are all nutrient-dense plant foods. It is impossible to claim one type of vegetable is better than another because each and every vegetable offers its own unique set of antiaging, disease-fighting antioxi- dants and phytonutrients. We separated dark leafy greens from other nonstarchy vegetables only because the dark leafy greens provide slightly fewer calories by volume along with boatloads of nutrients. Also it is important to eat raw vegetables every day, and compared to some other vegetables, green leafy vegetables taste really good as the foundation of a raw salad. But really, all vegetables are powerhouse super foods. Your best bet for getting a broad spectrum of all the good stuff vegetables have to offer is to think *kaleidoscope colors* and try to eat the rainbow of vegetables every day. The more, the better; and the more color variety you can get, the better. And don't play favorites or get confused thinking one vegetable is better than the other just because you hear a new study touting the benefits of say, artichokes as opposed to asparagus. The thing is you want to eat *all* types and *all* colors of vegetables because there's something special in each one.

The provitamin A compounds in bright red, yellow, and orange produce such as carrots help increase collagen production and thicken your dermis for more youthful skin. They also support a healthy immune system and offer protection from heart disease, cancer, cataracts, and other diseases. The vitamin C found in red bell peppers helps mop up free radicals, reduce arterial aging, aid in healing, boost your body's ability to absorb iron, and even helps protect against the effects of heavy-metal toxicity. Just hearing this might make you want to start eating nothing but carrots and bell peppers! But then you wouldn't have room for tomatoes! Luscious red tomatoes are famous for containing lycopene, a phytonutrient believed to be independently protective against heart attacks by the way,[14] but tomatoes are also rich in antioxidant vitamins C and E, potassium, folic acid, and beta-carotene. We can't even begin to scratch the surface of the healing, beautifying, anti-inflammatory, and anti-aging benefits of all sorts of vegetables in this one book because the benefits would be a set of books. The point is, like children, each and every vegetable is special. You don't want to eat so much of one type of vegetable (or one type of any food for that matter) that you don't have room left for others. Don't play favorites! As we discussed in Chapter 3, all vegetables are healthful; there is no added value in rating one over another for health benefits. The best strategy is to eat the widest possible variety of different vegetables over the course of several days. Although we have incorporated the following recommendations into our 8-week program (Chapter 9), here is an overview of what your goal for eating nonstarchy vegetables should be each day.

DAILY GOAL FOR EATING A RAINBOW OF NONSTARCHY VEGETABLES

- Eat *at least* 1 cup of any type of *raw* chopped vegetables each day. These can be added to your huge salad, if desired.
- Eat *at least* two additional servings of cooked or raw vegetables each day. One cup of raw vegetables is one serving, One half cup cooked vegetables is one serving.

TIPS FOR EATING A RAINBOW OF NONSTARCHY VEGETABLES

- Make a huge batch of veggie soup once a week (check out our veggie soup recipes in Part Four). Having a delicious vegetable soup on hand at all times guarantees you will eat more vegetables. Best of all, our soup recipes take no more than 30 minutes to prepare, and leftovers can be stored in the fridge for up to 4 days.
- Fresh tastes best, but there's nothing wrong with eating frozen vegetables either. We rely on frozen vegetables a lot because they can be thawed in the microwave in a matter of minutes. Thawing unwrapped vegetables in the microwave does not meaningfully change their nutritive value any more than any other type of cooking (all forms of cooking alter food molecules to some extent and destroy some enzymes, but there is nothing intrinsically bad with the microwave compared to any other type of cooking), nor does it in any way add toxins to the food.
- Keeping delicious sauces and toppings on hand at all times is the fastest way to boost the taste of just about any vegetable. You can completely elevate your vegetables to gourmet-quality restaurant status with a fabulous sauce. In fact, many times the sauce or topping is the chef's secret to making restaurant food taste so amazing. For example, steamed cauliflower can taste outrageous with a spoonful of our Indian pesto (page 354), and roasted asparagus is over-the-top delicious with a spoonful of our romesco spread (page 352). But, unlike restaurant-style sauces that are generally loaded with butter, cream, and empty-calorie oils, our Clean Cuisine sauces are made with healthy ingredients like fresh herbs,

nuts, seeds, and citrus that won't undo the good you do by eating the veggies in the first place! In addition, our sauces and toppers are very versatile too; use them to jazz up grilled tofu, cooked lentils, whole grains, baked potatoes, steamed fish, and the like. (For more ideas, see Sauces That Make the Meal in Part Four.)

MUSHROOMS:
A CATEGORY OF THEIR OWN

VEGETARIANS DEPEND ON mushrooms for their dense flavor and meaty texture. They are a good source of B vitamins, potassium, and vitamin D. Holistic healers place tremendous value on the therapeutic and healing benefits of mushrooms, and gourmet food enthusiasts relishes their culinary range—by the way, be sure to check out our Five-Star Portofino Portobello-Beef (or Buffalo) Burgers with Olive Tapenade on page 360, an innovative recipe with an abundance of umami in which ground meaty mushrooms blend right in with ground beef or buffalo, allowing you to enjoy full flavor while eating less meat. But as is the case with fine wine, mushrooms' flavors can vary tremendously. When it comes to health-promoting benefits, not all mushrooms are equal either. Although many mushrooms have therapeutic benefits, not all can be used for culinary purposes. The following four varieties are delicious to eat and therapeutic to boot!

- **Cordyceps:** This Chinese mushroom is used to promote energy and endurance as well as for issues related to kidney, immune system, adrenal, and respiratory health. You can buy whole, dried cordyceps in health food stores and add them to soups or stews; you can even drink tea made from them. Cordyceps also comes as a concentrate in liquid or capsule form.
- **Enoki:** This slender white mushroom looks almost like a mini squid with tentacles. It's delicious grilled. Just leave them in a little bunch and baste with a mixture of sesame oil and a good-quality soy sauce. Enoki mushrooms have significant anticancer and immune-enhancing effects.
- **Maitake:** This variety is available dried or fresh in many Japanese markets. Maitake is approved by the Japanese

government as an adjunctive cancer treatment and is used throughout Asia for just this purpose. They are especially good for counteracting the toxic effects of radiation and chemotherapy, including fatigue and nausea.

■ **Shiitake:** Ivy finds herself cooking mostly with these mushrooms not just because she loves their earthy, delicious flavor but also because they seem to be the easiest to locate at both the local health food store and our local grocery store. Shiitakes contain a substance called eritadenine, which encourages the absorption of cholesterol and lowers the amount of cholesterol circulating in the blood. In fact, Japanese researchers have reported that consumption of shiitake mushrooms lowers cholesterol by as much as 45 percent. Shiitakes also have potent antiviral and anticancer effects. What is more, 4 ounces of shiitake mushrooms provide a whopping 2,500 milligrams of potassium, an essential super mineral. Studies have shown that increased potassium intake can actually decrease the incidence of some forms of arterial aging. As an electrolyte, potassium helps regulate blood pressure and allows your heart and kidneys to function properly. Eat those shiitakes!

Super Whole Carb 3: Fruits

All fruits fit into the third category: açaí, apples, apricots, bananas, blackberries, blueberries, cantaloupes, cranberries, grapefruits, grapes, goji berries, kiwis, mangoes, nectarines, melons, oranges, papaya, peaches, pears, pineapple, plums, raspberries, strawberries, tangerines, and watermelons. As with vegetables, you want to think kaleidoscope colors; the more variety of color you get with fruits, the better. Remember, ruby-red cherries have a completely different nutrient, antioxidant, and phytonutrient profile than do slices of sunshine-yellow pineapples. Neither one is better than the other; they're both nutritious and delicious! Along with vegetables, whole grains, beans, and legumes, fruits are one of the very best sources of antioxidants in the world. The more antioxidants you can consume naturally from antioxidant-rich foods as opposed to isolated antioxidant supplements, the healthier you will be, the slower you will age, the less inflammation you will have, and the better you will look and feel. Eating your antioxidants in the form of fruit can be a sweet deal too! Even the picky palates of children love the taste of "Mother Nature's Candy." Who doesn't think a big bowl of fresh raspberries, blueberries, and strawberries sounds delicious? Who doesn't crave a fruit smoothie on a hot summer day? Who wouldn't love a slice of watermelon at a summer picnic? Not only does fruit naturally satisfy a sweet tooth craving but the availability of fresh fruit directly parallels the lengthening of the average life span. When you consider all the good stuff in fruit it's easy to understand why.

Before we go further we can just hear some of you wanting to know, "What about all the terrible sugar in fruit?" It is absolutely true fruits contain sugar—certainly more sugar than the ultra-low calorie dark leafy vegetables and the nonstarchy vegetables. But we don't want you to get hung up on the sugar in fruit because the kind of sugar in fruit (fructose) is converted into glucose, the type of sugar that causes insulin levels to rise, at a very slow rate. In other words, the sugar in fruit doesn't disrupt your blood sugar levels like the sugar from a lollipop or a can of soda pop. And if you avoid fruit juice and instead eat the whole fruit, which is what we recommend, you'll also consume plenty of blood sugar–blunting fiber, not to mention tons of nutrients too!

Just in case you are still worried about all the "fattening" sugar packaged with fruit, you should know the real world effects of fruit consumption have actually been shown to be inversely associated with BMI and body weight. In other words, people who eat fruit weigh less. In a study published in the journal *Nutrition*,[15] 77 overweight and obese dieters enrolled in a 6-month randomized controlled trial testing the effects of a computer-assisted dieting intervention program with the goal to decrease energy intake, increase fruit and vegetable consumption, and maintain a balanced diet. Although vegetable consumption increased as a result of the intervention, fruit consumption did not. However, after controlling for age, gender, physical activity, and daily macronutrient intake, higher fruit consumption was associated with a lower BMI both at the baseline and the end of the study. Although overall fruit consumption did not increase, those participants who did increase fruit consumption lost more weight. The results suggest that eating more fruit by no means reduces the likelihood of weight loss.

Besides, the vast majority of people don't eat anywhere close to the amount of fruit they should, so to worry about eating too much fruit is probably not where you should focus your energy. Instead, you should make sure you are eating at least three servings of fresh raw fruit a day along with all of the other foods we recommend. You shouldn't become a fruitarian and eat nothing but fruit, but to fear fruit because of sugar is also not sensible. The reason people are overweight and suffer so many degenerative diseases and accelerated aging is *not* because they are eating too many apples and pears! Besides, it's pretty hard to overeat whole fruit because whole fruit, such as strawberries, bananas, and plums, are high-volume foods that take up a lot of space in your stomach. Trust us, if you try eating three bananas (considered a high-sugar fruit) in one sitting you're going to feel pretty full, pretty darn fast! People don't binge on bananas, they binge on ice cream, cakes, and cookies. So don't worry about getting too much sugar from whole fruits; worry instead about how to eliminate empty carbs! Although we have incorporated the following recommendations into our 8-week program (in Chapter 9), here is an overview of what your goal for eating fruits should be each day.

DAILY GOAL FOR EATING A RAINBOW OF FRUITS

- Eat *at least* three different colored raw fruits each day. If you are particularly active, you should increase your consumption of fruit since fruit makes an excellent clean fuel for athletes.

- There's nothing wrong with frozen fruit! We buy frozen fruit in bulk and use it frequently—especially for our fruit smoothies. For the creamiest and richest-tasting fruit smoothies we like to peel and slice fresh bananas, freeze and then throw the frozen ones in our high-speed blender (we like the Vitamix brand) for the best-ever fruit smoothies. In addition, for smoothies we also love the creaminess of frozen açaí berries—look for Sambazon brand unsweetened frozen açaí smoothie packets. For smoothies and for just plain eating we buy plenty of other frozen fruits, including organic strawberries, peaches, mangoes, cherries, raspberries, pineapples, and blueberries. Look for frozen *wild* blueberries if you can find them because wild blueberries have considerably more antioxidants than their cultivated cousins; in fact, wild blueberries have more antioxidants and a greater free radical absorbance capacity than comparison fruits, offering more antioxidants per serving than pomegranates, blackberries, cranberries, strawberries, cherries, and raspberries!

- Organic dried fruits are just fine (but avoid canned fruits). In fact, we use organic dried fruits (which are considered raw by the way) in all sorts of ways all the time. Ivy especially likes to grind dried fruit, raw nuts, and dark chocolate chips in a mini food processor and sprinkle the crumbly mix on top of fresh fruit for a dessert topping. She frequently sweetens our smoothies with pitted dates. If you have a high-speed blender like a Vitamix, sweetening your smoothies with whole dried fruit is easy as pie and a much healthier option than adding sugar or syrup.

- Ivy even puts dried fruits in our pilafs and mixed into sautéed greens—one of our favorite ways to eat kale is with golden raisins, toasted pine nuts, and garlic. And nothing nips a sugar craving in the bud faster than the combination of a little bit of dried fruit eaten along with some raw nuts or seeds. When it comes to dried fruits think outside of the raisin box and look for variety such as goji berries, figs, and blueberries.

- End your meal with a fruit dessert. Another tasty, easy way to boost your fruit serving for the day is to have an after-dinner treat. Drizzling just a splash of liquor, such as brandy or amaretto, and letting your fruit marinate a bit has to be the very best way on earth to coax the most incredible flavor from just about any fruit. Or you could try baked bananas topped with a rum raisin sauce (recipe on page 429), or drizzle your fresh fruit with ribbons of luxurious extra dark chocolate sauce (page 427), or make a fruit crisp (page 430). The possibilities for serving fruit for dessert are endless.

TIPS FOR EATING A RAINBOW OF FRUITS

- Make eating a serving of raw fruit a breakfast staple (see page 305 for breakfast ideas).
- Make a fruit smoothie. Better yet, add some greens to your smoothie, too! (see pages 344–346 for recipe ideas).
- Satisfy a midafternoon sweet craving with some dried fruit and raw nuts, the combination is incredibly satisfying. If you want something all nice and neatly packaged look for Lärabars, our favorite fruit and nut bar. (Lärabars come in an assortment of flavors; Banana Bread is Ivy's favorite, whereas Andy prefers Key Lime Pie.) We also love Good Greens bars, made with a blend of

73

fruits, greens, and vegetables to provide antioxidants, and all sorts of good-for-you things. Both Lärabars and Good Greens bars make perfect pre- and postworkout snacks, and they are ideal for traveling. Ivy has one or the other stashed in her purse at all times.

- Make fruit-forward desserts (see page 425).
- Add fresh or dried fruit to your daily salad (or make one of our Salad Boosters with dried fruit; see page 318).

PESTICIDES: MORE THAN JUST PESKY TOXINS?

BECAUSE EATING LOTS of fruits and vegetables is absolutely an important part of our Clean Cuisine lifestyle we are often asked by our online readers and Andy's patients about our stance on buying organic produce. If we lived in a perfect world we would all consume only the highest-quality, freshest organic fruits and vegetables every day. But the reality of modern life is that it's practically impossible to eat 100 percent organic food 100 percent of the time. When it comes to eating clean produce, you are leaps and bounds ahead of the game simply because fruits and vegetables are very low on the food chain. They are automatically going to contain fewer toxins than foods high on the food chain, such as beef, dairy, chicken, and eggs. The higher up on the food chain you go, the greater the chance of acquiring toxins found in the environment. Still, the U.S. Food and Drug Administration estimates that roughly 20 pounds of pesticides per person are used every year. And of those pesticides, at least 59 are classified as carcinogenic. According to the Environmental Working Group (EWG), eating the 12 most-contaminated fruits and vegetables will expose a person to about 15 pesticides a day, on average. Eating the 12 least-contaminated will expose a person to fewer than two pesticides a day.

Sure, you might be telling yourself, pesticides can't possibly be good for you, but how bad can they really be? Considering that by definition pesticides are designed to kill living organisms we classify them as pretty darn bad. Pesticides are neurotoxins and among the worst offenders of all the potential environmental brain toxins because they target delicate nerve tissues and in the process promote free-radical production and inflammation. Anything that promotes free-radical production accelerates the aging process, and anything that promotes inflammation has the potential to worsen the symptoms of inflammatory conditions such as multiple sclerosis, asthma, arthritis, fibromyalgia, psoriasis, and even heart disease. The EWG points out that there is a growing consensus in the scientific community that small doses of pesticides and other chemicals can have adverse effects on health, especially during vulnerable periods such as fetal development and childhood. And, did you know pesticides even play a role in weight gain and make weight loss more challenging?

A study published in 2003 in the journal *Obesity Reviews* showed that, when released from our fat tissue where they are typically stored, organochlorines (a class of pesticides) can then "poison" our metabolisms. The study showed pesticides interfere with thyroid function (specifically lowering T3 levels) consequently slowing resting metabolic rate and inhibiting thermogenesis (fat-burning).[*] The researchers reviewed 63 scientific studies on the link between chemical toxins and obesity. The grim story is, because pesticides are toxins that are stored in our fat tissue, if you are already overweight, those toxins are constantly disrupting your metabolism and potentially thwarting your weight-loss efforts.

Another study has shown that the increase in toxins during weight loss reduced the subjects' ability to burn calories, thwarting further weight loss.[†] Yet another study, published in the *International Journal of Obesity,* found that individuals who released the most pesticides from their fat stores during weight loss had the slowest metabolism *after* weight loss.[‡] Collectively, these studies indicate pesticides can play a role in your metabolic rate, your body's fat-burning ability, and your thyroid function. Certainly the less pesticide exposure the better.

While we absolutely acknowledge the potential dangers of excess pesticides in our produce, we also can't ignore the tremendous research on nonorganic produce that shows the more fruits and vegetables a person eats, the healthier and slimmer he or she is with less risk of heart disease, less cancer, less diabetes, less inflammation, and less disease in general. The research on produce consumption showing these benefits has been done largely with conventional—not organic—produce. Without a doubt it is far better to eat conventionally grown apples, peaches, and kale than it is to eat refined calories from organic granola bars, cookies, and crackers. Don't lose the forest for the trees.

And again, do keep in mind there is significantly less exposure to toxic chemicals of all sorts on a plant-rich Clean Cuisine–style diet compared to an animal-rich diet. Fat-soluble pesticides and other harmful toxins climb up the food chain and congregate there. If a cow is fattened on a feedlot, the pesticide residues from all the corn and soy the animal eats end up concentrated in the fat of its meat. So, the higher up on the food chain you go, the more time, money, and effort you want to spend ensuring you are buying the cleanest food possible. Simply by eating more plants and less animals you will be making huge strides to reduce toxins.

So then, does our family buy 100 percent organic produce? No is the short answer. The reasons we don't buy 100 percent organic are cost and availability. The reality is produce is expensive and, because fruits and vegetables are not exactly calorie-rich foods, you need to eat a lot of them to fuel your body. If we were to buy only organic fruits and vegetables our grocery bill would be enormously high. Plus, our choices would be highly limited if we chose only organic because organic just isn't always an option for every single fruit and vegetable. Remember, variety is also important for health reasons, not to mention enjoyment! In light of all this we feel the sanest and most economical thing to do is to be aware of the Clean 15 and the Dirty Dozen. The EWG updates these two lists of fruits and vegetables yearly (www.ewg.org/foodnews). In our house, we do our very best to avoid conventional produce on the Dirty Dozen list. We save our pennies to buy exclusively organic strawberries, apples, peaches, and such. We then don't fret so much about buying non-organic foods that are on the Clean 15 list because we figure the health benefits of the fruits and vegetables on that list will far outweigh the negatives from the pesticides. By the way, you aren't just reducing your exposure to pesticides when buying organic. Because organic foods are grown in richer, purer soil they not only taste better but they are actually more nutritious. Studies have found organic produce to be higher in flavonoids, antioxidants, vitamin C, iron, calcium, magnesium, and chromium.[§]

In addition to being aware of and trying to avoid the Dirty Dozen you should also wash fruits and vegetables under running water before eating. One study even found spraying produce with a mixture of vinegar and water was an effective way to help wash contaminants away. For hard produce, such as apples, use a vegetable brush when washing.

---

* C. Pelletier, P. Imbeault, and A. Tremblay, "Energy Balance and Pollution by Organochlorines and Polychlorinated Biphenyls," *Obesity Reviews* 4, no. 1 (2003): 17–24.

† P. Imbeault, A. Tremblay, J. A. Simoneau, and D. R. Joanisse, "Weight Loss–Induced Rise in Plasma Pollutant Is Associated with Reduced Skeletal Muscle Oxidative Capacity," *American Journal of Physiology, Endocrinology and Metabolism* 282, no. 3 (2002): E574–79.

‡ A. Tremblay, C. Pelletier, E. Doucet, and P. Imbeault, "Thermogenesis and Weight Loss in Obese Individuals: A Primary Association with Organochlorine Pollution," *International Journal of Obesity and Related Metabolic Disorders* 28, no. 7 (2004): 936–39.

§ V. Worthington, "Nutritional Quality of Organic Versus Conventional Fruits, Vegetables, and Grains," *Journal of Alternative and Complementary Medicine* 7, no. 2 (2001): 161–73. L, Grinder-Pedersen, S. E. Rasmussen, S. Bügel, et al., "Effect of Diets Based on Foods from Conventional Versus Organic Production on Intake and Excretion of Flavonoids and Markers of Antioxidative Defense in Humans," *Journal of Agricultural and Food Chemistry* 51, no. 19 (2003): 5671–76.

More Good Carbs: Clean Cuisine Antioxidant and Fiber-Packed Whole Carbs

There is more to healthy carbohydrates than eating fruits and vegetables. Beans and legumes are just about the very best source of fiber and resistant starch on the planet. In fact, nearly half of the starch in beans comes from resistant starch, meaning the starch is not digested, thus making beans an incredibly powerful weight-loss ally. And for all the many health-promoting reasons we talked about earlier in the chapter, fiber is a super important health-promoting and detoxifying nutrient so the more fiber you can get from whole foods (*not* supplements!) the better. Although you will certainly be getting plenty of fiber eating fruits and vegetables, adding just ½ cup of beans or legumes to your diet daily will *dramatically* boost your fiber profile by approximately 8 grams. The National Cancer Institute recommends at least 25 grams of fiber a day; we believe you should eat a lot more fiber than that, but 25 grams is a good start.

But that's not all! Beans and legumes are truly a fountain of youth food, bursting with antiaging antioxidants and phytonutrients as well as a nutritional storehouse of vitamins and minerals such as folate, iron, potassium, and ultra-clean plant protein. Like all plant foods, each bean and legume has its own unique nutritional, antioxidant, and phytonutrient profile. So don't play favorites. All you need to know is that *all* beans and *all* legumes are healthful. Many public health organizations, including the American Diabetes Association, the American Heart Association, and the American Cancer Society, recommend legumes as a key food group for preventing disease and optimizing health. The 2012 edition of the *Dietary Guidelines for Americans* developed by the U.S. Department of Health and Human Services (USDHHS) and the U.S. Department of Agriculture (USDA) recommends 3 cups of legumes per week.

That old catchy rhyme that starts out "Beans, beans, they're good for your heart" also rings true. The resistant starch in beans can bind to cholesterol and other fats in your colon for removal. Regular bean consumption has been linked with reduced homocysteine levels and lowered blood pressure and, it's not surprising, reduced risk of heart disease. In a large study of almost 10,000 men and women in the United States, those who ate beans and legumes four or more times a week had a 22 percent lower risk of coronary heart disease and an 11 percent lower risk of cardiovascular events than those who ate them less than once a week. This heart health benefit was independent of other health habits. Bean eaters not only have healthier hearts but also have trimmer waistlines. There are many explanations for why beans are so slimming—for example, the fiber and resistant starch and the high nutrient to low calorie ratio. A Canadian study of 1,475 men and women found that those who consumed beans regularly tended to weigh less and have a smaller waist circumference than those who did not eat them. The regular bean eaters were also 23 percent less likely to become overweight over time.[16] Bean eaters weighed, on average, 7 pounds less and had slimmer waists than their bean-avoiding counterparts, yet they consumed 199 calories more per day if they were adults and an incredible 335 calories more per day if they were teenagers. It is important to note here that, as we discussed earlier, all calories are not equal. Fiber calories and resistant starch calories do not contribute to weight gain. Also, some foods increase cellular metabolism and encourage increased energy burn to a greater extent than do others. It is very possible to eat more calories yet still lose weight so long as you choose the right foods.

Beans and legumes are also one of the best foods you can eat for weight loss because they absorb water and expand in your stomach, keeping you feeling full and satisfied for hours. Beans and legumes are slowly digested too, so they slow the use of glycogen, thus improving insulin sensitivity and increasing your body's fat-burning potential.

Lentils, black beans, adzuki beans, cannellini beans, navy beans, white beans, red kidney beans, garbanzo beans, pinto beans, and black-eyed peas are all highly healthful. Every single bean and legume has something special to offer. So try to mix it up and eat a wide variety every week. Although we have incorporated the following recommendations into our 8-week program (Chapter 9), here is an overview of what your goal for eating antioxidant and fiber-packed whole carbs should be each day.

DAILY GOAL FOR EATING ANTIOXIDANT AND FIBER-PACKED WHOLE CARBS

■ Eat at least ½ cup to 1 cup serving of beans or legumes each day.

TIPS FOR EATING ANTIOXIDANT AND FIBER-PACKED WHOLE CARBS

■ Some of our favorite ways to add beans and legumes to our diet include the following:

- Make bean-based chilies (recipe on page 338).
- Scatter beans on top of your daily salad.
- Why not eat them for breakfast? That's what Ivy's grandfather, Earl Ingram, did every day for over 50 years. Grandpa Earl lived to be 97, maybe he was onto something.
- Use them in soups. Ivy especially loves to purée beans in veggie-based soups to create a rich and creamy texture (recipe on page 325). We use our slow cooker for making split pea soup but also for many other bean and legume recipes.
- Eat more hummus. Just about any bean or legume can be made into an incredible hummus.
- Try bean-based burritos. We spread beans on sprouted whole grain tortillas or between sprouted corn tortillas for meat-free Monday night dinners (enchiladas recipe on page 378).
- Use beans when baking. We mix beans in our pizza dough (recipe on the Clean Cuisine website) and in our cookie and brownie batters (also on our website).

■ If you buy canned beans to save time (and there's nothing wrong with that!), we do think it is important to look for brands that use

80

bisphenol A (BPA) free cans. Although more research needs to be done, BPA has been linked to health problems in humans and the National Toxicology Program has reported possible effects on brain and prostate development in young children and fetuses. We try to avoid BPA as much as possible. An alarming study in the *Journal of the American Medical Association* showed there was a whopping 1,221 percent increase in BPA levels among subjects who consumed canned soup (canned foods are a big source of BPA) for five straight days. Fortunately, levels dropped to normal when subjects switched to fresh soup. If you like to save time with canned beans instead of cooking dried beans from scratch we think it is important to look for BPA-free sources (one brand to look for is Eden Foods). Oh! To get rid of the "tin can" taste just do what chefs do, rinse your beans with water and drain well.

Clean Cuisine Satisfying and Energizing Whole Carbs

Eating the recommended amount of dark leafy greens, fruits, nonstarchy vegetables, and beans and legumes we have suggested so far in this chapter you will have eaten only about 450 calories or so, which is not a lot. You will have gobbled up a boatload of nutrients and eaten a large volume of food for those few calories, but you will still need to eat a lot more calories and a lot more food each day to satisfy your daily energy requirement. Now, you could of course meet the rest of your daily calorie requirements with protein-rich whole foods like eggs and chicken or high-fat foods like nuts, seeds, and oils but the thing is your body doesn't need tons of protein and fat and it won't run as efficiently if you feed it more protein and more fat than it needs. What your body *does* need for the many reasons discussed in the beginning of the chapter is more clean-burning whole carbs that are rich in phytonutrients and antioxidants. And if you exercise a lot you need even more whole carbs than someone who is sedentary. Men, who are more muscular than women, also need to eat more whole carbs; the more muscle you have, the more carbs you need—this applies to women too. Starchy, earthy vegetables (which include potatoes!) and whole grains fill in the calorie gap and supply your body with clean-burning, nutrient-dense fuel. They are also incredibly satisfying and very tasty.

Clean Cuisine Satisfying and Energizing Whole Carb 1:
Starchy, Earthy Vegetables

Carrots, beets, peas, butternut squash, parsnips, potatoes, sweet potatoes, and corn all fit into this category. Contrary to what low-carb diet gurus might have been leading you to believe, the truth is starchy whole carbs are absolutely healthful. And they are not fattening either! Yes, they are high in carbs, but your body *needs* carbs. If you don't eat enough carbs you will feel hungry, and you will most likely overeat foods that really *are* fattening. Then you *will* get fat! You are not going to get fat eating whole starchy carbs as long as you eat them whole, which means eating the skins on the potatoes, and you don't drown them with fatty cheeses, butter, and cream sauces. Starchy veggies take up a lot of bulk and space in your stomach; they work mechanically to fill you up. Nobody ever got fat eating too many peas and carrots! Even potatoes are hard to overeat. It is pretty darn hard to eat two whole potatoes, and even if you could manage such a feat you'd still end up eating only about 300 to 400 calories, not exactly calorifically stratospheric. Plus you will be getting all sorts of nutrients, including antioxidants and phytonutrients and lots of fiber with every starchy bite. Trust us, you won't have a lot of room left in your stomach for much else, nor will you have much hunger for much else.

The nutrients in starchy vegetables are pretty impressive. For example, did you know carrots provide more health-promoting carotenoids than any other vegetable? Beets are bursting with folate, iron, and fiber. We bet you also didn't know the betalain pigments present in beets have repeatedly been shown to support detoxification and many of the phytonutrients in beets have anti-inflammatory properties; the combination of detoxification and reduced inflammation will absolutely have a beauty-boosting and health-promoting benefit. Sweet potatoes are another sweet deal in the nutritional department; they are super rich in antioxidants, including beta-carotene and phytonutrients such as anti-inflammatory quercetin plus they pack in potassium; vitamins B6, C, and E; and even a dollop of calcium. Sweet potatoes are also rich in fiber and incredibly filling for the measly 100 calories found in one medium-size sweet potato. In fact, the sweet potato is one of the main carbohydrates eaten by the Okinawans, the healthiest, longest-lived population in the world. Even our favorite summertime party picnic food, good old corn on the cob, is incredibly nutritious providing vitamins B1 and B5, folate, and even a good amount

82

of plant protein. And, did you know corn on the cob contains a broad spectrum of phytonutrients including lutein and carotenoids plus tummy-filling fiber? The combination of protein and fiber in corn has been associated with better blood sugar control in diabetes. Fasting glucose and fasting insulin levels have been used to verify these blood sugar benefits. The point is, there is absolutely no need to relegate starchy carbs to the bad carb section. Starchy whole carbs are good carbs!

POMMES DE TERRE?

POTATOES—APPLES OF THE earth, or *pommes de terre*, as they say in France—were the low-fat power-food of the fitness-crazed 1980s. But they have come under increased scrutiny by fitness, health, and weight-loss experts in the last decade or so. Like leg warmers, potatoes have become very unfashionable among the health fad enthusiasts. Let's try to set the potato record straight. First, potatoes are not empty calories. If you eat potatoes whole—with their skins on the way we suggest you eat them— they are a nutrient-dense food filled with fiber, vitamin C, iron, B vitamins, antioxidants, phytonutrients, and potassium (almost double the amount of potassium per serving than bananas!). In fact, potatoes meet FDA requirements for the health claim, "consuming foods such as potatoes that are good sources of potassium and low in sodium may reduce the risk of high blood pressure and stroke." Potassium is a mineral that is part of every cell in your body. It helps regulate fluid and mineral balance and in doing so helps maintain normal blood pressure. Potassium is also vital for transmitting nerve impulses and helping muscles contract.

But what about being fattening? Will eating potatoes burst your pants button? Nope. Not if you can keep from piling on the sour cream, butter, bacon bits, and other fatty fixings. Potatoes are not fattening because they are not empty calories. Potato-bashers love to blame excess potato consumption for unwanted pounds, but according to the USDA Economic Research Service, potatoes make up only 2.5 percent of the U.S. per capita food supply. Maybe we shouldn't blame weight gain on potatoes after all!* Plus potatoes are an excellent source of resistant starch, so you don't even absorb all of the starch calories in the potatoes you eat. On top of this, potatoes are incredibly filling and satisfying. For years, researchers have studied satiety. While many things are known to influence satiety, including individual differences in endocrine levels from one person to another, one of the biggest factors is the type of food that you eat. Some foods fill your stomach faster or remain in your stomach longer, and therefore do a better job of holding off hunger. Potatoes happen to be one of those ultra-satisfying foods. One of the reasons potatoes (with their skins) are so satisfying is that they are a high volume food that can stretch your stomach. This process stimulates your digestive system's distension nerves sending the message to your brain that you are feeling full. Your hunger is then quieted and you feel satisfied.

---

* U.S. Department of Agriculture, Economic Research Service, "Loss-Adjusted Food Availability," www.ers.usda.gov/Data/FoodConsumption/FoodGuideIndex.htm

Clean Cuisine Satisfying and Energizing Whole Carb 2: Whole Grains

Buckwheat, oats, quinoa, amaranth, millet, brown rice, black rice, and other whole grains are also healthy carbohydrates. For the most part, whole grains are a very misunderstood group. On one side of the table you have people who are jumping up and down about how we need to eat more whole grains; 6 to 12 servings a day. At the other side of the table we are told that whole grains were not part of the human diet until as recently as 10,000 years ago, when agriculture was developed; this is the bunch at the table who like to say that because our early ancestors did not eat whole grains, we are not genetically designed to eat them and shouldn't eat them either.

Uggghh. Confusion! If we were sitting at such a table here's what we would have to contribute to the whole grain debate.

First, the average noncompetitive athlete living a moderately active lifestyle does not need to eat 6 to 12 servings of whole grains a day. If you ate this many whole grains you'd be getting anywhere between 600 and 1,200 calories a day and you would be pretty darn full and therefore have a hard time finding room for all the other healthful foods you should be eating.

> NOTE: If you are a growing teenage boy who happens to also be a competitive athlete or a well-muscled competitive adult athlete, you might do just fine eating 6 to 12 servings of whole grains each day simply because your calorie needs are far greater than those of the average person.

84

If you are an average person who exercises moderately (anywhere from 2 to 5 hours a week), eating massive quantities of whole grains can actually shortchange you in the nutrition department because you'll quickly meet your calorie needs but not have room left over for fruits and veggies. Although whole grains are absolutely healthful and have plenty of nutrients, calorie for calorie they are not nearly as nutrient-dense as vegetables, fruits, and beans so you shouldn't fill up so much on whole grains that you don't have room left for other super whole carbs.

As for the Fred Flintstone–era grain-free, semi-Atkins caveman (or Paleolithic) diet, we don't exactly consider early humans to have had the highest quality of lives; they certainly didn't have a long life span! The reason early humans supposedly did not suffer from the degenerative diseases we acquire today (heart disease, arthritis, cancer, and so on) is mostly because they died so young. The Paleolithic diet was lacking in antiaging phytonutrients because it did not contain enough fruits and vegetables. It was also a diet too rich in animal protein. And it's interesting to note our ancestors were a lot shorter than we are today too. And besides, whether early humans ate grains is irrelevant because our goal in Clean Cuisine is not to go back to the good old days of living without modern conveniences. And how can we even be sure of exactly what our ancestors ate anyway? While they might not have eaten whole grains, we really don't know *exactly* what their diet really looked like. Did they keep accurate dietary records dating back 2.6 million to 10,000 years ago? Doubtful. In addition, the animal foods our ancestors ate were distinctly different from the animals we eat today; their meat did not come from animals raised in feedlots and fed cheap and inferior foods; instead, they hunted animals that grazed on pasture and had significantly more omega-3 fat intake than the animals we eat today.

Instead of wasting time debating the Paleolithic diet, what we should try to do instead is move forward and learn how to optimize our health in *today's* world. We should also analyze modern, well-documented nutrition studies that look closely at whole grain consumption and human health. When we look in the nutritional medical literature we find studies on *humans* (not rats, not chimpanzees, not dogs, not cats) documenting that people who eat whole grains as part of their diet are healthier than those who don't. So in today's world, a moderate amount of whole grains should absolutely be part of our diet. Whole grains contain a broad spectrum of energizing B vitamins, antiaging antioxidants, disease-fighting phytonutrients, vitamin E, selenium, and magnesium. They supply a super-clean source of nutritious energy, and they help keep us feeling full and satisfied. Eating whole grains is also associated with longevity and good health; people who eat whole grains as part of their diet are less likely to develop heart disease, type 2 diabetes, and cancer. Whole grain eaters are also less likely to be overweight; studies show people who eat whole grains tend to weigh less and have less body fat than people who skip them.[17] In 2004, researchers at Harvard University published results of an analysis of more than 27,000 men over an 8-year period showing that those who consumed more whole grains consistently weighed less than those who consumed less whole grains.[18] Eating whole grains has also been associated with lowering blood levels of CRP, a marker for inflammation in the body that is associated with increased risk of heart disease.[19] Although we have incorporated the following recommendations into our 8-week program (Chapter 9), here is an overview of what your goal for eating satisfying and energizing whole carbs should be each day.

DAILY GOAL FOR EATING SATISFYING AND ENERGIZING WHOLE CARBS

- Eat *at least* one hearty serving of cooked starchy vegetables (about 1 cup) and one serving cooked whole grains (about ¾ cup) daily. If you are a man or you are a particularly active woman, you will most likely need to eat additional servings to get adequate calories.

TIPS FOR EATING SATISFYING AND ENERGIZING WHOLE CARBS

- Try roasting big batches of chopped starchy vegetables (carrots, beets, sweet potatoes, butternut squash, corn) in the oven and store in the fridge in sealed containers for quick use.
- Buy a rice cooker and get in the habit of cooking big batches of whole grains on a regular basis. You can cook any variety of whole grain in a rice cooker and doing so requires zero pot watching. Cooked whole grains will keep nicely for 2 or 3 days if stored in the refrigerator in a covered container or a self-sealing plastic bag. You can add cooked whole grains to soups, stews, and salads or serve them as an easy side dish. Whole grains make the perfect bed on which to nestle a medley of stir-fried veggies. They are great for breakfast when mixed with fruit and chopped nuts. And

just about any cooked whole grain can be turned into a delicious and elegant pilaf in a matter of minutes.

- Try making an all-veggie sandwich with toasted sprouted whole grain bread.
- Mix sprouted whole grain pasta with roasted spaghetti squash and top with a roasted root vegetable ragù.
- Give your regular rolled oats a break and try even more healthful steel-cut oats for your morning breakfast. Even though rolled oats are a healthful choice, they are still a bit processed—steel-cut oats are the superior choice from a nutritional standpoint. Plus they keep you feeling full longer because they have more soluble fiber. Steel-cut oats are a snap to make in a slow cooker: Simply combine 3¾ cups water (or hemp or almond milk), 1 cup steel-cut oats, and a pinch of sea salt in the crock, and cook on high for 2 hours. You can prepare the night before then refrigerate so it's ready when you are first thing in the morning.
- Buy some wheat germ and sprinkle it on top of your fruit.
- In a mega rush? Nothing wrong with raw oats! Try a morning muesli with raw oats (recipe on page 307) or simply lightly moisten raw oats with hemp milk, almond milk, or soy milk and add some fresh chopped fruit.
- Get exotic with your rice! It's hard to keep up with nutrition news, but in case you haven't heard, black rice is the new brown and considered to be the most healthful rice of all. Black rice is popping up everywhere. You can find black rice at Asian markets and natural foods stores, such as Whole Foods Market. Black rice can attribute a good deal of its health benefits to exceptionally high levels of antioxidants. Specifically, black rice is rich in a class of flavonoid antioxidants called anthocyanins (also found in blueberries, açaí, and grapes.) Exotic black rice has a mild but distinct flavor that pairs perfectly with a tremendous number of foods and flavors. Plus it looks beautiful and makes an impressive presence on any plate; it's the easiest ever side dish because it doesn't need to be all dolled up to look or taste exciting. You can cook black rice just like you cook any other rice—stovetop or in a rice cooker (which is how Ivy cooks all rice!).
- Add them to your soups.

We think it's important to eat a wide variety of different whole grains so we like to rotate our grains on a regular basis. Ivy generally makes a big batch of whole grains with the rice cooker then stores them in the fridge for up to 3 days in a covered container. She then uses the grains for hot breakfast cereal, to make pilafs, to add to salads, to eat with vegetables, to add to soups, and so forth. When the grains are gone she starts all over and makes a new batch with a new whole grain.

Going Gluten Free?

Do you find yourself wondering why gluten-free foods have suddenly become all the rage and why gluten-free diets are so popular? Why do we suddenly have such an unusually high percentage of the population who are unable to digest wheat and gluten? And why does it seem as if celiac disease were on the rise? It is interesting that the gluten-free trend comes at a time when there has never been more gluten in the typical American diet than now. Gluten is the protein found in foods like wheat and rye, and it is difficult for some people to digest. Symptoms of gluten sensitivity can be rather random (headaches, depression, fatigue, irritable bowel syndrome) and differ from one individual to the other. However, if you are truly allergic to foods that happen to contain gluten, your body will develop a true inflammatory response. For those with celiac disease, which is an autoimmune disease, eating gluten can lead to many serious health problems, including long-term damage to the small intestine and digestive system, and therefore absolutely must be avoided.

> NOTE: To get an accurate diagnosis of celiac disease, you need a blood test and an endoscopic examination, including biopsy, of the small bowel to determine if there is atrophy in your gut.

As a general rule, all foods containing wheat or wheat-related grains (rye, triticale, and kamut) contain gluten. Ancient grains such as spelt and barley are also on the gluten hit list, but they contain much less gluten than what is found in wheat. Oats remain a subject of great debate in the gluten-free community—oats don't actually contain gluten but they are often grown or processed right alongside wheat so there's the concern of cross-contamination. But because gluten is used as an all-purpose stabilizer and thickener, manufacturers add it to an astounding number of packaged food products ranging from marinades to coffees, packaged spices, and even multivitamins! Other hidden sources of gluten include fried foods, bacon bits and imitation bacon products, beer, brown rice, syrup, dairy substitutes, deli meats, hydrolyzed vegetable protein, imitation seafood, commercial salad dressings, and soy sauces. In addition, many processed vegan foods such as veggie burgers and fake meat—namely seitan—are specifically made from wheat gluten, which gives these foods their rubbery, meat-like texture. Needless to say, many of the foods that happen to be made with gluten, such as processed meat-like Fakin' Bacon or imitation seafood, are not exactly what we consider Clean Cuisine. It's not 100 percent fair to isolate the gluten and say the only reason these foods are unhealthful is because they contain gluten; they are unhealthful for numerous other reasons.

> NOTE: According to Dr. Peter Green, professor of clinical medicine and director of the Celiac Disease Center at Columbia University, the majority of people with celiac disease can tolerate oats.

But what about plain old wheat? What is wrong with that? The wheat we eat today is not exactly a completely natural food. Modern wheat has been encouraged to grow the way it does to produce a better crop yield. Today's wheat has been cultivated to produce more food on less land. The result has been higher levels of gluten in the wheat crop. To compound the problem, the typical American eating the typical American diet eats more wheat and consequently more gluten than ever before because wheat and wheat derivatives are found in many processed foods, most of which happen to be nutrient poor. The vast majority of gluten-containing foods made with refined wheat flour, such as packaged breakfast cereals, breads, bagels, English muffins, pretzels, white pasta, pizza crust, pastries, crackers, and the like are notoriously low in nutrition and high in empty-calorie starches. In fact, because refined carbohydrates are highly inflammatory foods, eating a diet high in processed empty-calorie carbohydrates can actually cause symptoms that mimic a food intolerance or food allergy. So, if someone who regularly eats a diet rich in refined carbohydrates (that happen to be high in gluten) complains of feeling bloated, tired, and depressed switches to a gluten-free diet and replaces their pizza and pretzels with nutrient-dense and naturally gluten-free carbs such as fruit, quinoa, and vegetables we wouldn't be surprised at all if they felt much better on their new diet. Is it because of the lack of gluten or is it because they are now eating an otherwise healthful diet low in refined carbohydrates? In most cases, with the exception of celiac disease patients, the improved diet as a whole is more beneficial than just going gluten free.

What about weight loss? Will going gluten free really help you lose weight? Not necessarily. Eating a gluten-free bagel or gluten-free Betty Crocker cake is not going to take off pounds any faster than eating a regular bagel or regular Betty Crocker cake. Loading up on gluten-free cakes and crackers will have about as much weight-loss benefit as eating fat-free SnackWell's cookies had back in the 1990s. In fact, if you avoid *only gluten*, rather than the empty-calorie, packaged carbohydrate foods gluten is often found in, you will likely be getting *more calories* with *fewer nutrients*. This is because many gluten-free substitutes end up being high in replacement empty-calorie starchy carbs (such as potato flour) and low in fiber. That's why people who go on prescribed gluten-free diets often see their body mass indexes increase, not decrease. While many people have erroneously concluded that gluten is bad, the truth is gluten is not bad for those who are not sensitive to it any more so than peanuts are bad if you are free of peanut allergy. Although naturally gluten-free unrefined whole grain foods such as quinoa and amaranth are absolutely healthful, gluten-free processed products are not exactly nutritional all-stars. Gluten-free processed products (such as breads, cookies, and crackers) actually tend to be lower in fiber, vitamins, and iron than are their wheat- and gluten-containing cousins. And finally, let's get real here, just because a cookie is gluten-free doesn't mean it's healthful!

So should you shun wheat and gluten from your diet? Unless you are truly allergic or sensitive to wheat or to gluten, we see no need for making unnecessary diet restrictions to otherwise healthful foods such as wheat germ, sprouted whole grain breads, and sprouted whole grain pastas. We also don't see any benefit to going out of your way to eat a wheat- and gluten-rich diet either! Think of it this way: You probably wouldn't eat eight bananas in a day so why would you eat eight servings of wheat a day? Aim for balance and variety. That's what we do. While we might eat sprouted whole grain pasta for dinner, we don't eat gluten-fortified crackers, pizza, cookies, and cake. We also think outside of the wheat box. There are plenty of other nutrient-dense, gluten-free grains to include in your diet, such as brown, wild or black rice; quinoa; millet; corn; buckwheat (we *love* soba noodles); and amaranth. No need to get stuck on wheat meal after meal after meal.

LOOK FOR FLOURLESS SPROUTED WHOLE GRAIN BREADS AND PASTAS

IT IS TRUE whole grain breads and pastas are considered whole carbs. However, when a whole grain is finely ground into flour it is absorbed into your bloodstream fairly quickly, and this can spike blood sugar levels and increase insulin response. The rapid rise of glucose and rise in insulin is undesirable for diabetics, people with heart disease, and anyone who is trying to lose weight. This means homemade whole grain hot cereals are a better choice than a boxed whole grain cereal that is made with whole grain flour such as whole wheat. The absolute most nutritious grains are those that are sprouted.

The process of sprouting releases all the vital nutrients stored within the whole grains and elevates whole grains from a healthful food to a power food. You can absolutely sprout your own whole grains by soaking them in water, but this isn't something a lot of people find particularly convenient. What is convenient is buying premade breads and pastas made with sprouted whole grains. We particularly love Manna Organics (made by Nature's Path) breads and muffins and the Food for Life sprouted whole grain sandwich breads, buns, and pasta lines. These brands are available in natural foods stores and larger supermarkets.

NOTE: You will find sprouted whole grain breads only in the frozen section of your supermarket because these breads are preservative-free, which is a good thing!

Eliminating the Bad Boy Empty Carbs

Unlike whole carbs, empty carbs are a nutritional nightmare. These foods are no longer nutritionally intact, the way nature designed them. They contribute to malnutrition (along with what we call the malnourished munchies), excess hunger, and out of control food cravings. The fiber and majority of naturally occurring nutrients have been removed during processing, and you are left with a low-volume, calorie-rich, nutrient-poor, empty-calorie food. Not exactly something you want to eat to reduce inflammation and look, feel, and age your best!

Because empty carbs are not bulky, they don't take up a lot of room or space in your stomach and you need to eat massive amounts of them to feel full. Empty carbs are rapidly absorbed, so they cause a sharp glucose surge into the bloodstream, which forces your pancreas to pump out the fat-storing hormone insulin. Whenever your blood sugar level spikes, your pancreas must produce insulin to bring the blood sugar level back down to a healthy level. The problem is insulin is your body's primary fat-storing hormone; it forces your liver to convert the excess sugar in your blood into fat. The more frequently you assault your body by eating quickly absorbed, blood sugar–spiking, empty carbs the more demand you place on your pancreas, the more fat you gain, and the greater chance you place yourself for developing type 2 diabetes. A diet rich in empty carbs is also linked to heart disease and even increased cancer risk. But that's not all! If you are not particularly active and the empty carbs you eat are not burned off for energy, your body can actually convert them into proinflammatory saturated fat, specifically a very dangerous type of saturated fat associated with an increased risk of heart disease called palmitic acid. The saturated fat your body manufacturers will increase inflammation in your body. Inflammation will not only negatively affect your appearance but will also exacerbate symptoms of inflammatory conditions such as MS, asthma, fibromyalgia, psoriasis, and arthritis. If that's not bad enough, did you know insulin also activates the main enzyme responsible for making cholesterol in your liver? What this means is that even if you eat a 100 percent cholesterol-free, animal-free diet your cholesterol can still increase if you eat too many processed empty-calorie carbohydrates.

Empty-calorie processed carbohydrates are easy to identify and easy to avoid if you know what to look for. Luckily, there really are only a few carbohydrates you want to avoid. Unfortunately, the following empty-calorie carbohydrate ingredients are ubiquitous in modern society and found in *numerous* processed food products. Keep your eyes open and avoid using the following processed empty-calorie carbs in the recipes you make and in the packaged foods you buy.

Empty Carb 1: Refined Flour

Refined flour is enriched flour, wheat flour, all-purpose flour, or any other flour that does not specifically have the word *whole* in front of it on the list of product ingredients. Refined flour is found in hundreds of processed food products. Refined flour is the nutritional equivalent of table sugar. The vast majority of flour and flour-based products sold in the United States are made from wheat. There is nothing intrinsically wrong with wheat, but in refining flour, the nutrient-rich wheat germ that contains antioxidant vitamin E along with a vast array of trace minerals and phytonutrients and the fiber-rich wheat bran are removed. This leaves behind nutrient-poor, fiber-free starch. *No nutrients equal empty calories.* Along with sugar, white flour is the ultimate empty-calorie carb. Enriched flours and all-purpose flours certainly sound more healthful than refined white flour, but they are all the same thing. Enrichment refers to the government-mandated processes of adding small amounts of synthetic vitamins and minerals to refined flour after it has been processed. As required by law, all refined flour is enriched. The only reason flour is enriched is because all the good stuff was removed during processing! Whole foods are not enriched, only processed foods are enriched. Enriched flour does not contain fiber, and *synthetic* vitamins and minerals that are added represent only a small portion of the nutrients that were removed during processing. Furthermore, your body does not recognize or use synthetic nutrients in the same manner it does naturally occurring nutrients. In addition, the disease-fighting phytonutrients are lost forever during the refinement process and are not added back.

FOODS LIKELY TO CONTAIN REFINED FLOUR
(Read the Ingredients List on All Foods You Purchase)

- Bagels
- Baked goods
- Breads
- Bread crumbs
- Breaded meats and vegetables
- Breakfast bars
- Cakes
- Cookies
- Crackers
- Muffins
- Pancakes
- Pasta
- Pizza
- Pretzels
- Rolls
- Waffles

WHOLE FLOUR IS OKAY TO EAT IN MODERATION

WHOLE WHEAT FLOUR and other whole grain flours such as stone-ground corn flour, barley flour, oat flour, and amaranth flour are acceptable in moderation as part of the Clean Cuisine lifestyle. However, keep in mind all flours, even whole grain flours, will be absorbed into your bloodstream more quickly than will the whole grains themselves, such as quinoa, steel-cut oats, and barley. Two versatile, relatively healthful flours Ivy uses most frequently and you should keep on hand at all times are:

Stone-ground corn flour: Stone-ground corn flour comes simply from grinding up dried corn. Ivy loves to use it to coat tofu for crispy pan-seared tofu nuggets or to make pan-seared scallops and fish. It's also delicious in corn muffins and even special-occasion crepes.

White whole wheat flour: White whole wheat flour is every bit as nutritious as its brown whole wheat flour cousin because it contains the nutrient-rich germ and the fiber-rich bran. However, white whole wheat flour bakes better and tastes more like the less-healthful all-purpose flour you might be more accustomed to. In comparison to regular whole wheat flour, which is made from red wheat, white whole wheat flour is made from a naturally occurring albino variety of wheat, which is lighter in color and has a sweeter, milder flavor, making it perfect for many baked good recipes, especially desserts. Best of all, white whole wheat flour offers the same nutritional goodness as its darker cousin. Because white whole wheat flour is less heavy than is traditional whole wheat flour, it can replace all-purpose white flour one to one in recipes.

Empty Carb 2: Sugar

We don't need to elaborate too much on sugar. Even a first grader can tell you eating too much sugar is not good. The problem is sugar is ubiquitous. Start reading labels, and you'll find sugar hidden in everything from spaghetti sauce to breakfast cereals to frozen food entrees. According to the USDA, the average American adult consumes more than 64 pounds of sugar every year! To put that in perspective, 64 pounds of sugar translates to a whopping 108,800 empty calories eaten per year. Ugh.

SUGAR BY ANY OTHER NAME IS STILL SUGAR

(Don't Be Fooled by Common Sugar Pseudonyms)

- Dextrose
- Fructose
- Glucose
- Sucrose
- Maltose
- Syrup
- Cane juice
- Raw sugar
- Evaporated cane juice
- Fruit juice sweetener
- Corn sweetener
- Corn syrup
- High-fructose corn syrup
- Modified food starch
- Honey
- Molasses

SWEET SORROWS

NOT ONLY IS sugar the perfect example of the ultimate empty calorie but it can also be a toxic age accelerator. In fact, diabetics are known to age on all levels significantly faster than nondiabetics largely due to the toxic effects of sugar. Eating excess amounts of sugar can wreak havoc with your cells on the *inside* but also damage your skin on the *outside* too. According to researchers sugar binds to the proteins collagen and elastin and works to make it harder for skin to repair itself.[20] In healthy, youthful skin collagen fibers twist together in linear strands, but when sugar gets clumped on to collagen the fibers can't pack together as tightly so the skin begins to look wrinkled and old. The older you get, after about age 35, the less resilient your skin becomes and the less capable it is of repair after repeated sugar attacks. So, while that cookie might look good today, it might not look so good 10 or 20 years from now.

Empty Carb 3: Fruit Juice

Okay, so maybe 100 percent fresh-pressed raw fruit juice (which is different in every way from the heated and pasteurized stuff you buy packaged at the supermarket) is not a totally empty-calorie carb, but it's not optimal either. Any way you pour it, juice provides a much more concentrated source of calories with fewer nutritional benefits compared to the whole fruit. It's also very easy to overconsume juice because it's fiber-free and therefore substantially less filling than the whole fruit. Fruit juice is especially undesirable if you are overweight or have diabetes.

The only juice that is really optimal to drink is whole juice, which is made from the *entire* whole fruit, pulp and all. When we make orange juice we peel an orange, quarter it, then put the whole orange segments in our blender and blend it up just like that for fresh whole orange juice; we do not squeeze the juice from the orange and throw out the pulp. In fact, a high concentration of the phytonutrients found in oranges is concentrated in the inner white pulp. Why on earth would you want to throw out the fiber-rich and phytonutrient-rich pulp and drink just the sugary liquid?

Empty Carb 4: White Rice

Just use brown rice, or better yet black rice. Short grain brown rice tastes basically the same as white rice, and black rice is just incredible. We really have no idea why on earth the white stuff was ever eaten in the first place.

Sweet Endings: How to Cheat and Have a Small Sweet Treat Each Day

Considering how much Ivy in particular loves sweets, we both wish we could tell you candy is dandy and that dessert should be a guiltless pleasure. But that would not be truthful (sigh). By definition, desserts are sweet and therefore contain sugar. So, while we unfortunately can't advise you to leave your dietary conscience at the back door once the dessert tray arrives (even if one of your favorite European chocolate tortes happens to be among the display), we can share some sensible strategies for how to incorporate sweet treats into your diet without causing too much harm. The overall strategy we find most helpful is to sneak in nutrition whenever and wherever possible (and we keep our dessert portions small too). If you have totally eliminated sugar elsewhere in your diet, and you otherwise eat nutrient-dense Clean Cuisine recommendations, then eating one *small* sweet treat each day is really not the end of the world. When you get to the 8-week program in Chapter 9, you will see some of Ivy's best tips for cleaning up your favorite dessert recipes and how to safely work sweet treats into your diet. And last but not least, the final part of the book includes several of our family's favorite *almost* guiltless sweet treats. Because life is too short to not be sweet!

5

CLEAN FATS:
Whole Plant and Marine
Sources of Essential Fats and
Some Good Oils Too

As a general surgeon who does a lot of weight-loss surgery for obesity, cancer surgery for colon and breast cancer, and gallbladder surgery and who happens to have a wife with MS—all conditions that are related to dietary fat intake—Andy has studied the role of fats from many different angles, including the role fats play in satiety and weight control, inflammation (the common thread linking seemingly unrelated conditions such as obesity, heart disease, fibromyalgia, arthritis, MS, asthma, and allergies), and heart health. The conclusion he has made after reviewing the available academic literature can be summed up as follows:

- *Unrefined* whole plant fats and marine omega-3 fats are the best fats for overall health and weight loss.
- Animal-based saturated fats and trans-fats are inflammatory, fattening, and disease-provoking.
- Eating fats in their whole form (walnuts instead of walnut oil) is best.
- Including the right types of fat in your diet is essential for appetite control and satiety.

- The omega ratio (ratio of omega-3 to omega-6) is critical for reducing inflammation, improving sensitivity to insulin (thus lowering risk of obesity and type 2 diabetes), and protecting against heart disease.
- Eating excess amounts of oils is unhealthy and fattening.
- Eating a very low fat diet is not necessary for good health or weight loss, but eating a right fat diet is essential for both.

From a culinary standpoint, and the fact that Ivy has spent close to 15 years experimenting in the kitchen trying to create the most healthful *and tastiest* whole food based Clean Cuisine possible, she can sum dietary fats up very simply:

- Fats are one of the most important conveyers of flavor in food. It is next to impossible to create fat-free recipes in which the food tastes good and is truly satisfying. If you want the food to taste good you have to add some fat. The trick to keeping your food tasty *and healthful* is to use the right fats in the right amount.

And so our goal is to eat the right types of fat in moderation for optimal health and satiety and to make our food taste good. This is an oversimplification for sure, so let's dig a bit and try to understand fats on a deeper level.

Our nutritional journey began over a decade ago with learning first about dietary fats. When Ivy was diagnosed with MS, her neurologist suggested she read *The Multiple Sclerosis Diet Book* by neurologist Roy Swank. Dr. Swank made the observation that in Norway an increased incidence of MS seemed to be correlated with groups that had a relatively high consumption of saturated fat from animal foods, particularly dairy products, and was lower wherever omega-3-rich fish intake was high. Dr. Swank's observational work dates back to the 1940s, long before modern disease-modifying MS drugs were available. To test his observation, in 1949 he enrolled 150 MS patients in an extraordinary 34-year study and recommended a very low saturated fat diet for these patients. With this study, Dr. Swank showed compelling proof that dietary modification could in fact reduce the frequency and severity of exacerbations in MS patients. A number of scientific papers resulted from this study, including publications in the *Lancet* (one of the world's premier medical journals), *New England Journal of Medicine, Nutrition,* and *Archives of Neurology.*

It was because of Dr. Swank's work and additional studies we reviewed pertaining to dietary modification for the treatment of MS that we became interested in nutrition in the first place. Even though Andy went to one of the top medical schools in the world (the University of Pennsylvania), he had never heard of nutritional therapy for the treatment of MS and was unaware of the research linking dietary fat to the disease. And, like other medical schools, the focus of his studies at the University of Pennsylvania was on medicine, not nutrition. Needless to say we *both* had a lot of learning to do on the subject of nutrition and dietary fat.

Early in the learning process we were fortunate to be introduced to the work of Dr. David Perlmutter, a highly regarded and innovative integrative neurologist and co-author of several books, including one of our favorites, *The Better Brain Book.* As a patient, Ivy went to visit Dr. Perlmutter at his clinic in Naples, Florida, and we were both highly impressed with the holistic approach he takes to promoting brain health for a broad range of very serious neurological conditions (such as MS, vascular dementia, Alzheimer's disease, Parkinson's disease, amyotrophic lateral sclerosis, and stroke) and boosting cognitive function in otherwise healthy people who simply want to enjoy better mental clarity, improved memory and quickness of thought, a better mood, and renewed mental vigor. Nutritional therapy, including consuming the right fats in the right amounts, is a key component of Dr. Perlmutter's integrative approach to improving brain health.

What we have learned is that the type of fat you eat can play a major role not only in inflammatory conditions such as MS, fibromyalgia, and arthritis but also in the management of obesity, heart disease, and type 2 diabetes. We learned that the same nutrition that is beneficial in the fight against one chronic disease will promote good health, protect against other diseases, and help you achieve a healthy body weight too. There is no such thing as a fat that is bad for heart health but good for MS. Nor is there a diet that is optimal for preventing cancer but harmful for diabetics. The Clean Cuisine whole foods–based, plant-forward, good fat, anti-inflammatory diet can help you achieve optimal health across the board. And it can dramatically slow the aging process and improve your appearance.

When it comes to fats, you need to know there are good, healing, anti-inflammatory fats and then there are disease-provoking, inflammatory, fattening fats. And even the good fats must be eaten in the right ratio to do good. If not, they can actually be harmful. Sounds complicated, we know. But fat science can be simplified; that's what we do in this chapter.

A Big Fat Primer

Fats are critical for helping your body absorb certain fat-soluble antioxidants such as lycopene and vitamins A, D, E, and K. Fats keep skin and cell membranes healthy, help repair tissues, provide cushioning to internal organs, and help make hormone-like substances that regulate a wide variety of important body functions, including sexual function. Depending on the type of fat you eat, your body produces either more or fewer inflammatory molecules, which affect metabolism, pain, and overall wellness. Fats also provide the structural components of cell membranes in the brain as well as myelin—the fatty insulating sheath in the central nervous system that surrounds each nerve fiber—enabling nerves to carry messages faster. Some fats must be obtained from food are are therefore called essential fats and are absolutely necessary for life itself. Your body can't make essential fats; you need to get these critically important fats from the foods you eat.

One thing is clear from the research: Not all fats are created equal. Natural fats come in three basic kinds: saturated, monounsaturated, and polyunsaturated. The polyunsaturated fats can be further subdivided into the oh so important essential omega-3 fats and omega-6 fats. Most foods that contain fat have a mixture of all three basic fat categories, saturated, monounsaturated, and polyunsaturated. For example, although olive oil is categorized as a monounsaturated fat, roughly 12 to 14 percent of the calories in olive oil actually come from saturated fat (but the plant-based saturated fat in olive oil is totally different from the animal-based saturated fat in foods like beef and cheese). Most animal fats contain a substantially greater portion of their fat in the less desirable saturated form; for example, butter is 63 percent saturated fat. There are a few plant-based foods that contain a high percentage of saturated fat, virgin coconut oil is a prime example. Virgin coconut oil contains a large amount of lauric acid, a saturated fat that actually provides health benefits. Furthermore, just because olive oil, coconut oil, and butter might all contain more or less the same calories from fat per tablespoon they are not nutritional equals.

Again, we know it sounds complicated, and to some degree it is, but keep reading and you will soon begin to understand.

Change Your Fat to Improve Your Brain, Heart, and Skin Health

As mentioned earlier, our interest in nutrition and dietary fat was driven by Ivy's MS diagnosis, so our research efforts initially focused on identifying the best and worst fats for brain (central nervous system) health. The brain is the most metabolically active organ in the body, and it's constantly replenishing and repairing itself. Much of the food we eat not only ends up being used by the brain for energy but ends up *in* the brain itself. By the way, your brain is actually made up of fat. Think of a marbled fatty burger frying in a puddle of grease. This is your brain on hamburgers. Gross, huh? Do you want all that animal grease going to your brain? Not us. But that doesn't mean fat free is best for your brain either. Your brain absolutely needs certain types of fat for optimal function. The good news is to a large degree you can control the health of your brain by controlling the types of fat you eat. And having a healthy brain doesn't just mean you'll improve symptoms of neurological diseases such as MS, you'll also improve your mood, sharpen concentration, and have a greater sense of overall well-being. The fats you eat have a huge impact on the levels of neurotransmitters, thus regulating all mental processes that affect how well we think and feel. But that's not all.

The foods and fats that are healthy for your brain are the same ones that are healthy for your arteries and heart. Your heart health greatly depends on the type of fat you eat. The bad fats, primarily saturated fat, trans-fats, and refined omega-6-rich vegetable oils not only promote neurological disease such as MS but also accelerate hardening of the arteries, thus making you more susceptible to a heart attack or stroke. Most strokes are caused by the same blood vessel process that causes a heart attack, except this time the organ under attack is the brain. The same fats that are associated with decreased risk of stroke and heart disease are the same fats associated with decreased incidence and severity of neurological disorders, including MS and depression—namely the omega-3 essential fats such as marine-derived docosahexaenoic acid (DHA). And there's more.

Your brain and skin are derived from the same embryonic tissue, called the ectoderm. There is a very close relationship between brain health and skin health. There is also an intimate relationship between the health of your blood vessels and your skin too. Your blood vessels supply nourishment to your skin, and if your blood vessels are in poor health you can rest assured you will look, and feel, older than your years. Eating fats that are healthy for your heart and brain will improve your appearance by making your skin glow. In addition, a deficiency in certain essential fats will leave you with dull, dry, and crepe-like skin. So the type of fat you eat matters on many levels for improving overall health, mood, and appearance. It matters a lot.

Fight Fat with Fat?

As a general surgeon and one of only a few hundred surgeons in the world currently directing an internationally certified Center of Excellence program offering weight-loss surgery, Andy has worked with thousands of significantly overweight patients. He has spent a good deal of time researching the science of appetite as well as the effect foods (including fats) have on body weight. And make no mistake, the amount and types of fat you eat *do* affect your body weight.

Fats provide a very concentrated source of calories for not a lot of bulk, so it makes sense that eating too much fat is not going to be as satisfying as eating bulky but low-calorie and fiber-rich foods. Plant foods that are low in energy density and high in water content, such as fruits, beans, soups, vegetables, and whole grains, are going to be more filling and allow you to eat more volume without gaining weight. But there's a caveat. If you reduce fat too much, you end up not feeling satisfied after your meal. Sure your stomach might be stuffed, but you don't feel psychologically *satisfied*. You don't need to rely on a scientific study to prove this either. You can conduct your own satiety experiment at your very next meal.

Suppose you eat a spinach salad with 2 cups of raw spinach tossed with 1 tomato and 2 chopped carrots. That's a lot of volume for only about 100 calories. So let's say you add in 100 calories of fat-free croutons made from toasted sprouted whole grain bread. Now you are up to 200 calories and more bulk. You then throw in ½ cup of beans for another 100 calories. Now you have a voluminous 300-calorie salad and your stomach should be feeling pretty full. But 300 calories is not a lot. And it's doubtful you are going to feel satiated with your salad, even though your stomach is technically full. And because fat is a critical culinary conveyer of flavor, it's also doubtful your salad is going to taste very good or provide much enjoyment either. Furthermore, all of the mostly carb-containing calories in your bulky salad are going to be digested rather quickly because compared with fat and protein all carbohydrates, even the good whole ones, are digested pretty fast. The carb-only meal will surely cause you to feel hungry again in no time. However, simply adding 100 calories worth of avocado or nuts and a drizzle of cold-pressed extra-virgin olive oil for another 40 calories or so will add tremendous flavor—for still not a lot of calories—and do wonders for making you feel full and satisfied. The fats will also delay stomach emptying, so you'll feel full longer. Plus adding important good fats will boost absorption of the fat-soluble vitamins and antioxidants (including the lycopene from the tomato) in your salad.

The secret to maintaining a healthy weight without deprivation is to eat in a way that is satisfying and enjoyable and keeps you feeling full for hours. Adding moderate amounts of healthy fats, especially whole fats such as nuts, seeds, and avocados, to your meals accomplishes all of this. Fats are the satiety macronutrient, and it is very difficult to feel satisfied without fat.

Further, eating the proper ratio of omega-3 to omega-6 fat (which we will show you how to do easily later in the chapter) will reduce inflammation and improve your body's sensitivity to insulin, thus making weight loss easier. Plus eating certain good high-fat foods—raw nuts and raw seeds in particular—is actually associated with a lower overall body weight. Studies show people who are allowed to eat as many raw nuts as they like on a regular basis are actually slimmer than those who do not eat nuts.[1] The consumption of nuts and seeds is believed to help improve insulin sensitivity and even help prevent type 2 diabetes, a condition intimately related to obesity.[2] In general, research suggests the consumption of nuts and seeds improves satiety and helps with weight management and weight loss. While we absolutely do emphasize the good fats and eliminate as much as possible the bad ones, rest assured Clean Cuisine is not a low-fat, tasteless, diet food way of eating.

The Big Fat Greek Olive Oil Myth

Here's the deal. Drenching your salad with olive oil and dousing your vegetables in several tablespoons of the stuff is not the best way to go about improving your heart health or slimming your waist. As we discussed in Chapter 1, the foundation of Clean Cuisine is to choose whole foods in their most natural and unrefined form, and while most oils are natural foods, they are not in an unrefined form. You don't see puddles of olive oil in nature. Olive oil comes from whole olives. Corn oil comes from whole corn. Soybean oil comes from whole soybeans. And so on. The thing is, the calories in *all* oils can add up quickly and *can* contribute to weight gain.

If you gain weight due to an excess intake of oil, the extra weight is going to negatively affect your health from a cardiovascular standpoint and also impair your immune system. It doesn't matter whether the extra weight comes from heart healthy olive oil or not; being overweight is not heart healthy. Furthermore, being overweight increases the toxic load in your body, accelerates aging, and increases inflammation, thus contributing to the chronic inflammation associated with diseases such as MS, fibromyalgia, arthritis, and so on. You will undoubtedly find it easier to reduce chronic inflammation and maintain your weight without hunger and without counting calories by eating a reduced-oil diet.

While there is clearly research showing that eating high-fat whole nuts and seeds is associated with reduced body weight, we have not been able to find research showing that people who eat oil-rich diets are slimmer. Again, oil of any kind is a more concentrated source of calories when compared to whole plant foods that happen to be rich in fat such as nuts, seeds, olives, and avocados. And of course oil is devoid of the fiber naturally packaged within the whole plant food. Many improperly processed oils are also devoid of the phytonutrients found naturally packaged in the whole foods. And, as we will explain later in the chapter, not all oil is processed in a healthful way either. Many oils, including vegetable oils such as corn oil and soybean oil, are processed with heat, solvents, and chemicals that make these oils downright dangerous.

Remember, we did not say follow a no oil diet. We know a little oil goes a very long way to making food taste fabulous, and a big component of the Clean Cuisine lifestyle is great-tasting food. So, yes, you can have some oil. We just want to stress not to go overboard. We'd rather you get most of your fat from plant-based whole fats such as nuts, seeds, coconuts, and avocados. Culinary oils such as olive oil should be added more as flavor-enhancers and eaten in moderation.

There are population studies of the Mediterranean-style diet showing people who eat monounsaturated fat–rich olive oil live longer and have less cardiovascular disease than people eating a diet that is high in saturated fat, refined vegetable oils, and refined carbohydrates, but a study comparing terrible diets with an olive oil–rich diet that also happens to have lots of plant-based whole foods and moderate amounts of fish does not constitute proof that the oil is the key factor in the differences in heart health.[3] Analyzing a population study on diet requires a close analysis of countless food substances and is an infinitely complex process. To say that the oil is the main reason the Mediterranean diet is heart healthy is too simplistic of an explanation.

After reading countless studies on nutrition, we believe if the Mediterranean-style diet were compared head to head against the Clean Cuisine diet, the Clean Cuisine diet would be the better choice for weight loss, heart health, and inflammation. The Clean Cuisine diet is devoid of trans-fats; is low in dairy, meat, and animal-based saturated fat; is low in sugar; and is relatively low in oil. At the same time, it is rich in unrefined plant-based whole foods, salads, vegetables, fruits; in whole fats from raw nuts, seeds, and avocados; in beans and whole soy; and in whole grains and legumes. The Clean Cuisine way of eating also contains moderate amounts of omega-3-rich fish, a healthful omega-3 to omega-6 profile, and a smattering of high-quality grass-fed animal foods. In other words, the Mediterranean diet is very good but could be even better and more slimming if there were less focus on the olive oil and an even greater focus on eating a wide variety of healthful whole plant foods.

A key point worth stressing emphatically is that eating more whole carb foods like vegetables, salads, and beans is going to make the biggest difference in how you age, look, and feel. Pouring tons of heart healthy olive oil on these foods is not going to do a thing to boost your health, and if you eat too much oil, it will negatively affect your health. So the take-home message here is to simply keep the health-promoting benefits of oil in perspective. Add oil more for flavor, not for health and certainly not for weight loss. Eating more oil is not going to help you lose weight. End of story. However, eating whole fats like olives, avocados, nuts, and seeds does play a role in weight loss and good health. We will discuss these good whole fats in more detail later in the chapter.

IS THE OIL IN OLIVE OIL HEART HEALTHY OR IS IT SOMETHING ELSE?

MEDICINAL USE OF olive leaves dates back to ancient Egypt and is referenced by Hippocrates and now in modern medical texts. And surely you have read about the health benefits of olive oil in countless magazines and have listened to the morning show personalities broadcast how olive oil is heart healthy. But, is it really the *oil* in olive oil that should get all the glory for olive oil's decades long untarnished heart healthy reputation, or is it something else in the olives themselves? The principal fat in olive oil is a monounsaturated fat called oleic acid, but some nutrition scientists are beginning to theorize the natural phytonutrient and antioxidant compounds in olives, the flavonoids, polyphenols, sterols, anthocyanins, and so forth, are the real key players and that it is these plant substances that provide the intrinsic health benefits of olive oil—*not the oil itself.* Could it be that olive oil is simply a delivery mechanism for these antiaging, anti-inflammatory plant substances? We can't say for sure just yet, but we have a hunch that the flavonoids, polyphenols, sterols, and anthocyanins are more beneficial to heart health and health in general than the oleic acid from the olive oil.

Let's put it this way, we would never routinely supplement our diets with a tablespoon of olive oil taken in medicinal spoonful form, but we *do* often supplement with olive leaf extract (Barlean's brand happens to be our favorite) because we know we are getting a concentrated source of phytonutrients, a super high oxygen radical absorbance capacity (ORAC) value (a measure of antioxidant power), and no extra empty and unwanted calories. On the flip side, the olive leaf extract is not taken for taste benefits because it does not taste particularly good, and it is guaranteed to ruin a recipe. Olive oil, on the other hand, contributes tremendous culinary benefits and a drizzle does wonders for making our salads, cooked veggies, beans, legumes, and whole grains taste delicious. So we don't exactly want to ditch our olive oil bottles either. Instead, we encourage you to think about the benefits of olive oil beyond the oil itself and to use olive oil in moderation because it enhances the flavor of our food. Olive oil is a healthful oil for use in recipes and for cooking, but it is not an essential nutrient.

The Bad Boy Fats You *Do Not* Need

Before we get to the good whole fats, let's get the two bad boy fats out of the way right now. There is absolutely no biological requirement for saturated fat or trans-fats. Both epidemiological studies and clinical trials have implicated saturated fats and trans-fats as dietary evils for humans.[4] Both fats promote inflammation and are directly linked to heart disease and cancer. Without question, eating a diet rich in animal-based saturated fat and trans-fats will accelerate aging and promote weight gain too.

Big Bad Fat 1: Trans-Fats

Trans-fats are trash can fats, the absolute worst fats on the planet and should not be eaten in any quantity. These terrible fats were created to extend shelf life, but they decrease human life. The good news is these bad boy fats are not nearly as prevalent as they once were and have been stripped from many processed foods, only to be replaced by cheap, highly processed empty-calorie vegetable oils! Still the fact that most people eat less trans-fat today than they did a decade ago is a big step in the right direction. But even a little teeny, tiny bit is still too much. The Institute of Medicine of the National Academies, the organization responsible for advising the U.S. government on health policy and responsible for determining the Reference Daily Intake (RDI) for vitamins concluded, "any incremental increase in *trans* fatty acid intake increases CHD risk."[5] Synthetic trans-fats are far more dangerous than the naturally occurring saturated fats found in animal foods like beef and eggs and are directly linked to heart disease. Terribly troublesome trans-fats are capable of altering your cholesterol profile toward the absolute most dangerous ratio in terms of risk for heart disease; trans-fats raise your bad low-density lipoprotein (LDL) cholesterol level *and* your total cholesterol level while simultaneously lowering your good, protective high-density lipoprotein (HDL) cholesterol. Your HDL cholesterol is the cholesterol that acts like a broom and sweeps your arteries clean, and a high HDL cholesterol is independently associated with a decreased risk of heart disease so anything that lowers good HDL cholesterol is bad.[6] If this weren't bad enough, trans-fats also increase triglyceride level and impair artery dilation, a one–two punch that further increases your risk for heart artery disease.

Because trans-fats are man-made fats they are toxic substances that are not recognized or properly digested by your body. Toxic, empty-calorie trans-fats increase inflammation, thus making for a nightmare fat that can make you look terrible and feel terrible. If you have an inflammatory condition such as MS, fibromyalgia, or asthma and you eat a lot of trans-fats you will undoubtedly worsen your symptoms. Trans-fats also contribute to insulin resistance by desensitizing your cells to the actions of insulin, thus making it necessary for your body to produce more of the fat-storing hormone than it should, and this dramatically increases your risk of obesity and diabetes. To cut to the chase, eating 100 calories of trans-fats is far more fattening than eating 100 calories of olive oil. And the bad gets worse. Trans-fat consumption is also associated with an increased risk of cancer. Ominously, in a study by the French National Institute for Health and Medical Research of almost 25,000 European women, it was determined that the risk of breast cancer almost doubles in women who have high levels of trans-fats in their blood.[7] And just when you've heard all the bad news to hear about these terrible fats, findings from an 8-year study following 18,000 women, led by researchers from the Harvard School of Public Health, showed the more trans-fats in the diet, the greater the likelihood of developing ovulatory infertility. The study saw an effect on fertility at daily trans-fat intakes of just 4 grams, far less than the average person eating a processed food–rich diet consumes in a typical day.[8]

HOW TO AVOID TRANS-FATS

THE BEST WAY to avoid trans-fats is to read the ingredients and avoid any food that lists hydrogenated or partially hydrogenated oil on the label. Even if the product label includes the words *zero grams of trans-fat,* that does not guarantee there is no trans-fat. That claim simply means there is less than 0.5 gram of trans-fat per serving. Because this fat adds up very fast in terms of harming health, you need to read the list of ingredients to make sure there is no hydrogenated or partially hydrogenated oil in the product at all. Trans-fats are often found in vegetable shortening, margarines, and processed foods such as crackers, muffin and cake mixes, packaged snack foods, frozen food entrees, breakfast cereals, soups, muffins, granola bars, and energy bars. You should also avoid any food fried in vegetable oil because heating, cooking, and reheating oils causes chemical changes that produce an effect similar to the hydrogenation process that creates trans-fat. Just remember, no amount of trans-fat is safe.

Big Bad Fat 2: Animal-Based Saturated Fat

Although everyone and their mother can now unanimously agree that trans-fats do in fact belong in the trash can, some people still try to argue that animal-based saturated fat is a natural fat and therefore not harmful. Well this just isn't true. Just because something is natural does not mean it is healthful. Many minerals, for example, are natural, like lead, cadmium, and arsenic, yet have no nutritive value and are quite toxic. Sugar and corn syrup are also all natural, but that doesn't mean eating these foods will make you healthy.

What is true is that nutrigenomics (the study of the interaction between genes and diet) does make a case for the fact that animal-based saturated fat is potentially much more dangerous for some people than for others. We all know the story of your neighbors' grandma who ate bacon, lard, eggs, and steak every single one of her 95 years and then died peacefully in her sleep. But these anecdotes do not constitute proof that the saturated fat in the bacon is therefore okay to eat. Grandma might have had a genetic advantage that allowed her to tolerate her bacon-forward diet, but that doesn't mean she wouldn't have been even better off had she eaten a Clean Cuisine–style diet her whole life. But she lived to be 95 years old, you argue! But did she live the absolute best-quality 95 years on such a diet? Was she free of arthritis and pain? Did she have tremendous zip, pep, and go? Did she maintain a trim figure? Was she mentally sharp? Maybe she was all of these things and was lucky to be in outstanding health her entire life. Maybe Grandma really was an anomaly and really could eat whatever she wanted with zero negative health or weight gain consequences. But we doubt it.

For now we stick with the science. When it comes to animal-based saturated fat, overwhelming scientific evidence shows that saturated fat has a powerful contributory link with artery disease (including heart attack and stroke) and cancer. The two substances most associated with substantial aging of the immune system and arteries are animal-based saturated fats and trans-fats. And remember, anything that ages your arteries will not only age your body on the inside but absolutely age your body on the outside too. There is no doubt about it, animal-based saturated fat is an age-accelerating and heart-disease promoting fat. Another way saturated fats are harmful to your heart health is that they increase triglycerides; elevated triglycerides are linked to arterial aging and are independently associated with heart disease. Less well publicized is that diets rich in saturated fat are highly proinflammatory and contribute to fibromyalgia, multiple sclerosis, asthma, vascular dementia, psoriasis, and other diseases. As a surgeon, Andy operates on *at least* one gallbladder every week and gallbladder disease is just another condition that is also linked to saturated fat–rich diets.[9]

Eating too much animal-based saturated fat can even disrupt your body's natural fat-burning capabilities and can cause metabolic syndrome. This syndrome is characterized by high blood pressure, an elevated fasting blood sugar, a large waist circumference, and abnormal cholesterol tests, in particular a low HDL level and high triglyceride level. Ultimately, metabolic syndrome leads to a significantly elevated risk for developing full-blown diabetes and heart artery disease. This is in part because saturated fats ignite the activity of a protein called NF-kappa-B, which prevents the transport of glucose to your cells, thus triggering hunger and promoting inflammation, which slows metabolism.[10] Not only will eating a diet rich in saturated fat make your body slow and sluggish but it has the same undesirable impact on your brain. Animal-based saturated fats negatively affect your mood by disrupting the levels of neurotransmitters and the structure of cells in our brains that regulate mental processes and affect how we think and feel.

> NOTE: *Omega-3 essential fats have the direct opposite effect of saturated fats and have been shown to improve mood and clarity of thought.*

Unlike with the essential omega-3 and omega-6 fats we discuss later, there is actually no biological requirement for saturated fat. In fact, your body can produce saturated fat on its own, if you eat a diet that is very low in fat with too many refined carbohydrates, your body can manufacture a saturated fat called palmitic acid. This manufactured saturated fat has the same negative consequences as saturated fat consumed in food, one of many good reasons to avoid the excess refined carbohydrates we discussed in Chapter 4. (And yes, there are different types of saturated fat. In general, animal-based saturated fats from foods like beef and cheese are the ones to limit most, whereas preliminary research suggests plant-based saturated fats from foods like raw coconuts and organic extra-virgin coconut oil can potentially be healthful in moderate amounts.)

HOW TO LIMIT ANIMAL SOURCES OF SATURATED FAT

Animal-based saturated fat is found in highest concentrations in foods like beef, lamb, pork, chicken, turkey, and dairy foods (butter, cheese, and full-fat milk). The easiest way to limit your animal-based saturated fat intake is to consume no more than one serving of one of these foods per day or no more than three or four times per week if you want to be more aggressive.

> NOTE: *We make an exception to the one animal food per day rule for organic pastured eggs. One pastured egg contains only 1.5 grams of saturated fat, so it is okay to eat one or two pastured eggs a day in addition to having one serving of another animal food such as chicken, beef, or lamb. If you don't know what a pastured egg is don't worry, we explain on page 167.*

This approach to limiting your animal-based saturated fat intake is a no-brainer way to keep its intake below 5 percent of your total daily calories, well below the 10 percent recommended by most nutrition authorities. Also, when it comes to animal foods, it is of utmost importance to choose the highest quality and cleanest food sources available; simply choosing cleaner animal foods such as grass-fed beef over feedlot-raised beef drastically reduces your saturated fat intake while improving the overall nutrient profile. For example, did you know feedlot-raised beef has an estimated 500 percent more saturated fat than grass-fed beef? (See page 165 for more details on choosing the cleanest and leanest animal-based foods.)

Keep in mind that although many saturated fat–containing animal foods, such as free-range chicken and their eggs and grass-fed beef, are a delivery system for important nutrients (such as vitamin B12), other saturated fat–containing animal foods such as bacon, sausage, and luncheon meats, have no place in your diet because they contain far too few nutrients to justify eating them. What this means in plain English is that we are okay with you eating a small serving of nutrient-containing pastured beef every so often, but we don't recommend you eat empty-calorie, saturated fat–rich foods like bacon and lard.

THE CHOLESTEROL CONUNDRUM

IN MANY DIETARY circles cholesterol is infamously recognized as saturated fat's bad brother sidekick. This is because animal foods that contain saturated fat also contain cholesterol, and as most of us know already, high blood cholesterol levels can make the inside of the arteries in your heart clog up. The higher your cholesterol, the more likely you are to have arteries clogged so badly that blood cannot get through, putting you at risk of a heart attack or stroke. **Understand very clearly though that simply reducing or eliminating cholesterol from your diet does not mean your arteries will be squeaky clean, not by a long stretch.**

First of all, it's not really the cholesterol you get from your food that is the main culprit when it comes to the amount of cholesterol in your bloodstream. High cholesterol in the bloodstream is mostly brought on by:

1. Eating too much animal-based saturated fat.
2. Eating trans-fat.
3. Consuming too many empty-calorie refined carbohydrates.

There are actually foods out there that are rich in cholesterol—eggs and shrimp are two excellent examples—but because they are relatively low in saturated fat they have little effect on your blood cholesterol level. Most people are surprised to hear carbohydrates can increase cholesterol levels, but if the empty-calorie carbohydrates you eat (bagels, crackers, soda) are not burned for energy, they can be converted by your body into saturated fat, which, as we now know, encourages the presence of cholesterol in the blood. Plus empty carbohydrate consumption stimulates your body to produce large amounts of insulin, and insulin activates the main enzyme responsible for manufacturing cholesterol in your liver. So yes, cholesterol is more complicated than just avoiding eggs.

Not that we want to pour more confusion into the mix, but the truth is cholesterol in itself is not the totally evil substance you might think it is. For one, cholesterol is a precursor to vitamin D, an anti-inflammatory superstar vitamin that plays a crucial role in how you age and feel. It is interesting that foods that provide vitamin D also tend to be high in cholesterol (eggs again come to mind). Your sex hormones and neurotransmitters can both be disrupted if your cholesterol is too low. In fact, cholesterol is a vital ingredient in proper brain function, and low blood cholesterol has actually been linked to depression and severe mood disorders. This is not surprising because the brain is the most cholesterol-rich organ in our bodies. In addition, cholesterol aids in the manufacture of bile acids needed to properly digest fat and forms a protective coating around the myelin sheath of our nerves, thus helping our brain communicate with the rest of our body in an efficient and uninterrupted manner. Cholesterol is such an important substance that it is contained in practically every cell in the human body and used for many essential functions. The point is, cholesterol is not all bad.

It is even possible to measure whether your body contains more good cholesterol or more bad cholesterol. The good cholesterol, called HDL, is so good that having a concentration greater than 60 milligrams per deciliter is considered a *negative* risk factor for coronary artery disease. Cholesterol is carried through your bloodstream attached to two different compounds called lipoproteins: low-density lipoproteins (LDL) and high-density lipoproteins (HDL). LDL is commonly known as the bad or lousy cholesterol because it is the cholesterol that gets deposited on arterial walls, thus creating hardening of the arteries. As mentioned earlier, HDL on the other hand, is known as the good cholesterol because it acts like a broom and sweeps your arteries clean. In most cases, the ratio of your total cholesterol to your HDL level is more indicative of good health than simply paying attention to your total cholesterol level. Total cholesterol should not be more than 3½ times greater than the HDL level.

The unrefined plant food–rich Clean Cuisine diet we recommend has been shown to lower cholesterol, particularly the bad LDL kind. A study published in the prestigious *Journal of the American Medical Association* showed that participants in a large randomized trial who ate less animal foods and added more plant-based foods rich in plant sterols and plant fats lowered their bad LDL cholesterol more than those who followed a diet low in saturated fats.*

Although there are many things you can do to improve your heart health and optimize your cholesterol ratio, you cannot deny genetics play a role. It's not fair, but some people simply process cholesterol better than others. Some people measure out better than others when they go to the lab to have their cholesterol level checked. That doesn't necessarily mean the folks with high cholesterol are all walking heart attacks waiting to happen simply because they have high cholesterol! Whether you get your total cholesterol down super low by following the Clean Cuisine lifestyle is not necessarily relevant because you will lower your body weight, blood pressure, CRP levels, body fat, and triglycerides on our plan and you will improve your cholesterol ratio as well. All of these offsetting health improvements are so intrinsically more beneficial to heart health and more beneficial to aging and inflammation in general that they offset the effect of a super-low total cholesterol level. **You have to realize that while your cholesterol level is important, it is absolutely not the only factor to be concerned with when it comes to heart health.**

An excellent review article we came across is "Cholesterol: Where Science and Public Health Policy Intersect." Published in the academic journal *Nutrition Reviews,* it summarizes the opinions of nationally recognized experts on diet and health as they relate to cholesterol intake from food.[1] It is interesting that the current U.S. policy as laid out by the FDA and the Committee on Diet and Health is at odds with the international community's policy. While the United States recommends specific limits on cholesterol intake (less than 300 milligrams per day for most people and less than 200 milligrams per day for persons with elevated blood levels of LDL), other countries' health policies make no specific recommendations. The World Health Organization (WHO), along with agencies representing Canada, Australia, and Great Britain, instead recommends reducing fat intake and the intake of saturated fat and trans-fat, in particular. The primary reason for this difference in opinion is the known stronger association between animal-based saturated fat intake and blood cholesterol levels than between cholesterol intake and blood cholesterol levels. In addition, not everyone responds to dietary cholesterol reduction in the same way; it is thought that as few as 7 percent of people would respond to substantially limiting dietary cholesterol by also showing a reduction in blood cholesterol levels.

After reviewing hundreds of academic studies here is our advice when it comes to cholesterol. Instead of worrying so much about how much cholesterol is in a food like eggs you should worry more about limiting your animal food intake in general and limiting your animal-based saturated fat intake in particular. You should also eliminate trans-fats and drastically reduce empty-calorie carbohydrates. And beyond that you should focus on doing all of the other things we recommend in this book that are proven to keep your heart healthy:

- Exercise regularly.
- Enjoy a glass of wine with dinner (this is optional but more than 100 studies suggest light to moderate drinkers have a lower risk of heart disease).
- Get most of your protein from plants instead of animals.
- Eat a broad spectrum of phytonutrient-rich plant foods, including beans, fruits, whole grains, nuts, seeds, and vegetables every day.
- Eat fatty fish two or three times a week and supplement with a pharmaceutical-grade fish oil daily.
- Achieve a healthful body weight (if you are overweight you will lose weight as a side benefit of following the Clean Cuisine lifestyle and losing even a modest amount of weight can lower cholesterol).
- Cook with lots of garlic and herbs and spices.
- Drink green tea regularly.

Common sense and hard science show it is *not* effective to ban eggs or shrimp from your diet with the intent of reducing cholesterol levels. Dietary cholesterol reduction is too simplistic of an approach for improving heart health and is not helpful.

> **NOTE:** For the record, we do allow eggs on the Clean Cuisine program and we are not advocates of the egg white omelet! We don't eat tons of eggs—maybe about three or four whole eggs a week each plus Ivy uses eggs in recipes, so we might get an additional egg here and there—but when we do eat eggs we eat the whole egg, including the cholesterol-rich yolk. The yolk has many important nutrients, including choline and lutein. And, as you will read in Chapter 6, the extra protein from the egg white is really not necessary as long as you are eating a healthy diet with enough calories. The type of egg you buy does matter for many reasons though, so

see page 167 for guidelines on buying the cleanest eggs, which are pastured eggs.

* D. J. Jenkins, P. J. Jones, B. Lamarche, et al., "Effect of a Dietary Portfolio of Cholesterol-Lowering Foods Given at 2 Levels of Intensity of Dietary Advice on Serum Lipids in Hyperlipidemia: A Randomized Controlled Trial," *Journal of the American Medical Association* 306, no. 8 (2011): 831–39.

† A. M. Brownawell and M. C. Falk, "Cholesterol: Where Science and Public Health Policy Intersect," *Nutrition Reviews* 68, no. 6 (2010), 355–64.

The Essential Clean Cuisine Fats You Really *Do* Need

Two diets associated with longevity, reduced age-related suffering, and illness-free living are the traditional Japanese diet and the Mediterranean diet; both diets have a favorable omega-3 to omega-6 essential fat ratio, as does the Clean Cuisine plan. (Both diets are also rich in plant foods and low in dairy and meat, and both diets include fish.) Essential omega-3 and omega-6 fats play an important role in how you age, look, and feel. They are also essential for the prevention and treatment of many chronic diseases. Ensuring that you get adequate omega-3 and omega-6 essential fats and that you get these fats in the proper healthful ratio is a key component of our Clean Cuisine lifestyle.

Omega-3 and omega-6 essential fats are unique in that they cannot be manufactured by your body. In other words, you have to get these fats from food. These fats play a wide number of vital roles in your body, including the production of eicosanoid hormones, some of which are inflammatory and some of which are anti-inflammatory. By modifying your diet, you can alter your body's balance of these hormones so that it makes more good anti-inflammatory hormones and fewer bad proinflammatory ones. The most direct way to do this is to eat the optimal ratio of omega-3 to omega-6 essential fats while also limiting animal-based saturated fat and eliminating trans-fats.

Although the public in general is unaware of the significance the omega-3 to omega-6 ratio has on overall health and well-being, established medical and nutritional journals have repeatedly reported the benefits derived from eating a balanced ratio of approximately 4 servings of omega-6 fats to 1 serving of omega-3 fatty acids. The average person eating the typical modern Western diet consumes 14 to 20 times more omega-6s than omega-3s! This out-of-whack ratio tends to place your body into a chronic state of inflammation, which contributes to heart disease, cancer, and numerous inflammatory and autoimmune conditions.[11] An imbalance of omega-3 to omega-6 fats can even increase your risk of obesity and type 2 diabetes by decreasing your cells' sensitivity to insulin. Because an out-of-whack omega-3 to omega-6 ratio increases inflammation, it will be considerably more difficult for you to lose weight. In a vicious circle, anything that causes inflammation predisposes you to gain weight, then the weight (fat cells) itself causes an increased amount of inflammation. For overall health, disease prevention, reduced inflammation, and weight management we can't emphasize the importance of the omega-3 to omega-6 ratio more emphatically.

Essential Clean Cuisine Fat 1: Omega-3 Essential Fats

Omega-3 essential fats support the health of your immune system, reproductive system, cardiovascular system, and central nervous system. These fats are the most powerful anti-inflammatory substances available without a prescription and are therefore beneficial to people suffering from seemingly unrelated conditions that all have inflammation as the common denominator, such as asthma, allergies, arthritis, multiple sclerosis, psoriasis, fibromyalgia, chronic pain, and even coronary artery disease. The omega-3 fats are also widely recognized for their triglyceride-lowering effects. Considered to be the beauty and brain nutrients, omega-3 fats play a vitally important role in supporting healthy skin, hair, and nails as well as improving your cognitive function, your attention span, and your ability to process and retain information. They even improve your mood and make you happier!

And did you know omega-3 essential fats are slimming fats? One particular type of omega-3 essential fat (EPA) binds to certain receptors in your cells that improve your body's ability to burn fat while also making your cells more sensitive to insulin. If you want to keep your weight under control, then you want to be insulin sensitive so your body needs to produce only a little bit of insulin at a time; the omega-3 essential fats help your body become more insulin sensitive. When omega-3 essential fats are missing from your diet, your body is less effective at using insulin and becomes less sensitive to its effects, thus weight loss becomes considerably more challenging. Unfortunately, modern diets are more deficient in the omega-3 essential fats than they are in just about any other nutrient. It's important to make sure you eat at least one serving of omega-3 rich food each day.

There are three types of omega-3 essential fats, and all three are important: alpha-linolenic acid (ALA), eicosapentaenoic acid (EPA), and docosahexaenoic acid (DHA).

NOTE: ALA is sometimes abbreviated LNA to avoid confusing it with alpha-lipoic acid, an antioxidant that is not an essential fat.

- **ALA** is found in vegan foods, including walnuts and hemp seeds, but two of the most concentrated sources of ALA are flax and chia seeds (when you get to Chapter 9, which outlines the 8-week program, you'll see that chia seeds are part of the daily Super-Green smoothie). Although eating the whole food in the form of nuts and seeds is the superior choice, you can also get your omega-3 ALA from *unheated cold-pressed* flax oil for drizzling on vegetables, salads, grains, and beans.

  NOTE: It is okay if the food on which the oil is drizzled is warm, but do not cook with flax oil.

- **EPA** and **DHA** are nonvegan sources of omega-3 fats. The richest sources of EPA and DHA are fatty fish and fish oil supplements. Egg yolks also contain DHA. Although it is true that your body can convert vegan ALA to EPA and then EPA to DHA, the conversion process does *not* happen optimally or reliably. For example, eating too much omega-6 fat, saturated fat, and trans-fats can interfere with the conversion process and create an omega-3 deficiency even if you are eating plenty of ALA from vegan foods, such as flax and chia seeds. So, even though a well-planned plant-rich whole foods vegan diet can contain plenty of ALA from food, we still recommend an EPA and DHA pharmaceutical-grade fish oil supplement for just about everyone because individuals differ in how well their body converts ALA to EPA and DHA and autoimmune conditions, metabolic issues, and numerous lifestyle factors can create a relative DHA deficiency even if the diet is rich in ALA. The greatest weakness of many otherwise very healthful vegan or nearly vegan, plant-strong diets is their lack of optimal amounts of omega-3 fat. These diets can be somewhat anti-inflammatory due to their very low bad fat content, but they are never optimal if they are deficient in EPA and DHA, as most are. Keep in mind the Okinawans are among the longest-living people in the world, and they traditionally consume approximately three servings of fish per week in addition to eating a clean plant-strong diet. To get optimal amounts of EPA and DHA we suggest you eat 2 or 3 servings (3 to 4 ounces each) of *fatty* fish every week (the fattier the fish, the better) and also supplement with a high-quality pharmaceutical-grade fish oil supplying at a minimum 1,000 to 2,000 milligrams of combined EPA and DHA daily (for specific fish oil guidelines see page 123). If you have an inflammatory condition such as MS, fibromyalgia, arthritis, or asthma, you could benefit from 1½ to 2 times this amount. If you are a strict vegan you could substitute the fish oil supplement with an algae-based DHA supplement though you will have to take a lot to attain optimal amounts of DHA.

NOTE: *It might sound fishy, but anchovy paste is a frequent ingredient in Ivy's day to day culinary vocabulary. It is salty for sure but not as strong in flavor as salted or canned anchovies. Instead, it has a rich, nutty flavor that contributes distinct personality to what otherwise might be a rather plain ho-hum dish. Over the years anchovy paste has become a go-to standby when Ivy wants to add a special savory, something-something quality to any number of dishes, including soups, vinaigrettes, tomato sauces, casseroles, pasta dishes, and even vegetables. Be sure to look for the best quality anchovy paste made only with extra-virgin olive oil, and avoid those made using less desirable vegetable oils such as soybean oil.*

IN THE KITCHEN WITH VEGAN SOURCES OF OMEGA-3 ESSENTIAL FATS

FLAX OIL

YOU CAN PURCHASE flax oil at any natural food store. However, you must be ultra-choosy when selecting it. Because flax oil has a limited shelf life it's important to choose a product with a pressing date no more than four months in the past. Be sure to look for high-quality refrigerated flax oil that has been protected from heat, light, and air during the packaging process. Heat, light, and air destroy the delicate essential fats found in flax oil. Spoiled, oxidized fats act like the bad fats we've discussed earlier and are actually counter-productive. Strictly observe any "best used before" date on the label. High-volume sellers usually stock fresh products, but it's still a good idea to check the date. Fresh flax oil should be nearly odor-less with a mild nutty taste. In contrast, rancid flax oil will smell and taste sort of fishy or chemical-like. It is important that you never cook with flax oil. Be sure to buy flax oil in small quantities and store it in the refrigerator. Probably the very best use for flax oil is on top of your daily salad as the oil base for a homemade vinaigrette. It is also fine to drizzle flax oil on a wide variety of foods after the foods have been cooked. Flax oil can top mashed potatoes, mashed sweet potatoes, cooked whole grains, beans, and even popcorn.

> **NOTE:** For over a decade, our family has come to fully trust and rely on the superior quality of Barlean's flax oil, which is widely available throughout the United States (see the appendix for more details).

FLAX SEEDS

GROUND FLAX SEEDS actually have a leg up on flax oil because they are fiber-rich and can be heated for use in baking. Ground flax seeds can be added to muffins, breads, whole wheat pizza crust, and even desserts. In addition to mixing flax seeds into all sorts of batters, you can also sprinkle them on hot whole grain cereals, add them to smoothies, mix them into meatballs, or sprinkle them on your salad. Flaxseeds are also nature's richest source of lignans, potent phytonutrients that fight free-radical damage and act as phy-toestrogens. Lignans and a few other naturally occurring phytoes-trogens provide protection against hormone-sensitive cancers such as breast cancer, ovarian cancer, prostate cancer, and even colon cancer.* Keep in mind, your body can't derive the full benefit of the omega-3 essential fats found within flax seeds unless they are ground, so eating them whole is not optimal. You can grind flax seeds yourself in a coffee grinder or you can buy them already ground (such as Barlean's Forti-Flax organic ground flax seed).

CHIA SEEDS

A TRUE SUPERFOOD, these itty-bitty, teeny-tiny seeds are compact powerhouses of nutritious energy. Containing a whopping 5 grams of fiber per 2½ tablespoons, chia seeds absorb up to 30 times their weight in water, which makes them exceedingly helpful if you are trying to lose weight without feeling hungry. Not only do chia seeds deliver a hefty dose of fiber and omega-3 essential fat, they are also surprisingly rich in calcium, B vitamins, easily digestible protein, and a broad spectrum of phytonutrients and antioxidants. Chia seeds are nothing new; they have been a staple food source for the Native American people for centuries; in fact the word *chia* is the Mayan word for "strength." Best of all, because chia seeds have a very mild, neutral flavor they are easy to mix into many of our Clean Cuisine culinary creations. Health-conscious foodies have found they can incorporate chia seeds into all sorts of decadent (but healthful!) desserts; use them as a substitute for other fats, binders, and thick-eners; or even mix them in hot whole grain cereals for nutritional oomph. Chia seeds give a delectable nutty crunch to salads, they are wonderful mixed in Mexican dishes like enchiladas, and they make the perfect French toast coating. You can even drink your chia! In fact, we include 1 tablespoon of chia seeds as a standard ingredi-ent in every single one of our SuperGreen smoothies (see Part Four). We like Barlean's brand organic chia seeds.

* K. Buck, A. K. Zaineddin, A. Vrieling, et al., "Meta-Analyses of Lignans and Enterolignans in Relation to Breast Cancer Risk," *American Journal of Clinical Nutrition* 92, no. 1 (2010): 141–53. C. L. Heald, M. R. Ritchie, C. Bolton-Smith, "Phyto-Oestrogens and Risk of Prostate Cancer in Scottish Men," *British Journal of Nutrition* 98, no. 2 (2007): 388–96.

Omega-3 Fish Oil Facts

Fish oil is the most validated supplement that exists, boasting over 19,000 121
studies having been conducted thus far. Research links the omega-3 fats in
fish oil with improved cholesterol profile and joint mobility; increased bone
density; reversal of metabolic syndrome; reduced risk of heart attack,
stroke, and congestive heart failure; healthy blood glucose levels and sexual
and hormonal function; protection against certain types of cancer, including breast and prostate cancer; and decreased inflammation. In a systematic review published in the *Archives of Internal Medicine*, fish oil was
found to be the most effective prevention for heart disease, and this includes
comparing fish oil head to head against all the fancy drugs.[12] The research
validating the tremendous health benefits of fish oil is simply irrefutable.
We thought we'd share some of the other benefits to the omega-3 fats found
in fish and fish oil you might not have heard of just yet.

FISH OMEGA-3S AS BRAIN AND MOOD FOOD

We learned about the importance of omega-3 fats over a decade ago when
Ivy was diagnosed with MS. MS is an inflammation-mediated disease of
the central nervous system and omega-3 fats from fish play an important
role in supporting a healthy central nervous system and slowing the progression of MS.[13] Because the central nervous system includes the brain,
the omega-3 fats, and in particular DHA, are often called *brain food*, and
for good reason! Did you know your brain is about 60 percent fat by weight
and that the fat you eat directly affects the way your brain functions?
Research supports omega-3 fats can dramatically improve your brain and
cognitive function by boosting mental clarity, improving quickness of
thought, and enhancing your ability to concentrate. The omega-3 fats
from fish oil have also been linked to reducing two of today's biggest
mind–body agers: stress and anxiety. And, if that were not enough promising news to put you in a good mood, you might want to consider trying
omega-3s to cheer up. It's true, consuming omega-3s is linked with being
happier. A tremendous amount of scientific data link low levels of EPA
and DHA to a number of mood disorders, including depression, suicide,
and learning disabilities. In an article published in the esteemed *Archives
of General Psychiatry*, researchers demonstrated an incredible 50 percent
reduction in the standard Hamilton Depression Rating Scale in the

majority of the research subjects taking an omega-3 fat supplement.[14] If you take the time to look, you'll find plenty of studies showing dietary supplementation with omega-3 fats as being effective and nontoxic therapy for bipolar disorder, postpartum depression, seasonal affective disorder, and attention deficit disorders.

FISH OMEGA-3S AS A BEAUTY BOOSTER

Did you know fish oils can even make you more beautiful? This is because omega-3 fats act as a natural lubricant for the skin and work from the inside out to help keep your skin soft and supple. Keep in mind no amount of externally applied high-end skin cream can compete with the natural internal lubricating benefits you'll get from a healthy diet containing adequate amounts of omega-3 fats. In fact, some of the symptoms of omega-3 fat deficiency include dry, itchy skin and brittle hair and nails. And if you battle with breakouts and acne you should notice improvement with these problems too once you start getting more omega-3s.[15]

FISH OMEGA-3S AS A SKIN-SAVING SUN BLOCKER

Omega-3s are also among the proven substances to reduce sun damage and provide protection from sunburn. Other protective substances are flavonoids, carotenoids, tocopherols, and tocotrienols. All of these substances have been proven to be orally bioavailable for the purpose of protecting your skin from the sun, meaning you can take them by mouth and levels will rise in your skin, where they do their work. Of these substances, the omega-3s seem to have the most research behind them; human studies show an approximate 35 percent increase in the amount of time it takes sunlight to redden the skin. While it is possible to get this protection from foods such as walnuts, flax, fish, and shrimp, omega-3 fatty acids should probably be supplemented because best results occur at doses as high as 4 grams daily (again, specific supplementation guidelines are given in Chapter 9). EPA alone or EPA and DHA together are effective. There is strong but not yet conclusive evidence that omega-3 fats can prevent skin cancer too. The bottom line is your skin just won't look as good, won't be as healthy, and won't stay as youthful as it otherwise could if you don't get enough omega-3 fish oils.

FISH OMEGA-3S AS FAT FIGHTERS

Just when you thought the fish fat benefits couldn't get any "phatter" there's more; eating more fish fats can potentially help you burn more body fat. Yup! It's true, folks. Fish fats help fight body fat for several overlapping and intertwined reasons. First of all, the latest obesity research recognizes inflammation is a primary offender leading to weight gain and that eating proinflammatory foods like trans-fats, butter, and sugar can make you gain weight. We have already explained that any weight you gain can cause more inflammation and potentially make you fatter still. The opposite is also true; anti-inflammatory foods—including omega-3 fish fats—can decrease inflammation and help you lose weight. Omega-3 fish fats also improve your body's sensitivity to insulin, thus creating a favorable fat-burning environment.[16] In addition, omega-3 fish fats are thought to bind to special receptors in your cells called peroxisome proliferator-activated receptors (PPARs) that actually turn on genes that cause your body to burn fat.[17] The omega-3 fats are also required for the production of thyroid hormones, and thyroid hormones stimulate your mitochondria to burn more fat for energy. All of this doesn't mean that simply downing some fish oil pills along with your morning doughnut is going to be the cure to your weight-loss worries. Instead, taking fish oil provides a safe weight-loss booster along with plenty of additional healthy fringe benefits. You have nothing to lose by adding fish oils to your diet . . . except for a few unwanted pounds!

ARE FISH OIL SUPPLEMENTS CLEAN?

WE REALIZE A lot of people interested in clean eating are concerned about the toxins in fish (and fish oil) these days. As a consumer, it's important to realize not all fish oils are created equal. Here's the deal: You get what you pay for. Without a doubt, some fish oils are purer (not to mention fresher and better tasting!) than others. If you buy a high-quality, pharmaceutical-grade fish oil that has been molecularly distilled and tested for purity by an independent third-party testing organization you can be pretty darn sure you are getting a clean product.

Freshness is a key factor in choosing a high-quality fish oil. The omega-3 fats in fish are extremely delicate and can easily be damaged by improper processing. You want to look for a supplement that does not include oxygen, excessive heat, or chemicals in its processing. A fishy taste is a tip-off that your fish oil supplement isn't up to snuff in the freshness department. If your fish oil supplement has a fishy taste, you absolutely don't want to take it. And keep in mind that a high-quality fresh fish oil should not leave any nasty fishy aftertaste, nor should you get that terrible fish burp (see Chapter 9 for specific recommendations on how to choose a fish oil supplement that won't give you fish burps).

Essential Clean Cuisine Fat 2: Omega-6 Essential Fats

Omega-6 essential fats are the other type of essential fat your body needs but cannot produce on its own. This means just like the omega-3 fats, you must obtain omega-6 essential fats from food. Omega-6 fats are broadly available in seeds and the vegetable oils extracted from them. Soy, wheat germ, corn, sunflower seeds, cottonseeds, peanuts, safflower oil, and many other plant-based whole foods contain large amounts of omega-6 fat (healthy whole sources of omega-6 fats are given later in this chapter). These omega-6 fats also build up in large amounts in the fat of *grain-fed* animal foods such as mass-market beef and chicken. For optimal health you need slightly more omega-6 fat than omega-3 fat, ideally no more than four times as much omega-6 fat as omega-3 fat. However, because the typical modern-day diet consists of such an overabundance of refined vegetable oils and so much grain-fed meat, and very little fatty fish and vegan omega-3-rich foods like flax and walnuts, the average person consumes a very unhealthful, unfit proinflammatory, fattening, and disease-promoting omega-6 to omega-3 fat ratio of about 14 to 1 or even 20 to 1.

The reliance on highly processed convenience foods is one reason so many people currently consume such an unhealthy ratio of omega-6 to omega-3 fats. Processed foods such as crackers, frozen foods, commercial baked goods, cereals, and snack bars often contain highly refined omega-6 fat from vegetable oils and are almost always completely devoid of omega-3 fats. This is a big problem because eating an unbalanced ratio of omega-6 fat relative to omega-3 fat increases inflammation, which exacerbates the symptoms of inflammatory conditions and makes your body less sensitive to the effects of insulin, which in turn contributes to obesity, type 2 diabetes, and heart disease. It's especially important when you consider that studies have linked diets rich in omega-6 fat to cancer.[18]

HEART HEALTHY VEGETABLE OILS LINKED TO HEART ATTACK AND OBESITY

ALTHOUGH VEGETABLE OILS have become popular for their ability to lower cholesterol, we can assure you eating a vegetable oil–rich diet will do nothing to improve your heart health or slim your waist. The Israeli paradox illustrates this point perfectly. In Israel, cooking techniques rely heavily on omega-6-rich vegetable oils and margarines. Even though the people living in Israel are noted for having one of the lowest cholesterol levels in Western countries and even though Israelis eat much more polyunsaturated fat than saturated fat, they also have exceedingly high rates of heart attack and obesity.[*] The simple take-home point is that *all* polyunsaturated fats, whether they are omega-3 or omega-6, have the power to reduce your cholesterol level, but only by eating more omega-3s can you personally reduce your risk of cancer, heart disease, and obesity.

[*] G. Dubnov and E. M. Berry, "Omega-6/Omega-3 Fatty Acid Ratio: The Israeli Paradox," *World Review of Nutrition and Dietetics* 92 (2003): 81–91.

Based on all this you might be questioning why omega-6 fat is even necessary to eat at all. The reason is your body still needs omega-6 fat and, as mentioned earlier, you actually need *slightly* more of it than omega-3 fat. Furthermore, whole non-oil sources of omega-6 fat (whole grains, nuts, and seeds) contain other important nutrients. Too little omega-6 fat and too much omega-3 fat can put you at risk of bleeding and some types of stroke and may also make it harder for you to fight off certain forms of infection. We *do not* recommend ever limiting omega-3 fat, however, because this problem almost never occurs in modern society.

Unfortunately, if you eat a diet rich in processed and packaged foods you are going to get most of your omega-6 fat from highly refined empty-calorie vegetable oils, such as corn oil, pure vegetable oil, peanut oil, soybean oil, sunflower oil, safflower oil, grape seed oil, and cottonseed oil. Even if you buy healthful-sounding packaged foods labeled organic, all-natural, gluten-free, and so on, you are still likely to be consuming too many vegetable oils and too much omega-6 fat. Remember, these vegetable oils are super cheap and therefore highly profitable for food manufacturers. Despite their healthful-sounding names, vegetable oils, even if they are organic or all-natural, are anything but healthful and here's why:

- **Standard vegetable oils are processed improperly.** Mass-marketed vegetable oils are refined at very high heat temperatures, processed, and then deodorized to make their taste acceptable. For the most part, vegetable oils on the mass market are made from omega-6-rich grains and seeds like corn kernels, sunflower seeds, and soy beans. While omega-6-rich foods are healthy in their whole and unadulterated state, they are harmful when processed and handled improperly. Like the omega-3 fats, omega-6 fats must be protected from heat, light, and air, otherwise they become damaged, unhealthful fats. Conventional processing techniques used to refine grains and seeds into oil actually damage the highly heat-sensitive and delicate omega-6 essential fats found within the whole food. Omega-6-rich vegetable oils, like all essential fats, by their very nature, are unable to withstand high temperatures without oxidizing and going rancid, yet high temperatures are exactly what these fats are exposed to when processed into oil. The vast majority of vegetable oils are not processed properly because it costs more money to cold press and expeller press these oils.

- **Vegetable oil is an empty calorie food.** The typical innocent-looking bottle of vegetable oil squatting on the supermarket shelf contains an empty-calorie food. Because we are already eating too much omega-6 fat as it is, we do not need to eat more omega-6 oil. At least if you are eating an omega-6 seed you're getting fiber and other phytonutrients. If you eat only the oil, you get nothing useful at all except for more calories, which is the last thing most of us need.

- **Vegetable oil has the wrong omega-3 to omega-6 ratio.** In addition to most vegetable oils being a source of empty calories, these oils are a highly concentrated source of excess omega-6 fat. The more of these oils you eat, the worse your omega ratio will be. The only widely available oils that naturally contain a better than average, healing, omega ratio are canola oil, flax oil, walnut oil, and hemp oil. Flax oil, walnut oil, and hemp oil are very fragile and cannot be used for cooking at all. Canola oil does contain omega-3 fat, but not nearly as much as the other three. Unfortunately, mass-market processing of canola oil destroys most of the good fats (as described earlier). Thus it is better to use heat-safe healthful oils such as extra-virgin olive oil than canola oil, and it is also better to purchase products made with extra-virgin olive oil instead of with canola oil.

The easiest way to avoid eating too much empty-calorie omega-6 fat is to ban processed vegetable oils from your diet and to avoid eating processed foods, convenience foods, and salad dressings that contain these oils. Instead, read the ingredients on all of the foods you buy, and when you prepare food at home use healthier oils that contain either more omega-3 fats or more monounsaturated fats.

You should also make every effort to purchase meat from grass-fed animals rather than grain-fed because grass-fed animals have a more optimal omega-6 to omega-3 ratio. Finally, to be certain you are obtaining the small amount of omega-6 fats your body does need in their freshest, most nutritious form you want to eat clean and nutrient-dense whole food sources of unrefined omega-6-rich foods daily. Read on to learn some excellent sources of high-quality omega-6 fat from plant-based whole foods.

ARACHIDONIC ACID, AN ANIMAL-BASED OMEGA-6 FAT TO LIMIT

ARACHIDONIC ACID (AA) is an omega-6 fat that is a direct contributor to inflammation. The foods we eat are our most direct source of AA, and this type of omega-6 fat is found only in animal foods. In addition to contributing to inflammation, high blood levels of AA are associated with increased platelet aggregation (or stickiness) in the bloodstream, which is a major contributing factor to heart disease. As bad as AA sounds, it is important to realize we do need some omega-6 AA (in balance with omega-3 EPA and DHA) to maintain optimal health and a well-functioning immune system. For example, it is no accident that AA is present in breast milk because our bodies do need some of it; we must make sure we don't overdo it. AA is found in animal foods, including meats, egg yolks, and fish. However, you can dramatically reduce your AA consumption simply by choosing animal foods that are fed the way nature intended the animals to eat. For example, meat from grass-fed cattle has less AA than does that from conventional grain-fed animals. Pastured hens and their eggs have less AA than do factory farmed chickens and eggs. When it comes to fish, the difference is rather astounding. For example, 4 ounces of Atlantic farmed salmon contains 1,306 milligrams of AA compared to just 303 milligrams of AA found in 4 ounces of wild Atlantic salmon. We can't emphasize enough the importance of eating only the highest quality animal foods.

Clean Cuisine Whole Sources of Omega-6-Rich Foods

To ensure you get adequate amounts of omega-6 essential fats you want to eat one serving of one of the following foods each day.

- Whole soybeans, such as edamame (serving size one half cup)
- Raw nuts like almonds, pecans, pistachios, pine nuts, and macadamia nuts and all-natural raw nut butters (serving size one ounce)
- Raw seeds like sesame seeds, pumpkin seeds, and sunflower seeds and all-natural raw seed butters (tahini, for example) (serving size one ounce)
- Wheat germ (serving size two tablespoons)
- Tofu (serving size 4 ounces)
- Tempeh (serving size 4 ounces)
- Hemp seeds (serving size two tablespoons)

> NOTE: *Raw nuts and seeds are also a good source of heart-healthy monounsaturated fats.*

Omega-6-Rich Processed Vegetable Oils to Trash

There is no reason to eat any foods containing the following ingredients because you are merely eating excess empty calories and are making yourself sicker by worsening your omega ratio.

- Corn oil
- Oil marketed as pure vegetable oil (usually a mixture of soybean oil and corn oil)
- Peanut oil

- Soybean oil
- Safflower oil
- Sunflower oil
- Cottonseed oil
- Grape seed oil

GOT HEMP?

AND NO, WE aren't talking about the hemp you smoke. Hemp seeds are actually an incredibly nutrient-dense super fruit that deliver a hefty dose of omega-3 and omega-6 essential fats. Tiny and round, they have a pleasing, mild, and slightly nutty flavor and aren't crunchy. Hemp seeds are similar to sesame seeds but even softer in texture. They taste sort of like pine nuts with an even mellower, milder taste. We love them. And they really, really are *so* exceptionally healthful! Hemp seeds contain a fabulous source of biologically available and easily digested protein (3 tablespoons of hemp seeds provide 11 grams of protein) in addition to vital nutrients, such as calcium, phosphorus, magnesium, and potassium. By the way, whenever we get e-mail from our Clean Cuisine readers asking for our recommendation for the best protein shakes on the market (and we get such e-mail all the time!) we always tell them to skip the fancy processed packaged protein powders and instead just add hemp seeds to water and blend up with some frozen fruit. A hemp shake is about the best antioxidant, superfood, protein-rich smoothie on the market! And it's cheaper and tastier too.

Hemp seeds and hemp seed oil have a highly favorable omega-3 to omega-6 ratio of three times more omega-6 than omega-3 so they possess potent anti-inflammatory properties, thus making hemp a great food for anyone with inflammatory conditions such as asthma, multiple sclerosis, eczema, psoriasis, and seasonal allergies. Along with borage oil, spirulina, black currant oil, and evening primrose oil, hemp seeds and hemp oil are two of only a very few sources of gamma-linolenic acid (GLA). Although we discuss GLA in more detail in the 8-week program in Chapter 9, for now, just know GLA is a special type of highly anti-inflammatory omega-6 fat that you can't really overdose on. GLA supports a healthy metabolism and facilitates fat burning. Some people who struggle with weight loss despite eating a healthful diet get a weight-loss boost simply by adding GLA. This special omega-6 fat can even help reduce hormone-mediated nuisance symptoms (bye-bye PMS!) and give you healthy hair and nails and glowing skin too.

As for how to eat hemp—it's amazing the culinary creations you can concoct with just a little bit of imagination! Ivy makes rich, luscious, and creamy vinaigrettes (and a to-die-for Caesar salad dressing; see page 320) with hemp seeds puréed in extra-virgin olive oil. She also mixes them right into vegan chili, hot whole grain cereals, smoothies, whole grain muffin batter, and whole grain pizza dough as well as puréed bean dips and vegetable soups. Probably the easiest way to eat them is just to sprinkle them right on top of a salad or on top of fresh fruit.

You can also buy hemp milk as a much more healthful substitute for dairy milk. Unlike soy milk or almond milk, hemp milk has a richer consistency similar to dairy milk and we prefer it as our milk of choice. Although we often buy hemp milk ready-made, Ivy also makes fresh hemp milk and even hemp cream too, both of which are incredibly tasty! Here's a quickie recipe:

HEALTHFUL HOMEMADE HEMP MILK

Yields 2½ cups

½ cup hemp seeds
2 cups water
3 pitted dates
1 teaspoon pure vanilla extract
Pinch unrefined sea salt

IN A HIGH-SPEED blender (such as a Vitamix), purée all ingredients until smooth, about 1 minute. It is okay to store in a covered container in the fridge for up to 2 days. Shake well before drinking. Variation: If you want to make hemp cream simply reduce the water to about 1½ cups.

What About Omega-9 Fats?

We've already talked about the essential omega-3 and omega-6 fats but what about those omega-9 fats you have surely read about in a health magazine or two or seen splashed on a supplement bottle of something or other? Here's the deal, omega-9 fats are nothing more than monounsaturated fats. Olive oil is an omega-9 fat, as is the fat contained in avocados. We like to nickname the omega-9 fats the "Mediterranean fats" because they are the primary fat in olive oil, the purported linchpin to the successful Mediterranean diet. Yes, the omega-9 fats are absolutely healthful, but they are not required for life itself. Remember, if you don't get any omega-3 fat or omega-6 fat at all you will die. That is not the case with omega-9 fat.

In nutrition circles you'll also hear people talk about oleic acid. Oleic acid is nothing fancy either, it's just a special type of monounsaturated fat. Monounsaturated fats are most popular for being the heart healthy fats associated with the Mediterranean diet because they have the ability to increase the good HDL cholesterol that helps clean your arteries. Monounsaturated fats also help prevent bad LDL from oxidizing, which is a good thing because LDL cholesterol is responsible for clogging blood vessels primarily after it is oxidized. In addition, studies have shown replacing processed omega-6-rich vegetable oils with monounsaturated fats can help decrease blood pressure. These plant-based fats are particularly rich in antiaging and disease-fighting antioxidants and phytonutrients. When used in place of saturated fat and omega-6-rich processed vegetable oils, monounsaturated-rich oils have been associated with decreased risk of diabetes and cancer, including breast cancer. These good fats help slow digestion, control blood sugar levels, and increase satiety. When used in moderate quantities they can also be helpful for weight management. In one study, researchers found that your body burns more fat energy in the 5 hours after a meal high in monounsaturated fats than after a meal rich in animal-based saturated fats.[19] Monounsaturated fats also have the unique ability to boost your body's capability of using the super antiinflammatory omega-3 essential fats most people don't get enough of in the first place. In other words monounsaturated fats can indirectly improve your omega ratio by making the omega-3 fats you eat work better.

Although olive oil is one of the best sources of monounsaturated fats, this healthful fat can also be found in whole foods such as avocados, whole olives, and in a large variety of nuts, including peanuts, almonds, pistachios, pecans, hazelnuts, and macadamias. Unlike the very fragile omega-3 and omega-6 essential fats, the sturdier monounsaturated fat–rich oils are able to withstand rancidity at higher temperatures and are therefore considered to be clean cooking oils at low to moderate levels of heat.

The thing you need to keep in mind with the omega-9 fats is that they are absolutely healthful but they are not essential. There is no need to pour globs of olive oil on your salad or to sauté your veggies in a quart of the stuff in an effort to improve your health or lose weight. Instead, use *all oil* in moderation, including the monounsaturated-rich oils like olive oil and try to get more of the fat you eat from whole foods such as avocados, nuts, and seeds.

A Clean Cuisine Oil Change

Now for our general philosophy on fats and oils as a whole: We do *not* advocate a low-fat diet. We encourage healthy whole foods that contain fat. But as we stated earlier, oil is not a whole food; nutrients and fiber are removed when pressing plant foods into oil. Although a fairly high fat diet rich in good fats is acceptable, nobody should be eating an oil-rich diet. Even if the oils you eat are considered to be more heart healthy than eating the bad fats and the bad oils, it is still not good for your heart or any other part of your body if you eat any oil in excess. Oil is a condiment, a flavoring, and a means to cook food. Oil is not a meal, nor is it a necessary nutrient.

If you swap whole plant-based fats such as nuts, seeds, and avocados for excess oil you'd be getting a lot more fiber, phytonutrients, plant sterols, and a number of other nutrients that would be much more useful at protecting your heart and your health compared to consuming heart healthy oils alone.[20] Also, the more oil you eat, the more weight you are likely to gain. The truth is you could absolutely go oil free from a culinary standpoint and get all of the fat you need for health purposes simply by eating whole fats such as nuts, seeds, avocados, and fatty fish.

> NOTE: *If you are a vegan, we highly recommend algae oil and flax oil supplementation to obtain optimal omega-3 fat intake.*

At Clean Cuisine we could of course just tell you to avoid oil completely and let that be the end of the story. And we would do that, *except* for the fact that it is next to impossible to go oil free if you also want your food to taste good! As we have mentioned many times in this book, Clean Cuisine is every bit as much about enjoying good tasting food as it is about healthful food, after all *cuisine* is part of the title. Take, for example, a marinara sauce; anybody who cooks regularly will tell you there is just no other way to make a marinara sauce taste good if you don't add some olive oil. That's why both chefs and skilled home cooks cringe and wrinkle their noses at fat-free cookbooks. The bottom line is an oil-free kitchen is likely to be an unexciting, bland, not-so-tasty kitchen. Even if you can manage to make your kitchen oil free and tasty, it is likely to take too much time, preparation, and thought in doing so. But fret not, we believe you can have your oil and eat it too. Our goal is to strike a balance, not veer off into extremes. The judicious use of *superior-quality oils* that have been produced and handled in such a manner that their natural flavors and nutritional components have been left intact can do wonders for boosting the flavor of your food without causing any damage and even adding a few nutritional perks here and there.

There really are only four things you need to keep in mind with oil:

- Avoid omega-6 oils such as corn oil completely and instead choose primarily omega-3 oils like flax oil or monounsaturated oils like extra-virgin olive oil. Plant-based saturated fat oils like extra-virgin coconut oil can be used in moderation for high-heat cooking.
- Be choosy and select only the absolute highest quality oils.
- Be very careful when cooking with oils and use only heat-safe oils, otherwise you risk damaging the oil and generating toxic byproducts. Heat-safe oils are monounsaturated oils and plant-based saturated fat oils.
- Always use oil in moderation and use some common sense. Less oil is generally better. Zero oil is going overboard.

Choosing the absolute highest quality oil is crucial for both the taste of your food and your health. Low-quality manufactured oil is one of the most harmful foods that can be consumed, and unfortunately, it lurks everywhere in the packaged food and convenience food world, including, and especially, at restaurants. The thing is high-quality oils are not as easy to come by as you might think; they are pretty much never found in processed foods, and they are even difficult to locate in higher-quality natural and organic packaged foods. Top-quality oils are also considerably more expensive than lesser-quality oils, which is why food manufacturers and most restaurants don't have a penchant for using them. You get what you pay for when it comes to oil.

134

You want to look for oils that are cold-pressed and unrefined. You specifically want to avoid refined oils that have been processed with chemicals, exposed to high heat (refined oils are often heated up to 470°F, which damages them significantly), or deodorized. The best-quality cold-pressed oils are expeller pressed in a heat-controlled environment to keep temperatures below 120°F. It's important to note that although Europe has rigorous standards in place for the terminology of cold pressing (fully *unrefined* oil extracted at temperatures below 122°F), the phrase *cold pressed* has been used erroneously in the United States for a number of years and is often employed as a marketing technique. You really have to do a bit of homework on the oil brands you choose and not just grab one from the shelf because the company has invested in a splashy marketing campaign or pretty packaging.

Processing can damage even healthful oils. When it comes to buying olive oil and coconut oil, you want to buy only cold-pressed, extra-virgin brands that are made from the very first pressing and thus have more nutrients, more antioxidants, and superior flavor. We always use extra-virgin olive oil and extra-virgin coconut oil for this reason.

CLEAN CUISINE OILS

OUR FAVORITE CLEAN CUISINE OILS FOR COOKING

Extra-Virgin Olive Oil

The acronym EVOO might have been made popular by cooking personality Rachel Ray, but extra-virgin olive oil has been a mainstay of the Mediterranean diet and is one of the oldest known culinary oils. Extra-virgin olive oil contains predominately monounsaturated fat. It also contains antioxidants and flavonoids that help prevent bad LDL cholesterol from oxidizing and becoming particularly dangerous to your blood vessels. Extra-virgin olive oil *cannot* be heated to extremely high temperatures or it will spoil, so be careful to cook on low heat, such as low-heat sautéing. You can roast vegetables with extra-virgin olive oil and even bake with it, but again, keep the heat low. By the way, a good test for any oil is that if it smokes, the heat is too high.

Finding extra-virgin olive oil is not as easy as you might think. *Consumer Reports* even did a feature on extra-virgin olive oils in September 2012 and reported that their taste testers decided many olive oils labeled extra-virgin simply don't make the grade. We were happy to discover the one that we use, Costco's Kirkland brand, was rated "very good." We consider this one the best quality and taste for an incredible value. *Consumer Reports* also rated McEvoy Ranch, Trader Joe's California Estate, Whole Foods 365 Everyday Value 100% California Unfiltered, and Lucini Premium highly.

Extra-Virgin Coconut Oil

Pressed from the fruit of the coconut palm tree, a superior-quality extra-virgin coconut oil will *not* make your food reek of some tropical-smelling sunscreen. It is surprising that a high-quality extra-virgin coconut oil has almost no smell when used for cooking. Instead, it delivers a luxurious richness that can compete head to head with butter. In fact, in the vast majority of recipes that call for butter, extra-virgin coconut oil can be used as the perfect Clean Cuisine substitute. You can even bake with it. We love how it can withstand high-heat temperatures without oxidizing. We don't fry many foods, but when we do we use only extra-virgin coconut oil because it is so heat stable that it can even withstand the high heat associated with frying without spoiling and without any risk of creating trans-fats. Do keep in mind that extra-virgin coconut oil is rich in saturated fat (albeit the mostly healthful plant-based saturated fat), so it is best to use it in moderation. Our favorite brand is Barlean's, made from hand-selected, freshly picked coconuts.

Macadamia Nut Oil

Part of the popularity of macadamia nut oil stems from the fact that it is richer than any other oil in monounsaturated fat, even richer than olive oil! This nutritious oil finds favor with chefs all over the world for its versatility and practicality of use. With a rich, nutty flavor it's absolutely amazing drizzled on salads, beans, and whole grains. Note too that macadamia nut oil has a high smoke point of around 425°F, which is higher than that of olive oil. Because it has such a high smoke point, macadamia nut oil does not break down into toxic by-products that are harmful to your heart and overall health. All in all, it's a very practical addition to your Clean Cuisine cabinet, especially for occasions when olive oil can't be used due its lower smoke point.

OUR FAVORITE CLEAN CUISINE OILS FOR RAW FOODS RECIPES, DIPS, DRESSINGS, AND FOR DRIZZLING ON COOKED FOODS

Flax Oil

WE LOVE GOLDEN flax oil for its uniquely hefty dose of omega-3s (in the form of LNA) just as much as we love it for its earthy, nutty flavor. It's perfect for making pesto, hummus, and vinaigrettes, but we also love dipping our sprouted whole grain bread in little bowls of flax oil with a bit of fresh rosemary, freshly ground pepper, and salt. You do have to be very choosy about the flax oil you buy because for whatever reason many brands are not fresh. Our favorite brand for consistently and reliably fresh flax oil is Barlean's.

Walnut Oil

A CULINARY TREAT delivering a nearly optimal omega-3 to omega-6 ratio, walnut oil is sensational for adding the finishing flavor touch to many vegetable, pasta, and whole grain salad dishes. It's also the perfect delicately flavored oil base for vinaigrette and is particularly delicious in raspberry and lemon rind vinaigrettes.

Hemp Oil

DARK GREEN WITH a smooth, rich, and nutty flavor, hemp oil has nearly an ideal ratio of omega-3 to omega-6 fats. Best of all, some of the omega-6 fat in hemp oil is from the super useful GLA fat that your body appreciates more than any other omega-6 fat. As a matter of fact, GLA is just as good as the omega-3 fats for the purposes of fighting inflammation and improving health. GLA is not readily available in most foods and generally must be taken in supplement form such as evening primrose oil capsules or borage oil capsules. Use hemp oil drizzled on top of salads and cold grain and pasta dishes. Toss hemp oil into a vegan sandwich filler; one of Ivy's favorite sandwiches is a combination of finely chopped parsley, carrots, red peppers, and basil tossed together with a bit of hemp oil and eaten as a sandwich between two slices of sprouted whole grain toast.

Truffle Oil

ALONG WITH ANCHOVY paste, truffle oil is another one of Ivy's secret Clean Cuisine culinary ingredients. Truffle oil can be made by infusing the flavor of truffles into any oil, but for health reasons we prefer to buy truffle oil infused into olive oil. As with other oils, not all truffle oil is created equal. Some truffle oils are made from an organic compound called 2,4-dithiapentane—derived either naturally or from a petroleum base—mixed together with olive oil. It is not surprising that those oils don't taste so good. Our favorite brand is Roland. This stuff is not cheap, but believe us, an itsy bitsy, teeny tiny little bit goes a very long way toward creating intense culinary bliss. We especially love black truffle oil drizzled on baked potato fries, roasted vegetables, whole grains, salads, and any dish with mushrooms.

Coconuts

It is very important to understand that just as not all fats are created equal, all saturated fats are not created equal either. Just as there are good fats and bad fats, there are also good saturated fats and bad saturated fats. Plant-based coconut fat is absolutely rich in saturated fat, but it's not the same as the saturated fat found in animal foods. Just like you cannot consider grocery store orange juice the same as whole orange juice squeezed with the pulp, rind, and all, you cannot haphazardly clump lard and coconuts in the same category either.

We consider *unrefined* whole coconut meat, coconut milk, and high-quality *extra-virgin* coconut oil to be good saturated fats. When you dive into the nutritional science, you will read about epidemiological studies showing that the saturated fats found in animal foods such as dairy, beef, turkey, and chicken, is absolutely correlated to impaired heart health, whereas the saturated fat found in *unrefined* and *unprocessed* coconut foods is not harmful.[21] Studies conducted in the early 1980s showed that the traditional Polynesian diet consisted of between 34 and 64 percent of total calories from coconuts, yet even this large amount of plant-based saturated fat had no negative health or coronary heart disease consequences.[22] The coconut-eating islanders not only had healthy hearts but had healthy, lean, and otherwise disease-free bodies too. Additional research shows that even though the saturated fat in coconuts might raise cholesterol levels, it raises the good protective HDL cholesterol and does not raise triglycerides, which helps explain why populations eating coconut-rich diets do not suffer from heart disease, as you might expect on a high saturated fat–rich diet.[23] It would be irresponsible not to point out that studies showing a coconut-rich diet to not be harmful were done on people who were eating otherwise healthy, unrefined whole foods diets. The native islanders in the studies we mentioned were not eating Oreos made with coconut oil!

Still, how, you wonder, can the saturated fat from coconuts be handled by the body differently from the saturated fat from beef? For one, not all saturated fats are created equal. Even though coconut oil is exceptionally rich in saturated fat, it is a *plant-based* saturated fat, which means it offers a delivery agent for disease-fighting and antioxidant-acting phytonutrients that are not found in animals. Those phytonutrients give coconuts a tremendous advantage over animal-based saturated fats. Furthermore, plant-based saturated fat from coconuts is biochemically different from the saturated fat found in butter, beef, and lard. Coconut oil is rich in medium-chain triglycerides (MCTs), a form of saturated fat that is metabolized and used differently from the longer chain saturated fats found in most animal foods. Unlike long-chain animal-based saturated fats that are deposited within cells and organs and are responsible for clogging arteries, MCTs are easily digested, quickly transported to the liver, and very quickly burned for energy; MCTs are not easily stored in your arteries as cholesterol, and thus they are not easily stored as body fat either.

Although we are not suggesting you start eating globs of coconut oil as a way to lose weight, there are studies suggesting the MCTs in coconut oil might be helpful for reducing body fat. According to a 2001 study published in the *Journal of Nutrition*, long-term clinical trials revealed that eating MCTs resulted in less body fat accumulation in humans as compared to consumption of other fats.[24] What is more, about half of the fat found in coconuts is lauric acid, a particularly good fat linked to immune health and improved insulin sensitivity.

Just like all saturated fats are not equal, all coconut foods are not created equal either. You'll notice we've been stressing that the coconut foods eaten in the population studies we cited have been *unrefined* and *unprocessed*. The importance of eating unrefined and unprocessed *fresh* coconut foods cannot be overemphasized. Most coconut foods found in commercially prepared products have been highly processed and are not at all the same as the unrefined coconut foods eaten by the heart-healthy native islanders. For example, refined coconut oils found in convenience items such as microwave popcorn, artificial coffee creamers, nondairy whipped toppings, and vegetable shortenings, have been highly processed, stripped of innate nutrients (including the naturally occurring vitamin E and carotene found in unprocessed coconut oil), and exposed to chemical solvents. We can't overstate that eating processed coconut oil is absolutely harmful. In fact, any studies that have ever shown coconut oil to have a negative effect on health have all been on *processed* coconut foods. If you look at population studies of people eating diets based on unrefined, natural coconut foods you don't see health problems, but you *do* see health problems occur when people (and animals!) eat processed and refined coconut foods. Specifically, many processed coconut oils contain hydrogenated oils and we now know it is the hydrogenated oils (which contain trans-fats) that are harmful to your health, not the *unrefined* coconut.

CLEAN CUISINE COCONUT TIPS

■ **Clean Cuisine swap: replace butter with extra-virgin coconut oil.** Extra-virgin coconut oil is the tastiest and healthiest butter substitute because it is one of the only unrefined nutrient-containing vegan fats that does not oxidize at high heat temperatures.

> NOTE: *When substituting coconut oil for butter you'll want to use 25 percent less extra-virgin coconut oil because it has a lower water content and is more concentrated.*

■ **Eat clean: choose only the highest-quality coconut foods.** It is extremely important you choose the absolute highest-quality, unrefined coconut foods. A fresh coconut is obviously the superior choice. But when buying coconut milk look for organic, when buying shredded coconut look for organic and unsweetened, and when buying coconut oil don't settle for anything less than organic extra-virgin. Avoid coconut oils labeled virgin or simply coconut oil. We've come to rely on Barlean's organic extra-virgin coconut oil for supplying the best-tasting coconut oil on the market.

> NOTE: *Barlean's uses only hand-selected and fresh-picked coconuts for their oil; coconuts that are immature or overripe or that*

have fallen to the ground are nutritionally inferior and not used. Barlean's oils are also carefully cold pressed to preserve nutrients from the whole coconut, and they are processed without the use of chemical solvents or hard mechanical filtration.

- **Be mindful of how much saturated fat from coconuts you are consuming.** If you are familiar with our first book, *The Gold Coast Cure*, you'll recall we recommended keeping your saturated fat intake to less than 15 grams a day. This recommendation was based on the research we did on diet and multiple sclerosis as outlined in Dr. Roy Swank's *The Multiple Sclerosis Diet Book* and scientific journals such as the *Journal of Neurology*. Limiting your saturated fat intake to 15 grams or less per day was the only counting we encouraged in our book, and we still stand by that recommendation. However, you can eat a good amount of coconut-based foods and not go over that limit, especially if you are otherwise limiting saturated fat intake by avoiding animal sources. Note that ¼ cup of fresh coconut meat contains about 6 grams saturated fat. And keep in mind a little bit of coconut oil goes a very long way.
- **Coconut oil beyond the kitchen and into the bathroom.** For whatever it's worth, you'll find extra-virgin coconut oil not only in our kitchen pantry but also in our bathroom. That's because we have yet to find a more luxurious and more effective moisturizer and shave cream on the market. If you want the best body exfoliator in the world just mix a bit of brown sugar with your coconut oil and scrub away.

Wholesome Whole Fats That Boost Flavor, Improve Health, and Stimulate Weight Loss

We've talked a lot about oils, yet we've sort of skimmed over wholesome whole fats such as avocados, nuts, and seeds. From a health standpoint, the healthiest fat choice will almost always be raw whole fats instead of the oils made from those foods. For example, ground flaxseeds offer health benefits such as fiber and lignans, those cancer-preventing compounds mentioned earlier, both of which are missing in the oil. It's not that flax oil is bad, it's just that ground flaxseeds are an even better choice.

Whole fats offer unpolluted, clean sources of essential fats plus healthy monounsaturated fats packaged with antioxidants, vitamins, phytonutrients, vegan protein, and minerals, so it is no surprise that when you dig through the medical journals on nutrition science you see these foods are closely associated with disease resistance and life extension. A review of epidemiological studies such as the Adventist Health Study, Iowa Women's Health Study, Nurses' Health Study, Physicians' Health Study, and CARE Study show eating whole fats in the form of raw nuts and seeds increase the lifespan and decrease the risk of dying from *all* causes.[25] In a study published in the *Archives of Internal Medicine,* men who ate raw nuts had an astonishing *half* the risk of sudden cardiac arrest compared to men who did not eat nuts.[26] In a study published in the *American Journal of Clinical Nutrition,* researchers documented that walnuts could reduce total cholesterol and bad LDL cholesterol levels, even when no other dietary changes were made.[27] Macadamia nuts have been shown to produce similar benefits, and pecan-enriched diets have been shown to favorably alter blood lipid profiles in healthy men and women.[28]

But aren't nuts fattening? Apparently not. In fact, epidemiological studies actually show an inverse relationship between nut consumption and BMI and a study published in the *American Journal of Clinical Nutrition* showed that people who are allowed to eat as many nuts as they liked on a regular basis were actually slimmer than their non-nut-eating peers.[29] Additional research shows regular nut and seed consumption is closely correlated with long-term weight loss. Even your risk of developing diabetes, a condition intimately related to obesity, is reduced by eating nuts and seeds.[30] Keep in mind whole fats like nuts and seeds are going to be more filling and satisfying than the same number of calories and the same amount of fat grams from oil. The whole fats come packaged with necessary nutrients and tummy-filling fiber too. So if you are trying to lose weight it makes sense to get more of your fat from whole foods like nuts and seeds rather than from the oils made from them.

Obviously it would be impossible to study each and every nut variety on the face of the earth, but a review of the nutrition research clearly shows regular consumption of nuts and seeds is unarguably associated with a healthy, trim body. As far as we are concerned, it really doesn't matter which nut you choose to eat either. What *does* matter is that you choose the cleanest and healthiest nuts. Undressed, unfancy, naked, *raw* nuts are the superior choice. Dry roasted nuts are second best, but you specifically want to avoid the nuts and seeds roasted in any type of oil. The ingredients list for packaged nuts should not include any oil at all. And remember, freshness is key!

Nuts and seeds can go rancid if exposed to too much light and if left sitting around for too long. Eating rancid fats can be harmful and can increase inflammation in your body. To keep your nuts and seeds ultra-fresh it is generally best to store them in airtight containers in the refrigerator or in self-closing plastic bags in your freezer (this is what we do).

BOOSTING NUTRITION FROM NUTS AND SEEDS

SOAKING NUTS AND seeds is an easy way to improve their digestibility and increase their nutritional profile. Harder nuts like almonds should be soaked for 6 or 8 hours; cashews, for 4 hours; and softer nuts like walnuts, pecans, macadamias, and pine nuts, for 1 or 2 hours. Even if you don't have time to soak them for the full length of time, soaking them just a little can still result in significant benefit. If you want to speed the process up a bit you can use warm water, but if you are soaking nuts and seeds overnight, be sure to refrigerate them to avoid spoilage. Once they are soaked simply drain, rinse with cool water, and store in the refrigerator for 2 or 3 days, making sure to rinse them daily. Soaking your nuts and seeds might seem like a whole lot of extra work for nothing, but it really does boost nutrition and it takes barely any time.

Creating Clean Cuisine with Nuts, Seeds, and More

It is one thing to read about all the health benefits associated with a particular food but it's another thing altogether to work that food into your daily life and your recipes. Luckily, whole fats like nuts and seeds are incredibly versatile in any Clean Cuisine kitchen. Sure you could just grab a handful of nuts and seeds and eat them just like that, but there are so many other creative and tasty ways to work these superfoods into your diet. Here are some of our favorites.

- **Nut crumbs and salad boosters.** One of our favorite ways to eat nuts and seeds is in crumb form. This is primarily because nuts and seeds are ultra-filling; therefore, it's difficult to eat too many of them at once; if you try boosting your nut consumption in a recipe by simply tossing a handful into the pot you aren't going to get as much flavor or satisfaction as you would if you dispersed the nutty goodness throughout the recipe in crumb form. Nut crumbs lend remarkable texture and flavor to countless recipes, and they make the best-tasting, most nutritious replacement for traditional bread crumbs sprinkled on casseroles, tossed on top of stir-fries, blended into pesto, and sprinkled on top of whole grains. By the way, pine nut crumbs make an amazing substitute for Parmesan cheese scattered on top of a plate of pasta with marinara. We also love nut crumbs as a base to our Salad Boosters (see page 318). Nothing beats a simple breakfast of a big bowl of fresh fruit sprinkled with nut crumbs and a drizzle of raw honey. Best of all, nut crumbs are beyond easy to make: Simply place dry nuts in a food processor and pulse several times until they are crumbly. It takes all of 30 seconds to make nut crumbs, and they can be stored in big batches in self-sealing plastic bags in your freezer for up to 2 months.

NOTE: *Nut crumbs are more likely to go rancid than are whole nuts so be sure to store them in the freezer to prolong freshness.*

■ **Raw nut butters.** Although they can get a little pricey, we think raw nut butters are absolutely worth the price. The ultimate fast food, they are super convenient, too. By all means you want to avoid any nut butters made with any added oils. Especially bad are those nut butters containing added hydrogenated oil. Also check the ingredients list to make sure there are no added sugars. The purest, most nutritious nut butters are raw. Even though peanut butter is by far the most popular nut butter it is practically impossible to find raw peanut butter, and in fact, many, but not all, peanut butter brands contain unhealthful added oils and sugars. The best tasting and healthiest peanut butter is the fresh stuff you can grind yourself at the supermarket. Our favorite commercially available raw nut butters are almond butter, cashew butter, and macadamia butter. If you have a high-speed blender like a Vitamix you can go online and learn to make your own raw nut butters using just about any nut. Nut butters are a delicious spread on sliced fruit such as apples and pears, and they make the most decadent mayonnaise alternative in sandwiches. Three of our favorite super

144

simple vegan nut-butter sandwich creations made on sprouted whole grain bread are almond butter, sliced heirloom tomatoes, and arugula; peanut butter with banana, shredded carrots, and cinnamon; and cashew butter with leftover roasted vegetables and watercress. We also use nut butters to thicken sauces and vinaigrettes or as a milk replacement in shakes and smoothies (see Part Four for no-milk shakes).

- **Raw seed butter.** Raw tahini is made from sesame seeds, and it's unbelievably versatile. We use it in hummus, roasted eggplant dip, vegetable spreads, and creamy salad dressings. Like the sesame seeds it is made from, tahini is rich in calcium and a great vegan protein source. It's also got a hefty dose of fiber, potassium, iron, and magnesium.

- **Cashew cream and cashew milk & pine nut cream and pine nut milk.** These are secret and magical ingredient that make living without cream (except for the bit Ivy still puts in her coffee!) easy, doable, and tasty. Cashew cream originated in the raw foods world and is used to make some of the most outrageously decadent raw desserts. But it's also a vegan chef's staple, and steps in for dairy in a variety of creative ways, including cheese fillings for ravioli, ricotta, and rich whitesauces, for Ivy's decadent creamy pasta dish), and as a heavy cream for soups. As far as we know, pine nut milk is not used in the raw food community, but Ivy uses this too frequently when preparing our meals. Pretty much anytime a recipe calls for cream or full-fat milk, you can use cashew cream or pine nut cream or thinned out cashew/pine nut milks instead. Cashew and pine nut cream/milk can be stored 2 days in the fridge, and each takes less than 5 minutes to make. The trick when making them is to use raw cashews or raw pine nuts for the best flavor and texture. You can play around with the consistency to make it thicker for cream or thinner for milk. Here's the basic recipe.

cashew cream (or pine nut cream)

½ cup raw cashews or pine nuts, ideally soaked for 4 or more hours
1 cup filtered water
Pinch of unrefined sea salt

In a Vitamix or equivalent high-speed blender, blend the nuts and water on high speed for about 2 minutes. Add the salt and blend again.

cashew milk (or pine nut milk)

½ cup raw cashews or pine nuts, ideally soaked for 4 or more hours

2 cups filtered water, use less water for a more full-fat version and more water for a light version

Pinch of unrefined sea salt

In a Vitamix or equivalent high-speed blender blend the nuts and water on high speed for about 2 minutes. Add the salt and blend again.

■ **Other assorted nut milks and nutty no-milk shakes.** Nut milks and nut shakes are dairy-free milks made from raw nuts. It sounds crazy, but trust us, when you blend raw nuts with water in a high speed blender you end up with a rich, creamy, and luxurious milk that tastes even better than cow's milk. If you're used to cow's milk and try to swap it with a low-fat alternative such as soy milk or even commercial almond milk (which is very low in fat), the lack of fat is going to throw the flavor and texture off completely, and you'll end up feeling like you are being short-changed eating such diet foods. The reason nut milks and shakes made with nuts taste so decadent is because the healthy fat in nuts contributes a velvety milk-like creaminess. Low-fat soy milk just can't compete. You can make nut milks from just about any common raw nut, including macadamias, pecans, walnuts, and almonds. In general, fresh nut milks will keep for 2 days in the fridge if stored in a covered container. Check out the recipe for cashew milk above, then use the same general guidelines for making other nut milks. For nut-based shakes made with whole fruits check out our recipes in Part Four.

■ **Avocado:** Technically a fruit, avocados are brimming with antioxidants, vitamins C and E, folate, potassium, and numerous antiaging phytonutrients. Avocados also contain lutein, a potent antioxidant that helps keep your eyes healthy and your skin glowing. Even though avocados are rich in fat, they actually depress insulin production and help keep you feeling full and satisfied for hours, which is a great formula for weight management. And by the way, avocados are also rich in fiber. One avocado contains approximately 10 grams of fiber! We use avocados in all sorts of ways in the kitchen; here are some ideas.

- **Classic guacamole.** Nothing beats homespun guac!
- **Creamy avocado-based vinaigrettes.** See our recipe ideas at cleancuisine.com.
- **Fruit and avocado salsas.** Play around with combinations such as mango and avocado and grilled pineapple, jalapeño, and avocado.
- **Straight up!** Cut one ripe avocado in half and remove the pit. Squeeze a bit of fresh lemon or lime juice into the bowls the pit leaves behind, add a dash of unrefined sea salt and eat right out of the skin with a spoon.
- **Toast topper.** Lightly mash a ripe avocado in a bowl with lemon juice, unrefined sea salt, crushed garlic, and red pepper flakes. Spread over toasted sprouted whole grain bread.
- **Slivered salad slicers.** Did you know adding avocado to your salad helps your body absorb nutrients from the rest of the vegetables? Try adding slivered sliced avocado strips to any salad, squeeze a bit of lemon juice on top, and drizzle with a tad of oil.
- **Chilled avocado soup.** Nothing beats cold, creamy avocado soup made by puréeing avocados, lime juice, cilantro, water, garlic, a bit of cayenne, and unrefined sea salt.
- **Avocado smoothie.** Avocados yield creamy decadence to fruit smoothies. We especially love avocados blended with frozen pineapple, coconut water, lime juice, and mango. Mmmmm....

You really do need to get to know your fats. Educate yourself on the good, healing whole fats; make sure you get enough omega-3s; reduce your intake of all types of culinary oil; and get rid of or drastically reduce your intake of highly refined oils, butter, and animal fats. If you get the vast majority of your fat intake from plant-based fats in their unrefined, whole form and you get enough omega-3s, you'll be in good shape. Fat science is really not much more complicated than that, folks.

6

CLEANING UP YOUR PROTEIN ACT
Do You Really *Need* All of That Protein?

Protein is an essential nutrient. It helps rebuild body tissue and forms the framework of your body, including the muscles, organs, and connective tissue. In the form of enzymes, proteins help you digest your food, and as antibodies, proteins protect you from illness when viruses and bacteria attack. No doubt protein is really important stuff. But, protein is *not* the wonder macronutrient many people think it is. There *is* such a thing as getting too much protein, eating unclean sources of protein, and getting fat from eating too much protein-rich food. There is absolutely no reason to eat above and beyond the protein your body needs for maintenance and repair.

It is interesting that of the three macronutrients—carbs, fats, and proteins—the only one that seems to get off scot-free when it comes to being blamed for its potential role in degenerative diseases—and weight gain— is protein. Nobody ever seems to want to blame protein, for anything harmful. Carbs and fats get blamed for obesity, heart disease, type 2 diabetes, and so on, yet somehow protein has remained unscathed in the eyes of the general public. In fact, protein is the stuff everyone still seems to be scrambling to get *more* of! We've never heard of someone saying, "Oh no, I can't have more chicken, I'm trying to limit my protein intake."

And of course some big hunk of protein still takes center stage on most modern dinner plates. Protein is also the stuff dieters make a mad dash to the nutrition store to buy in bulk. You don't see many carb bars or fat shakes on the nutrition store shelves, but processed protein bars, protein powders, protein shakes, and protein supplements are bountiful. It's as if we were all in some sort of enormous protein emergency. But, of course, we are not. We are in anything *but* a protein emergency. In reality we eat far too much of the stuff than our bodies really need.

> NOTE: *So many of the protein supplements out there have been processed so heavily that they have had pretty much all of their other nutrients removed, leaving behind pure protein and usually some filler fats and carbs. These are, of course, not natural whole foods.*

You Can Still Get Fat (and Accelerate the Aging Process and Promote Inflammation) if You Eat Too Many Skinless Chicken Breasts

Regardless of what certain diet gurus and fitness trainers would like you to believe, protein is not a free food. If you eat more protein than your body needs, the extra protein doesn't just magically evaporate into thin air; it gets stored as body fat. That means the protein calories in that extra piece of chicken don't just vanish. Eat too many skinless chicken breasts or too much whey protein powder or too many egg whites, and your jeans can soon be too tight. Eating more protein (or any other macronutrient for that matter!) than your body needs will also accelerate the aging process by increasing oxidative stress.

Although many people are no doubt confused about the facts on protein, if you took a random poll picking any John or Jane Doe off the street, that person would tell you protein and animal foods such as beef and chicken go hand in hand. This means if you are eating a diet high in protein you are most likely eating a diet rich in animal foods. One of the problems with an animal-food-rich, protein-packed diet is that your stomach can hold only so much food in one day; if you are filling up on animal foods, you are basically just pushing all the other phytonutrient-rich, anti-aging, and disease-fighting plant foods such as fruits, vegetables, whole grains, beans, nuts, seeds, and avocados right off your plate. People aren't eating nearly enough unrefined whole plant foods as it is, so the last thing we need is to displace plant foods with large portions of protein-packed beef, chicken, milk, and protein shakes. We don't need more protein, people! What we really need to be eating are more unrefined plant-based foods. Plant foods are the foods we are deficient in; we are not deficient in skinless chicken breasts.

Keep in mind, protein-packed animal foods contain none of the disease-fighting phytonutrients found in plant foods that are essential for reducing inflammation, preventing DNA damage, helping us stay youthful, and protecting against disease. In addition, animal foods are lacking in important substances that protect against cancer and heart attack, including fiber and phytonutrients, and they are rich in substances that are directly associated with degenerative diseases, such as saturated fat. It's not that animal foods don't come packaged with other nutrients that are absolutely essential, such as the omega-3 EPA and DHA found in fish, the vitamin D in eggs, or the vitamin B12 found in all animal foods. These are all very important nutrients that are pretty much impossible to get adequate amounts of if you don't eat some animal foods or take supplements. But you do not need to be eating animal foods just to get enough protein. As we'll discuss in more detail later in the chapter, you actually can get plenty of protein from a well-balanced plant food diet.

We can see the meat lovers closing this book right now. But don't get nervous! Just because we tell you that you can get plenty of protein from plants doesn't mean we are trying to convince you to convert to a vegan diet (Andy, in particular, isn't about to give up his salmon burgers and he still loves a sirloin steak now and then too!), instead we are trying to drive home the point that protein should come as a whole package deal. There are far too many nutrients that we need from plant foods, and if we over-consume animal foods just because we are under the misguided impression we will be protein-deficient if we don't, then we end up shortchanging ourselves in overall total nutrition. Instead, the vast majority of our protein should come from unrefined whole plant foods, which come packaged with phytonutrients. Animal foods should be consumed in much smaller quantities than what is standard in the modern-day diet. So yes, you can still have some steak (preferably pastured and organic steak, but more on that in a bit), but you should keep your portions moderate. And you don't need to eat animal foods at every meal either.

How Much Protein Do You Need Each Day? A Lot Less Than You Think.

There is still some gray area as to the exact grams of protein per kilogram of lean body mass a person needs each day. Some experts estimate the amount to be 1 to 2 grams of protein per kilogram of lean body mass. The Institute of Medicine recommends that we ingest 0.8 gram of protein for every kilogram that we weigh.[1] For example, a 120-pound woman would need to eat only about 44 grams of protein a day. This isn't a whole lot! (See page 152 to see how quickly protein adds up in a day.)

It's not that you have to be tallying up precisely how much protein you eat each and every day, a tiresome bore of a chore if there ever were one, but it is good to have a general idea of how much protein you need. Because metric measurements aren't second nature for many of us, we like to say a good rule of thumb is to know you should consume roughly 0.5 gram of protein per pound of body weight. If you are overweight you should calculate your protein needs based on your *ideal* body weight, not your current weight. Any excess amount of protein over this amount is more than likely going to be empty calories (the exception to this is if you are recovering from a major surgery or you exercise *intensely* for more than 6 hours a week). Based on this guideline, a healthy weight 120-pound woman could have about 60 grams of protein per day.

When you start to look at the protein content in your food you soon realize it is *extremely easy* to get 0.5 gram of protein per pound of body weight, and it's even easier to get 0.8 gram of protein per kilogram! In fact, because of our animal-foods-rich diets, the average American consumes 100 to 120 grams of protein per day. According to the Institute of Medicine, that amount should really be eaten only by people with *ideal body weights* of between 275 and 330 pounds. And according to our more lenient 0.5 gram of protein per pound of body weight calculation, 100 to 120 grams of protein should be consumed only if your *ideal body weight* is between 200 and 240 pounds. Trust us, the prevailing nutrition problem with modern society is not that we are not getting enough protein; instead, we aren't getting enough unrefined whole plant foods! If anything, people eat way more protein than they should.

Where's the Protein?

Even if you decided you wanted to eat 100 percent vegan and never ever touch a piece of chicken or beef again, you could still actually get all of the protein you need from unrefined whole plant foods, assuming you ate enough calories. For example, did you know that 52 percent of the energy in spinach comes from protein? Broccoli contains 38 percent protein; black beans, 26 percent; quinoa, 14 percent; and walnuts, 10 percent. And don't worry about the outdated advice that you need to mix and match your foods to get a complete protein. Your body cannot use protein directly from the food you eat anyway; it must convert food protein into amino acids and then use the amino acids to repair your body, regulate hormones, and so on. Because your body stores and releases the amino acids it needs over a 24-hour time period, it is totally unnecessary to go to the hassle of combining foods to achieve protein completeness. While it is true some plant foods have more essential amino acids than others, in the end your body gets the protein it needs from the foods you eat on a long-term basis, not from a single meal. For example, legumes like cooked dried beans, dried peas, and lentils are low in sulfur-containing amino acids such as methionine but they are high in another amino acid called lysine. Grains are just the opposite. So if you eat both foods during the course of a day or even a couple days apart, you still get all the essential amino acids your body needs. What is more, certain plant foods, such as soy, contain adequate amounts of all essential amino acids so no specific effort to combine proteins is required at all. In fact, even the American Dietetic Association has stated that:

> *Plant sources of protein alone can provide adequate amounts of the essential and non-essential amino acids, assuming that the dietary protein sources from plants are reasonably varied and that caloric intake is sufficient to meet energy needs. Whole grains, legumes, vegetables, seeds and nuts all contain essential and non-essential amino acids.*[2]

VEGAN FOR THE DAY

NOT LONG AGO, as an experiment, Ivy decided to add up her protein intake on a day when she didn't eat any animal foods whatsoever. Take a look; she still got a good amount of protein.

Breakfast: Strawberry Banana Split No-Milk Shake (see page 312), containing 2 tablespoons hemp seeds (8 grams protein), 1 frozen banana (1 gram of protein), and 1 cup frozen strawberries (1 gram of protein).
Total: 10 grams protein

Snack: SuperGreen Smoothie: Ginger-Berry Cocktail (see recipe on page 345), containing 2 handfuls of romaine lettuce (2 grams protein), 1 cup frozen blueberries (1 gram protein), 1 tablespoon chia seeds (2 grams protein), and 2 dates (negligible).
Total: 5 grams protein

Lunch: Large mixed green salad with 2 tablespoons pumpkin seeds, chopped red bell peppers, and lemon-hemp oil vinaigrette (7 grams protein) with 1 slice sprouted whole grain bread made into croutons (4 grams protein) along with 1 cup lentil vegetable soup (13 grams protein) and 1 whole grain corn muffin (see CleanCuisine.com for recipe; 4 grams protein).
Total: 24 grams protein

Dinner: 6 ounces grilled tofu (23 grams protein) with grilled vegetable kabobs (3 grams protein), ¾ cup black rice (4 grams protein), and dessert of ½ cup coconut ice cream dessert (2 grams protein) and sliced peaches (1 gram protein).
Total: 33 grams protein

The food Ivy ate during the sample day contained 72 grams of protein, even without any animal foods at all. If Ivy swapped the grilled tofu for 6 ounces of chicken breast she would add an additional 12 grams of protein and therefore be up to 89 grams of protein for the day. If she had eaten just 3 ounces of shrimp for lunch instead of the bread she would have added an additional 15 grams of protein. It doesn't take a lot of animal foods to quickly contribute a lot of protein to your diet, but getting more protein than you need isn't exactly desirable.

Protein and Exercise?

Don't you need more protein if you exercise? Yes and no. On the day Ivy recorded her meals (page 152) she happened to *not* exercise, but if she had exercised, she surely would have been hungrier and would have eaten more calories; if she ate more calories some of those calories would have almost certainly contained protein and so she would have increased her protein intake just by consuming more calories. If you exercise, your body needs more of *all* macronutrients—carbs, fat, and protein. You don't need just more protein. If you regularly work out, you want to make sure you get enough total calories; enough carbs to fuel muscles; optimal amounts of essential fats; and a wide variety of amino acid–containing plant-based whole foods such as nuts, seeds, green vegetables, beans, and whole grains. You can still have moderate amounts of protein-rich animal foods too, but the thing is you don't need to go out of your way to stockpile skinless chicken breasts in your freezer either. As long as you eat enough good clean calories, including fats and carbs, and get a nice mixture of amino acid–containing whole foods, your body will have the raw material it needs to repair itself and build lean muscle mass after a workout. And do keep in mind, intense exercise substantially increases your need for carbohydrates, not just for energy to fuel your workouts but also for replenishing muscles post-exertion.

If you exercise for weight management or your workout goal is to lose weight, eating more protein isn't going to help you trim down any faster. In fact, eating more protein and increasing total caloric intake while maintaining the same exercise level will build an equal amount of additional fat and muscle mass, according to a study published in 1992 in the *Journal of the American Geriatrics Society*.[3]

In general if you are a moderate exerciser (and we hope you will try the fitness program we recommend in Chapter 8), you really don't need to modify your diet much at all. Maybe you'll need to add a modest-size snack, such as a smoothie or some fruit and nuts before or after your workout, but you certainly don't need to refuel with laboratory-created protein powders. However, if you exercise intensely you *do* need to eat more calories. And again, by eating more calories from whole foods you will, by default, be getting more protein. Let's take beans as an example here. Suppose you don't normally exercise very much, so you eat only about a ½ cup of beans at a single sitting. On average, most ½ cup servings of beans will give you 7 to 10 grams of protein. If you suddenly start a rigorous workout program your appetite is going to increase, so when you sit down for your next dinner, you may consume 1 cup of beans, which means you will be getting 14 to 20 grams of protein total or 7 to 10 grams more protein than what you got from your usual serving of beans. The point is you don't need to consciously go out of your way to single protein out as the one macronutrient to eat more of; if you are active, you simply need to eat more food and more total calories in general.

Instead of worrying so much about protein, if you exercise a lot it is especially important to make sure you get more antioxidants and phytonutrients to combat the exercise-induced oxidative stress that is inevitable with an intense fitness training program. And the more hardcore your workout is, the more cell-protecting antioxidants and phytonutrients you need to ingest. Keep in mind, unrefined whole foods are the best sources of antioxidants, and plant foods are the only sources for phytonutrients.

> NOTE: *If you are an endurance athlete or serious body builder, we encourage you to consult with a sports nutritionist to tailor a nutritional program unique to your increased calorie needs. In general though, you would then need to eat relatively more dense carbs than our fruit- and veggie-forward Clean Cuisine diet recommends, not necessarily more protein-rich foods.*

Clean Protein from Plant Foods

Because protein is an essential part of plant cells, at least some protein is found in *all* plant foods. We bet you didn't know that *per calorie*, cooked spinach has more than twice as much protein as a cheeseburger. It's not that we don't eat meat, it's just that we don't eat meat specifically for the protein because we know we can get protein from plant foods if we eat enough calories.

When it comes to eating clean, it's important to remember plant foods are lowest on the food chain and therefore contain considerably fewer toxins than animal foods. Keep in mind that for every step you climb up the food chain ladder, there is a greater chance of accumulating and concentrating toxins found in the environment; toxic overload can tip the body's balance toward inflammation, illness, and accelerated aging. While it would be ideal to eat 100 percent organic food, if this is not possible, and it usually isn't, it is important to know you will still get far fewer toxins choosing *nonorganic plant* foods over even *certified organic animal* foods.

And let's not forget that animal foods are not just pure packages of protein. Although meat lovers have an affinity for championing the Meat Is Protein and Protein Is Meat notion, the reality is animal foods also contain saturated fat. While it is of course true that some animal foods contain more fat than others, all animal foods contain fat. It's not that fat per se is bad, but most animal food sources deliver a high percentage of saturated fat and animal food sources of saturated fat are not healthy. Even skinless chicken breasts, which are considered very low-fat animal foods, contain most of their few fat calories from undesirable saturated fat. If you are getting omega-3 fats from an animal food such as fish, then it is good fat, but the vast majority of the fat we get from animal foods is not from omega-3-rich fish, it's from four-legged animals that contain a large amount of saturated fat and very minimal amounts of omega-3 fat. And, as we discussed in Chapter 5, saturated fat from animal foods is pro-inflammatory and harmful to your health in many overlapping ways. Unrefined fat eaten as part of a whole plant food—even if it's plant-based saturated fat from coconuts—is considered clean healthy fat.

Not only do plant foods supply plenty of amino acids and protein, but they come packaged with all sorts of antiaging and health-promoting perks in the form of antioxidants, fiber, and phytonutrients that are not found in animal foods. Choosing to eat a variety of the following foods will supply your body with adequate protein containing all the essential amino acids.

NUTRIENT-DENSE, PROTEIN-RICH, CLEAN WHOLE PLANT FOODS
- Nuts and nut butters
- Seeds and seed butters, such as tahini
- Beans
- Legumes
- Lentils
- Tofu
- Edamame
- Tempeh

CONFUSED ABOUT SOY?

IN ANDY'S GENERAL surgical practice, one in which he sees a large number of patients with cancers of the breast, colon, and thyroid, conditions that have been rumored to be correlated with soy, he is frequently asked about whether soy is in fact healthful. Well here's the deal: soy in its *natural* whole traditional form, such as tofu, black soybeans, and edamame, and especially in its fermented form, such as tempeh, miso, nama shoyu, and natto are absolutely healthful foods but soy made to imitate other foods, such as soy cheese, soy chicken nuggets, tofurky (we still can't figure out why on earth anyone would eat such a food), commercial soy burgers, and other processed foods made with textured vegetable protein, hydrolyzed vegetable protein (usually made from soy), and soy protein isolates and concentrates are not healthful and are not whole foods. Soybean oil is also a terrible soy-derived food for all the reasons we discussed in Chapter 5.

We are well aware of the claims against soy such as how soy contains bad phytoestrogens that can lead to cancer (more on this in a bit) and that enzyme inhibitors in soy prevent proper digestion. But when you dig around into reputable research, you discover an overwhelming amount of scientific evidence supports the fact that whole traditional soy is absolutely safe and is a nutritious food when eaten in reasonable quantities. We don't suggest you start soy-spiking your diet by any stretch because doing so would shove other healthy foods right off your plate. So then, what is a reasonable quantity? One or two servings of soy a day—which is about ½ cup of edamame or black soybeans, 4 ounces of tofu or tempeh, or 1 cup of soy milk. To avoid the pesticides sprayed on conventional soy, we do suggest you buy organic soy products.

The real deal with soy consumption is that whole soy intake in moderate amounts is associated with longevity and good health. Opposite what the naysayers claim about the phytoestrogens in soy leading to hormone-sensitive cancers, studies show whole soy is actually associated with reduced risk of two of the most prevalent hormone sensitive cancers: breast and prostate cancer. In fact, a study showing the benefits of soy for breast cancer patients recently appeared in the *Journal of the American Medical Association*, one of the most prestigious medical journals in the world.* But you are kidding yourself if you think chomping down on a processed veggie burger made with isolated soy protein is going to give you the same health benefits of sipping miso soup. It's important to realize most of the nutritional power of soy is found in the phytonutrients that whole soy foods contain, and these substances are largely absent in processed soy foods like tofurky and soy dogs.

Here are seven reasons we have always recommended whole soy products, and we continue to recommend them:

- **Soybeans are a nutrient-rich whole food.** Soy is a vegetarian source of complete protein. The World Health Organization has established soy protein eaten alone, even if no other complementary foods are eaten, contains high enough concentrations of all the essential amino acids necessary to meet human requirements so long as soy protein is consumed at the recommended level of daily intake.† By recommended level of daily intake, we mean that you are indeed getting all of the protein your body needs, 0.5 gram per pound ideal body weight per day and are therefore not protein deficient. In addition to being protein-rich, soy is also a good source of essential fat and important micronutrients such as vitamin K, magnesium, and iron.
- **Whole soy is low in saturated fat.** Soy is a superb alternative to animal protein, providing your body with the complete protein you'd get from animal foods minus the negatives associated with eating too much saturated fat. If you have heart disease, or any inflammation-mediated condition such as multiple sclerosis, asthma, arthritis, or fibromyalgia, replacing saturated fat–rich animal protein with anti-inflammatory whole soy is especially beneficial.
- **Whole soy contains essential fat.** About 50 percent of the fat in soybeans is omega-6 fat, and 7 percent is omega-3 fat. The omega-6 essential fat found in whole soy foods (but not in processed soybean oil) is the healthful, unrefined, unheated type of omega-6 fat your body needs for optimal health. Eating whole soy regularly ensures you get both omega-3 and omega-6 essential fats.

- **Whole soy protects your heart.** Soy protects your entire cardiovascular system by altering your cholesterol profile for the better. In human studies, soy has been proven to lower bad LDL cholesterol levels, decrease overall cholesterol absorption, and increase cholesterol excretion. The American Heart Association states, "There is increasing evidence that the consumption of soy protein may help lower blood cholesterol levels in some people with elevated total cholesterol levels, and may provide other cardiovascular benefits."[‡] In the *New England Journal of Medicine,* one of the most respected medical journals, researchers report, "the consumption of soy protein rather than animal protein significantly decreased serum concentrations of total cholesterol, LDL cholesterol and triglycerides."[§] Replacing some of the animal protein foods you currently eat with whole soy is an effective way to reduce your overall saturated fat intake without decreasing your protein intake. The end result will be better cardiovascular health.
- **Whole soy is slimming.** Whole soy is a nutrient-dense food providing loads of satiety in a low-calorie package. Because it's slowly digested, it has minimal effect on blood sugar and insulin levels. Many soy foods, including soybeans and tempeh, are also exceptionally rich in tummy-filling fiber.
- **Whole soy contains health-preserving, health-enhancing phytonutrients.** Phytonutrients are substances found *only* in plant-based foods. Phytonutrients possess disease-preventing qualities. Many phytonutrients also have antioxidant and anti-inflammatory properties. Scientific evidence proves phytonutrients help prevent and treat at least four leading causes of premature death: cancer, diabetes, hypertension, and cardiovascular disease.[**]
- **Whole soy is one of the richest food sources of health-promoting phytoestrogens.** Phytoestrogens are natural plant compounds capable of exerting estrogen-like and anti-estrogenic actions in the body, which can be of benefit to women and men alike. Phytoestrogens partially inhibit the activity of excess bad human estrogens. Studies also suggest whole soy foods have a beneficial role in protecting against hormone-sensitive cancer, such as breast cancer, as well as

osteoporosis and menopausal symptoms.[††] The phytoestrogens in soy behave as natural estrogen-receptor modulators, also referred to as SERMs. Other SERMs you may be familiar with are tamoxifen, a powerful medicine used to treat breast cancer, and raloxifene, a drug that has been used to slow the effects of osteoporosis. The phytochemicals in soy possess many desirable SERM effects without causing side effects such as hot flashes, blood clots, and uterine cancer.

BOTTOM LINE: HOW MUCH SOY SHOULD YOU EAT EACH DAY?

As with all things, moderation is key. Yes, whole soy is healthful. No, you probably shouldn't eat soy for breakfast, lunch, and dinner. There are too many other healthful foods out there to eat! Studies show health benefits from eating just 11 grams of soy protein per day. We think that's about right. Try to eat one serving of whole soy several times a week.

---

* X. O. Shu, Y. Zheng, H. Cai, et al., "Soy Food Intake and Breast Cancer Survival," *Journal of the American Medical Association* 302, no. 22 (2009):2437–43.

† FAO/WHO/UNU Expert Consultation, *Energy and Protein Requirements,* WHO Technical Report Series 724 (Geneva, World Health Organization, 1985).

‡ J. W. Erdman Jr., "AHA Science Advisory: Soy Protein and Cardiovascular Disease: A Statement for Healthcare Professionals from the Nutrition Committee of the AHA," *Circulation* 102, no. 20 (2000): 2555–59.

§ J. W. Anderson, B. M. Johstone, and M. E. Cook-Newell, "Meta-Analysis of the Effects of Soy Protein Intake on Serum Lipids," *New England Journal of Medicine* 333, no. 5 (1995): 276–82.

** R. H. Liu, "Health Benefits of Fruit and Vegetables Are from Additive and Synergistic Combinations of Phytochemicals," *American Journal of Clinical Nutrition* 78, suppl. 3 (2003): 517S–20S.

†† X. O Shu, Y. Zheng, H. Cai, et al., "Soy Food Intake and Breast Cancer Survival."

Consider Pushing Protein to the Side of Your Plate

We realize pushing meat to the side of the dinner plate is a radical deviation from the way many people have grown up eating. And we totally understand that the thought of deemphasizing animal protein has sort of an undesirable new-age health movement ring to it, one that sounds like it means self-denial and deprivation. We get it. We also understand that a change in diet requires considerable creativity and a bit of behavior modification at first. But even with all of this in mind, we are going to ask you to rethink your standard dinner plate anyway. And in doing so, we promise to broaden your appreciation of food in general. Think of the less meat thing as a culinary journey—a journey that will awaken your senses to all the incredible other foods and flavors that you miss if you eat a meat-heavy diet. Just browse through our recipe collection in Part Four, and you'll see our less-meat recipes are anything but boring or blah.

And really, we just have to ask, is eating baked skinless, boneless chicken breasts as the main dinner entrée night after night truly exciting? By the way, it's not your imagination that we've been digging on skinless chicken breasts throughout this chapter; we've been doing so because we know many people think they are a great clean food. There is nothing inherently wrong with eating a bit of pastured chicken, but people eat too much of it. According to the USDA the average American eats 80 pounds of chicken each year. That's a lot of chicken, people! Is all that chicken really that tasty? Do you think you could get by eating a smidgen less? And maybe you could also eat a bit less than the 65 pounds of beef and 60 pounds of pork the average person consumes each year *on top of the 80 pounds of chicken*. You have to ask yourself, Is all this animal protein making us healthier as a nation? Leaner? Just some food for thought.

The rest of the world is actually way ahead of the United States in terms of incorporating smaller amounts of meat as a supporting cast member to the plate as a whole. A plate that is often bubbling over with flavor from spices, herbs, and vegetables we might add. But even here in the good old U.S.A., where visions of Texas ranches and steakhouse restaurants dance in our heads, there is a growing audience of people who declare themselves omnivores yet have begun to trim back on animal foods. This would include us. We consider ourselves to be "flexitarians," or part-time vegetarians. We still eat animal foods, but we really do limit our intake of them. We know to purists being part-vegetarian is like being half-alive, but after doing the research, we cannot find proof that being either vegetarian or vegan is the healthiest way to eat. Limits for the sake of limits is not our style.

161

Vegan the Best Way to Go? Not Necessarily.

The primary factor that makes some people believe a vegan or vegetarian diet is healthier than more conventional diets containing animal foods is that the vegan or vegetarian *supposedly* consumes first and foremost more nutrient-dense fruits and vegetables followed by unrefined whole foods in the form of beans, whole grains, and nuts and seeds. We emphasize *supposedly* because the reality is not all vegan or vegetarian diets are fruit- and veggie-forward and not all vegan and vegetarian diets are based on unrefined whole foods. Simply being vegan does not mean you are optimizing your health. In fact, the vegan or vegetarian who eats a diet based on nutrient-poor foods such as bagels, pretzels, processed breakfast cereals, French fries, and white rice will be far worse off than the nonvegan who eats most of his or her calories from fruits, vegetables, beans, nuts, whole grains, and seeds but also includes small amounts of animal foods too, such as eggs and lean cuts of beef and chicken. And we just can't find scientific evidence to support health reasons for anybody eliminating fish from their diets. Furthermore, even though studies do show that vegetarians have fewer heart attacks, less incidence of cancer, less obesity, lower weight, less high blood pressure, and longer life spans in general, if you dig deep into the research you'll see even those who are not super strict at avoiding animal foods enjoyed equally impressive health benefits across the board, as long as the bulk of their calories came from unrefined whole plant foods with plenty of fruits and vegetables.

The take-home message here is that science supports that you can reap the health and weight-loss benefits of a vegan diet without being 100 percent vegan. Even Colin Campbell, Ph.D.—one of the biggest champions of vegan diets in the medical community, co-author of the best-selling book *The China Study*, referred to as the "Grand Prix of epidemiology" by the *New York Times*—states in his book that it has not been proven that a zero animal food diet is best. We agree, it has not been proven. We would go further as to say we believe a slightly less than vegan diet, one that contains omega-3-rich seafood and is more like Clean Cuisine, is the most healthful. Our goal is not to set the bar for dietary purity so high that it guarantees failure; instead we want to help you learn to eat in a way that fits into your lifestyle, a way of eating that is doable, tasty, *and* healthful. Less than 0.5 percent of the population is vegan, meaning they eat no animal foods whatsoever; you don't need to go to these extremes to improve the way you age, look, and feel. Clean Cuisine is not about exclusivity or making people think they can't measure up to nutritional idealism. And to repeat, going to vegan extremes is not necessary or proven for optimizing health.

So then, how many animal foods do we actually eat? As a general rule we don't eat more than one animal food per day (with the exception of eggs); typically we are ovo-vegetarians until dinnertime. At least two thirds of the few animal foods we do eat are fish or shellfish. On a few days each week we eat a completely vegan diet, such as meat-free Mondays. When we do eat animal proteins, we choose the absolute cleanest sources.

NOTE: *We've included some of our family's favorite dinners for meat-free Mondays in Part Four.*

WHY WE EAT ANIMAL FOODS

AS STATED EARLIER, we don't eat animal foods so much for the protein they provide because we know we can get the protein we need from plant foods, assuming we eat enough calories and enough variety. Instead, we eat animal foods because animal foods contain certain nutrients that are difficult to get in adequate amounts from plant foods. Nutritional supplements are an option for strict vegans, but it is best to use supplements as just that, supplements. It is always far better to get the nutrients your body needs from whole foods. Some of the nutrients found in animal foods that are difficult to obtain in adequate quantity from plant foods are the following.

- **Vitamin B12.** Strict vegans absolutely must supplement their diets with B12 or choose vegan foods to which supplemental B12 has been intentionally added. There are no nonfortified vegan sources of vitamin B12.

NOTE: If you supplement with vitamin B12 look for methylcobalamin (the methylated form) because it requires no additional metabolic steps to be used by the body.

■ **Iron.** Good plant sources of iron include cooked dry beans, leafy green vegetables, hemp seeds, flaxseeds, and tofu. However, iron from plant foods is not absorbed nearly as well as the heme iron found only in animal foods. If you do not eat any animal foods at all you really need to pay extra special attention to eating iron-rich plant foods. We do not suggest iron supplements unless under a physician's supervision because iron supplements can be toxic and free-radical forming.

NOTE: Eating foods that contain vitamin C along with iron-rich foods will boost the body's absorption of iron from a meal.

■ **Docosahexaenoic acid (DHA).** Considered the most beneficial of all the omega-3 fats, DHA is for the most part found only in fatty fish and egg yolks. Even if you are not vegan and you eat fish and egg yolks we still think everyone should take an omega-3 fish oil supplement containing DHA. Strict vegans who do not eat fish or take fish oil should supplement with an algae-based DHA supplement.

NOTE: Algae-based DHA supplements contain less DHA than do fish oil supplements. See Chapter 9 for a more complete discussion of omega-3 supplements.

■ **Vitamin D.** Whether you eat animal foods or not, getting enough vitamin D should be a concern for everyone. If you are overweight you need more vitamin D than the average person because body fat traps this fat-soluble vitamin and makes it unavailable for your body to use. Unfortunately vitamin D is found in very few foods naturally so it's hard to get optimal amounts. Although cow's milk and dairy products are well known for being good sources of vitamin D, dairy foods contain synthetic vitamin D; natural vitamin D is found in fatty fish and eggs. Fatty fish is a far richer source: 6 ounces of salmon contains 900 International Units of vitamin D compared to 160 International Units found in 2 large eggs. In the plant kingdom, portobello mushrooms exposed to ultraviolet light contain approximately 400 International Units of vitamin D. But other than those few sources, vitamin D is not readily available from the food you eat. Although your body can make vitamin D from sunlight exposure, we feel eating a vitamin D–rich diet and taking vitamin D supplements are important for everyone (see Chapter 9 for specific recommendations). And, we should add, you should step outside without sunscreen on a regular basis too. A little sunlight and fresh air will always do a body good.

■ **Zinc.** One of zinc's major roles is to allow the body to use dietary protein as building blocks for the regeneration of muscle as well as support a healthy immune system. However, because zinc from plant foods is poorly absorbed, it is important for vegans to eat plenty of zinc-rich plant foods such as peanuts, soy foods, wheat germ, sesame seeds, and cocoa powder. Animal food sources of zinc include dark meat turkey, fish, eggs, oysters, crab, and red meat.

■ **Calcium.** Calcium sort of stands in its own category because, although it is certainly true calcium is found in dairy foods, dairy foods actually cause your body to release even more calcium than you take in. In fact, your body absorbs calcium from plant foods far more efficiently than from animal foods such as cow's milk. Did you know only about 30 percent of the calcium in milk is absorbed? Drinking milk for the calcium is a scenario tantamount to winning a new house but then being told the house is in Greenland. It's not worth it. Canned sardines and salmon, packed with small bones, are far superior animal food sources of absorbable calcium than is dairy. And while it is true a vegan diet based on vegan junk foods could potentially be too low in calcium, if you eat a plant-forward diet rich in a variety of whole foods, including dark leafy vegetables, beans, nuts, and seeds you will get plenty of calcium without ever taking another sip of milk again. Dairy-free, vegan sources that are particularly rich in calcium are sunflower seeds, green leafy vegetables, parsley, chickpeas, almonds, figs, prunes, sesame seeds, flaxseeds, broccoli, and tofu.

Clean Protein from Animal Foods

You would naturally assume organic animal foods would be the cleanest source of animal protein. And it is absolutely true that by choosing organic animal foods you are taking one giant step toward quality and one big leap toward eating healthier animals. Eating organic animals in comparison to conventionally raised animals will lessen your exposure to pesticide residues, synthetic hormones, antibiotics, and toxins in general. Yet, when it comes to buying the cleanest and highest-quality animal foods it's really essential to think about going *beyond* organic and consider the diet of the animal. This is because the animal's diet reflects the health of the animal, which ultimately affects the health of the person who eats it.

It's important to understand modern conventional farming is designed to grow and fatten animals at an unnaturally rapid rate; the animals eat a calorie-rich, grain-based diet rather than the nutrient-rich, grass-based diet they would naturally consume in the wild. Cows are ruminants, meaning their digestive systems are designed for eating grasses. Inappropriately feeding animals a deviant diet of dry grain is a direct contributor to those animals developing pathogens such as *E. coli* (in cattle) and salmonella (in poultry). Did you know that mad cow disease is unknown among cattle fed entirely on pasture and hay? When cows eat the foods nature intended the cows to eat, they are healthier. You simply can't separate the health of the animal you eat from your own health.

In addition, when factory-farmed cows eat grains, they aren't as healthy as they would otherwise be, and unhealthy cows get sick (and need antibiotics). So, even if ranchers feed cows organic grain, that doesn't mean grain per se is optimal for cow health. Ultimately, grain-fed beef is not desirable for you either. The same logic applies to sugar; if push comes to shove, we suppose it's better to eat organic sugar over conventional sugar, but eating organic-stamped sugar cubes will never be what the doctor ordered for optimal health.

Grain-fed animals and the milk from grain-fed animals are less nutritious than grass-fed, pastured animals. For example, compared with grass-fed meat, grain-fed meat has only one quarter as much vitamin E and one eighth as much beta-carotene. And because the composition of the fats present in eggs, chicken, meat, and dairy directly reflects the foods the animals consume, animals raised on conventional, commercial grain feeds (even *organic grain feed*) have less than desirable fat profiles.

Conventionally raised animals fed grain-based diets have far more pro-inflammatory omega-6 fat and much less anti-inflammatory omega-3 fat. The balance between these two types of fat is essential to our overall health. And as we discussed in Chapter 5, most people eating a modern-day diet already consume far too many omega-6 fats and far too few omega-3 fats. Too much omega-6 fat and not enough omega-3 fat can disrupt the body's immune system, exacerbate inflammatory conditions such as asthma and allergies, decrease the body's sensitivity to insulin and increase the risk of type 2 diabetes, and even contribute to obesity and heart disease. Eating conventionally raised animals containing high amounts of omega-6 fat is one of the major contributing factors as to why our omega fat ratio is so out of whack. The fat in grass-fed animals is much closer to a healthy balance.

Keep in mind, it really doesn't matter whether the animal is fed ordinary grain, genetically modified grain, or organic grain. Feeding large amounts of *any* type of grain to a grazing animal will negatively affect the quality of the animal's meat and milk. So, while organic meat may be free of unwanted toxins, it is still nutritionally inferior to grass-fed meat. Pastured chickens that are raised on fresh pasture and are free to roam and forage for a naturally healthful chicken diet of insects, worms, grass, and wild plants are also nutritionally superior to caged chickens fed an unnatural diet of grains alone. A chicken allowed to consume a natural chicken diet has a more balanced ratio of omega-6 fat to omega-3 fat, and the chickens themselves are leaner because they get to exercise. The eggs from pastured chickens are also more healthful.

The bottom line when it comes to animal foods is to realize there is more to choosing a healthful animal food than simply picking organic. And do keep in mind that the two diets most associated with longevity and reduced cardiac morbidity are the traditional Japanese diet and the Mediterranean diet, both of which are noted for incorporating only small amounts of animal foods (including fish) and for having a balanced omega-3 to omega-6 fat ratio (plus plenty of vegetables and minimal amounts of refined foods). Our general advice when it comes to animal foods can be summed up as follows:

- Always look at the animal's diet; choose only animals that were fed the diet nature intended the animal to eat.
- Choose organic whenever possible.

- Find a dairy-free substitute for milk; there is no nutritional reason to drink milk, and there are plenty of tasty milk substitutes. We prefer hemp milk and hemp cream and cashew milk and cashew cream, for example.

- Eat cheese as a special treat and in very small quantities; cheese isn't healthful, but we have found it absolutely impossible to find a cheese substitute that actually tastes good.
- Recognize that fatty fish will give you the most nutritional bang for your animal food buck owing to its omega-3 fats (EPA and DHA), and nutrients (vitamins B12 and D, iron, and zinc).
- Eat animal foods in moderation; consider being an ovo-vegetarian until dinnertime and then eating animal foods only as a modest part of your dinner, not the main attraction.

THE MOST HEALTHFUL ANIMAL FOOD TO EAT HANDS DOWN
- Fish, the fattier the better!

ANIMAL FOOD PROTEIN SOURCES TO EAT IN MODERATION
- Pastured eggs
- Shellfish like shrimp and scallops
- Pastured lamb
- Pastured beef
- Pastured chicken
- Pastured duck

ANIMAL FOOD PROTEIN SOURCES TO EAT VERY SPARINGLY, IF AT ALL
- Organic, pastured cheese (preferably raw)
- Organic, pastured kefir

Free-Range Chickens and Eggs? Let's Chat about Them.

More than 90 percent of U.S. eggs come from caged hens. These birds have a space smaller than the size of a sheet of paper to move around in and they live in filthy conditions. Not only are caged hens dirty, they (and their eggs) aren't as nutritious as the hens raised on pasture. Pastured hens are raised outside on land where they can do what hens *naturally* are supposed to do: roam free and forage around for bugs and grasses. A study from Pennsylvania State University published in *Renewable Agriculture and Food Systems* found that pastured hens boasted higher vitamin and omega-3 fat levels when compared to their commercially fed, battery-cage-kept counterparts.[4] Eggs from pastured hens contained twice as much vitamin E and almost three times more total omega-3 fats as the eggs from caged birds.

In an ideal world you would purchase your eggs and chicken from a local farmer in your area where you could *see* the chickens roaming on pasture and you could *see* plenty of open space per bird. Or you could just raise your own chickens as some are doing. Okay, all right, so the idea of raising your own chickens might be a little out there. So then, your second best bet is to buy your chicken and eggs from a natural foods store or other market where they are clearly labeled *pastured*. Pastured eggs and chickens should be housed on grassland in portable shelters that are periodically moved to give the chickens fresh pasture. It is sad that there is no third-party inspection required to ensure that's what's really happening. By the way, the label *free range* or *free roaming* is not as good as *pastured* because the free-ranging chickens aren't guaranteed any specific amount of time outdoors or even exposure to sunlight, for that matter. Again, there is no third-party inspection.

USDA organic chickens (and their eggs) do have third-party inspection, and these animals were not kept enclosed in battery cages. Organic chickens are *offered* access to the outdoors, but that doesn't mean they actually ever go outside. They are, however, fed certified organic feed and they are free of antibiotics. But just being organic is still not as good as pastured.

Clearly we do not live in an ideal world when it comes to selecting clean eggs and chicken. The bottom line is your best bet is to try to get as close to the source as possible and try to find out *exactly* where your chicken and eggs come from and what they eat. That's what we do.

NOTE: As far as we are aware, Vital Farms is the only company that sells pastured eggs that are nationally distributed.

EGG WHITE OMELETS ARE *NOT* ALL THEY HAVE BEEN CRACKED UP TO BE

WE'VE NOW SAID it a bunch of times, but it's worth restating: We don't eat animal foods so much for their protein; instead, we eat animal foods, in moderation, because they come packaged with other nutrients that are not as readily available in plant foods and they add variety and flavor to our diet. When it comes to eggs, throwing out the yolk is equivalent to throwing the baby out with the bathwater. Yes, eggs have cholesterol, but if you read the facts on cholesterol (see page 111), you'll see why we are not overly concerned with the cholesterol content of our food and especially not concerned about the cholesterol in eggs. It's also worth taking into consideration the results of a study on real people and egg consumption. We're not just talking a study with 10 or 12 people but rather a study involving 188,000 people that showed those who ate five or six whole eggs a week actually had less heart disease than those who ate less than one egg per week.* The study was published in the prestigious *Journal of the American Medical Association* in 1999. In the well-known Framingham Study, researchers analyzed 912 subjects over a number of years and found there was no significant relationship between egg consumption, blood cholesterol levels, and coronary heart disease.†

The thing is, eggs, yolk and all, are a very nutrient-dense food that happen to also be low in saturated fat. One whole large egg is only 70 calories with just 1.5 grams of saturated fat, neither of which is high at all. And for those 70 calories you get a lot of bang for your paltry calorie buck. Much more bang we might add than if you ate 70 calories from just egg whites or 70 calories from the mother chicken. In fact, we would far prefer you eat one whole egg with the yolk rather than the calorie equivalent of chicken or egg whites because the whole egg has way more to offer nutritionally. That's one of the reasons eggs are the exception to our "one animal food per day" rule. Compared to egg whites and chicken itself, whole eggs steal the nutritional show. Here are just a select few of the egg-ceptionally important nutrients you get in a whole egg with the yolk. (Yes, the *egg-ceptionally* part was a little corny!)

■ **Vitamin D.** Vitamin D is an important anti-inflammatory nutrient that has recently been associated with decreased risk of cancer and heart disease. Additional research suggests vitamin D provides protection from hypertension, psoriasis, and several autoimmune diseases such as multiple sclerosis and rheumatoid arthritis. Vitamin D also boosts your body's natural healing response. This super vitamin even acts like an antioxidant, both internally and externally. In fact, getting enough vitamin D is essential for healthy, younger-looking, and smoother skin. Some preliminary research even links vitamin D deficiency to weight gain. It is important to remember that vitamin D is not readily available *naturally* in very many foods other than eggs and fatty fish.

> *NOTE:* Dairy foods are fortified with vitamin D, but vitamin D is not found naturally in dairy.

■ **Omega-3 fats.** The *pastured* eggs we recommend are a good source of anti-inflammatory and immune-supporting omega-3 fats. These fats are particularly important for heart health, protection against cancer, reduced inflammation, improved sensitivity to insulin, and smooth, supple skin.

■ **Lutein.** Lutein is an incredible antioxidant especially for eye health and the prevention of age-related eye diseases such as macular degeneration. Lutein is a gold-star member of the carotenoid family. While lutein is found in dark leafy greens such as spinach and collards, a human study published in the August 2004 issue of the *Journal of Nutrition* shows that lutein is much better absorbed from egg yolks than from lutein supplements or even spinach.‡ This is probably because carotenoids are always better absorbed with fat, and lutein is a carotenoid. So even though there is slightly less lutein in eggs than in fat-free spinach, the lutein from the eggs is absorbed by your body better. In addition, the whole egg comes packaged with another antioxidant, zeaxanthin, which works synergistically to boost the bioavailability of lutein.

■ **Choline.** Eggs are one of nature's richest sources of choline, an essential micronutrient that supports cardiovascular health and brain function in addition to reducing inflammation. In fact, people whose diets supplied the highest average intake of choline have levels of inflammatory markers such as C-reactive protein and interleukin 6 at least 20 percent lower than those with low to average choline intake.[§] Choline also helps transport fat and cholesterol to your cells, thereby preventing their accumulation in your liver. Furthermore, choline converts to trimethylglycine, which helps reduce your homocysteine level, thus lowering your risk of stroke, heart disease, cancer, Parkinson's disease, Alzheimer's disease, and many degenerative diseases.

> *NOTE:* Soybeans, wheat germ, and salmon are also good sources of choline.

- **Lecithin.** Lecithin actually helps the body digest fat and cholesterol.
- **Vitamin A.** Fat-soluble vitamin A is well known for the role it plays in vision, but it is also essential for healthy skin and immune function, fertility, and cancer prevention. Less well known is the importance vitamin A plays in keeping bones and teeth strong. It is important to know that vitamin A works in synergy with vitamins D and K2.
- **Vitamin K2.** Pastured eggs are among the very few readily available sources of the vitally important vitamin K2. Although vitamin K2 doesn't get a lot of media buzz, it plays a critical role in bone health and heart health. Vitamin K2 funnels calcium into bones and teeth where it is needed and away from arteries where it can cause dangerous arterial calcification. In addition, it has important antioxidant-like actions and contributes to the production of myelin, the protective coating that surrounds brain cells and nerves.[**]

> *NOTE:* Vitamin K2 is different from the vitamin K1 you get from dark leafy greens.

We aren't suggesting you start going overboard eating eggs for breakfast, lunch, and dinner. Eat them in moderation (four to five a week is totally fine). When you do eat eggs, please eat the whole shebang. No more egg white omelets. *Please.*

* F. B. Hu, "A Prospective Study of Egg Consumption and Risk of Cardiovascular Disease in Men and Women," *Journal of the American Medical Association* 281, no. 15 (1999): 1387–94.

† T. R. Dawber, R. J. Nickerson, F. N. Brand, and J. Pool, "Eggs, Serum Cholesterol, and Coronary Heart Disease," *American Journal of Clinical Nutrition* 36, no. 4 (1982): 617–25.

‡ H. Y. Chung, M. Rasmussen, E.J. Johnson, "Lutein Bioavailability is Higher from Lutein-enriched Eggs than from Supplements and Spinach in Men." *Journal of Nutrition* 164, no. 8 (2004): 1887–93.

§ P. Detopoulou, D. B. Panagiotakos, S. Antonopoulou, et al., "Dietary Choline and Betaine Intakes in Relation to Concentrations of Inflammatory Markers in Healthy Adults: The ATTICA Study," *American Journal of Clinical Nutrition* 82, no. 2 (2008): 424–30.

** H. H. Thijssen and M. J. Drittij-Reijnders, "Vitamin K Status in Human Tissues: Tissue-Specific Accumulation of Phylloquinone and Menaquinone-4," *British Journal of Nutrition* 75, no. 1 (1996): 121–27.

Fresh Catch of the Day?

The romance associated with Moby Dick and a fisherman's life, a life on the sea filled with excitement and peril, has, for the most part, been replaced with fish farms. As wild fisheries are overexploited, fish farmers have stepped up to the plate to help meet the worldwide demand for finned culinary staples. The reality is there just aren't enough fish in the sea to keep up with demand, so today about half the seafood consumed around the world comes from fish farms.

Farmed seafood can be inferior to wild fish in taste, and in many cases the nutritional value of the fish is also compromised. For example, nature did not intend salmon to be crammed into pens and fed soy, poultry litter, and hydrolyzed chicken feathers. As a result of a deviant diet, farmed salmon is lower in vitamin D, lower in anti-inflammatory omega-3 fats, higher in proinflammatory omega-6 fats (specifically, farmed salmon is particularly rich in proinflammatory arachidonic acid we discussed in Chapter 5), higher in saturated fat, and higher in overall contaminants (such as PCBs, carcinogens, and pesticides like dioxin and DDT). We also find it disturbing that farmed salmon would be gray in color if it weren't for pink chemical dye. We feel it is absolutely worth the extra price to pay for wild salmon. If you want a budget-friendly option go for sockeye (red) salmon that is often sold in cans; sockeye salmon is the variety that cannot be farmed. Sockeye salmon is not only inexpensive but it's delicious in casseroles and makes a fabulous salmon burger (see Ivy's favorite recipe on page 365) while remaining high in omega-3 fats.

Another unsettling fishy fact is that only 5 percent of the farmed sea-food eaten in the United States comes from domestic fish farms, and only 2 percent of the imported fish consumed in the United States is inspected in this country. Not only does importing seafood leave a big carbon foot-print, but overseas fish farming is not exactly clean. Most of the seafood we import is sourced from locations where health, safety, and environ-mental standards for raising and catching fish are weak or nonexistent. Many fish farmers pack their ponds too tight, leading to disease and pol-lution from fish waste. And just like cattle are given antibiotics and other drugs, fish in farms are given the same things. Then there's the concern about what the fish are eating. Just like with cows, if fish don't eat the foods they would naturally consume in the wild, then the fish are not going to be healthy; this suboptimal health of the fish will directly impact the health of the fish eater, you. Many fish farms are no doubt a muddled mess of murky water.

When we visited the Monterey Bay Aquarium on our 2011 California family road trip, we learned that their Seafood Watch program mostly discourages consumers from choosing farmed fish, both for health reasons and because of concerns over the environmental impact of fish farming. However, we haven't totally ruled out eating farmed fish because when it is done properly it can be safe. We buy our farmed fish from Whole Foods Market and from a local fish market because we know they set the bar high for quality standards. If you buy farmed fish, you want to buy it from a reputable place. Ask the fishmonger what the fish eats and where it swims.

The big picture of course is that fish (and fish oil supplements) are the most readily available, most ample source of the long-chain omega-3 EPA and DHA fats we all desperately need. The omega-3 fats are a nutrient most people in first world nations are deficient in. And the research showing fish eaters are healthier than nonfish eaters is solid. The American Heart Asso-ciation recommends we eat fatty fish such as salmon and trout at least twice a week. These recommendations are made because a number of studies published in some of the very best medical journals have repeatedly proven that eating fish can prevent, reverse, and even cure cardiovascular condi-tions including atherosclerosis, cardiac arrhythmias, stroke peripheral vascular disease, high blood pressure, and even sudden cardiac death.[5]

No other dietary therapy is more effective at lowering triglycerides than a diet containing EPA- and DHA-rich seafood, which has been shown to reduce triglycerides by up to 65 percent. Of course you can't eat fish sticks fried in recycled oil and expect to improve your health, but research has shown that when fish is prepared healthfully there is a 50 percent decrease in death due to heart disease among persons who eat fish three or more times per week.[6] People who consume fish on a regular basis have also been reported to have low risks of cancers of the pancreas, colon, thyroid, and prostate. It's also interesting to note that three populations who consume fish at least three times per week, the Okinawans, Japanese, and Inuit, have very low incidence of breast cancer. Fish consumption is even associated with enhanced weight loss when dieting.[7] Furthermore, recent studies suggest eating fish will make you feel happier too; studies on omega-3 fat consumption have linked low fish intake to an increased incidence of psychological problems, including depression, bipolar disorder, postpartum blues, and suicidal tendencies.[8]

Taking all this into consideration and weighing the pluses with the minuses, we are left with the question of what fish to eat. It's easy to feel lost in a sea of confusion when trying to figure out the cleanest fish to buy, but there are some simple guidelines you can follow to choose the best fish. You should also know that the toxin content of many fish depends on size: Bigger fish have more toxins, so it's better to eat smaller fish. Sardines and anchovies are particularly good choices because these small fish are not only low in toxins but also super rich in omega-3 fat. Here are the guidelines we follow for choosing the best fish for our family:

- Go for small fish.
- Choose local over imported.
- Choose wild fish when possible.
- Choose wild Alaskan salmon or sockeye salmon over farmed.
- If you do choose farmed fish find out how it is farmed and find out where the fish were raised and what they ate.
- If you are lucky enough to live near the coast, go native and buy locally caught wild fish.
- Look for the blue Marine Stewardship Council (MSC) ecolabel. To get the highest quality fish of any variety, you want to look for sustainable fish that have met the independent environmental standards of the MSC, the world's leading certification and eco-labeling program for sustainable seafood.
- Avoid fish labeled *fresh from frozen*, which means it has been

previously frozen; these fish may look fresh but their taste and texture will have been compromised. Sometimes these fish sit for days before selling. Not a fresh catch.

- For the best tasting fish, look for fresh fish and buy it from a reputable source. Frozen fish is also a good option. Keep in mind, because the journey from sea to market may take a week or longer, frozen fish can actually end up tasting fresher than fresh fish. This is because thanks to modern freezing techniques, many fish are now frozen on the boat, just minutes after being caught, with flash-freezing units that maintain a temperature far below the typical home freezer. (But see our fresh from frozen warning in the previous bulleted item).

- Avoid fish that has been given antibiotics and added growth hormones.

- Avoid fish that has been given poultry or mammalian by-products in its feed.

- Avoid fish containing preservatives such as sodium bisulfite, sodium tripolyphosphate (STP), and sodium metabisulfite. Seems logical enough.

- Prepare your fish healthfully! If you drown your fish in béarnaise sauce or fry it in vegetable oil, you might as well eat a doughnut.

- Get to know your fishmonger! Ask questions. Where does the fish swim? What does the fish eat?

- Go for quality over quantity. You don't need to eat massive amounts of fish so you can afford to spend more for better quality. Three to five modest total servings, perhaps about 4 ounces each, per week provides essentially *all* of the health benefits.

A SUSTAINABLE CATCH!

OYSTERS, MUSSELS, AND SCALLOPS may be the filters of the sea, but these bottom-dwelling bivalves are some of the most sustainable seafood choices on the market. They are low on the food chain and very low in mercury. Definitely a good animal source of protein.

What about the Mercury in Seafood?

We've addressed this issue in our previous books but will briefly touch on it here. While it is true people who eat fish have higher levels of mercury than people who do not eat fish, multiple studies performed on *real people* (not animals) in real life have proven beyond a doubt that fish eaters live longer and suffer fewer heart attacks than people who do not eat fish.[9] Furthermore, the largest scientific study performed to date has specifically shown there to be no harmful relationship between either prenatal or postnatal mercury exposure and developmental outcomes in either 5-year-olds or 9-year-olds. In these studies, childbearing women ate an average of twelve servings of fish *weekly*, far more than what we recommend per week and far more than most people would ever choose to eat.[10]

Does Milk Do a Body Good? And Do You Really *Need* All That Calcium?

Dear Dairy Council,

I wanted to show my heartfelt appreciation for your billion-dollar industry doing all you do to help educate the public on the virtues of milk, yogurt, and cheese. With millions of Americans suffering from asthma, allergies, obesity, type 2 diabetes, osteoporosis, heart disease, cancer, and so many other devastating conditions, it is so crucial you do your part to educate us on nutrition and to continue to get your 3-Every-Day of dairy message out. Especially because we all know that milk does a body good, an idea I learned primarily from you! The millions of dollars you allocate each year for the purposes of marketing dairy are doing such a wonderful job convincing us we really do need more milk.

I also wanted to congratulate you on creating some of the most iconic images in the history of advertising, including the 1950s era Drinka Pinta Milka Day campaign and of course the celebrity-driven Got Milk? mustaches we see splashed all over magazines today. I appreciate all that you do to help educate us on how to stay healthy and of course how to maintain strong bones and teeth, mostly by drinking milk! I know you have a tough job to do and that you work hard providing nutritional expertise to the industry, proactively pro-moting the nutritional benefits of dairy, and protecting dairy from inaccurate and unfair publicity. This is so thoughtful of you!

However, because we have some readers on our Clean Cuisine website who are suspicious of the good work you do I was hoping you might help answer just a few of their questions. I pulled together 10 of the most frequent questions we get on our site. Can you please help answer the following:

1. *Even though dairy contains a lot of calcium, is it true that the animal protein in milk and cheese pulls calcium from our bones?*
2. *Does drinking milk prevent osteoporosis?*
3. *Are there any good nondairy, plant sources of calcium?*
4. *Does milk naturally contain vitamin D?*
5. *Is it true that 75 to 80 percent of the world's adults are lactose intolerant?*
6. *Is it true that dairy is the most common food allergy?*
7. *Has milk consumption been linked to autoimmune diseases and cancer?*
8. *Is it true that one glass of milk can contain 180 million white blood cells (pus cells) and still be considered safe to drink?*
9. *Is it true that many nonorganic dairy cows are given a hormone called bovine somatotropin (BST), also known as rBGH, to increase milk production?*
10. *Is it true that the vast majority of dairy cows, including organically raised dairy cows, are fed a deviant diet of grain and are not free to pasture and graze the way nature intended?*

I so look forward to hearing back from you so I can share your answers with our readers. I cannot thank you enough for your time.

Warmly,
Ivy Larson

This was a real letter Ivy sent to the National Dairy Council. Nobody responded so we decided to dig a little deeper into some of these questions. We had to do a bit of research because to be honest, we had never really researched milk much until we started getting questioned about it. We never believed milk was a superfood, but we also didn't think it was all that bad either as long as it was low fat or skim, of course. But, after digging around a bit here's what we found out.

1. **Even though dairy contains a lot of calcium, is it true that the animal protein in milk and cheese pulls calcium from our bones?** Dairy foods are complex mixtures; they have some components that promote calcium retention, such as magnesium, vitamin D, and potassium, but they have other components, primarily animal protein, that promote calcium excretion through the urine.[11] Epidemiological studies actually link osteoporosis *not to low calcium intake* but to other nutritional factors, primarily a diet high in animal protein, which cause excess calcium loss. It is interesting that, although plant foods do contain protein, plant protein is not associated with increased calcium excretion.[12]

2. **Does drinking milk prevent osteoporosis?** No. In fact, studies show the exact opposite. People who live in parts of the world where cow's milk is not a staple of the diet are less likely to develop osteoporosis than in places such as the United States, where dairy is a dietary staple. Countries that have the highest consumption of dairy happen to have the highest incidence of hip fractures. A major finding from the Nurses' Health Study, a prospective study of 121,701 women ages 30 to 55, was that milk consumption *does not* protect against hip or forearm fractures.[13]

3. **Are there any good nondairy, plant sources of calcium?** Yes! One cup of cow's milk provides 291 milligrams of calcium, but remember, not all of that calcium is actually absorbed or used by your body because milk comes packaged with animal protein. There are so many other nutrient-dense plant foods containing comparable amounts of absorbable forms of calcium. Dark leafy greens are one of the most outstanding sources of calcium because they result in far greater net calcium retention than you'd get from dairy, and they come jam-packed with all sorts of nutritional perks in the form of fiber, phytonutrients, antioxidants, and vitamins for a fraction of the calories found in dairy! Dark leafy greens are also one of the very best sources of vitamin K, a vitamin that does not get nearly the attention it

deserves for its vital role in improving bone health. In fact, in the Nurses' Health Study, women who got more than 109 micrograms of vitamin K a day were 30 percent less likely to break a hip than women who got less than that amount.[14] But back to the calcium: Although 1 cup of milk contains 291 milligrams of calcium, did you know 1 cup of cooked collards has 358 milligrams of calcium? Or that 1 cup of cooked spinach has 244 milligrams of calcium? One cup of cooked kale has 94 milligrams, 1 cup of cooked mustard greens has 150 milligrams, and 1 cup cooked Swiss chard has 102 milligrams. The point is, milk is not the only source of calcium. On the Clean Cuisine program you should be eating one huge serving of greens every day anyway, so you will automatically be getting plenty of *absorbable calcium* from eating dark leafy greens. Other foods such as beans, tofu, sesame seeds, almonds, bok choy, broccoli, and even raisins and figs contain calcium. Regardless of the message the National Dairy Council has tried to convey, you do not need to drink even one sip of milk to get the calcium your body needs.

4. **Does milk naturally contain vitamin D?** No, the vitamin D added to milk is not naturally occurring like the vitamin D you get from fatty fish, egg yolks, or mushrooms exposed to ultraviolet light, and it's not nearly as much as your body can manufacture readily from sunlight. This is an important distinction because it is always best to get nutrients naturally from food (or, in the case of vitamin D, from the sun) rather than from supplements. The vitamin D you get from milk can easily be replaced by a vitamin D supplement and a little bit of sun exposure. And you can eat some fish, egg yolks, and mushrooms too.

5. **Is it true that 75 to 80 percent of the world's adults are lactose intolerant?** Yes. Lactose is a sugar consisting of glucose attached to galactose; when you are a baby you have an enzyme called lactase that can break lactose apart but, after the age of weaning the vast majority of people in the world lose that enzyme and are therefore lactose intolerant.

6. **Is it true that dairy is the most common food allergy?** Yes! In fact, cow's milk protein, not nuts, is the leading food allergy in children.[15] Cow's milk consumption has been linked to environmental allergies in general too.[16]

7. **Has milk consumption been linked to autoimmune diseases and cancer?** Yes. A number of studies point to the idea that the proteins in milk can cause the body to have an immune reaction and make antibodies to the milk protein. The link between type 1 diabetes is well documented in respected medical journals such as the *New England Journal of Medicine*.[17] In the medical literature, when autoimmune diseases are studied in relation to nutrition, the consumption of animal foods, especially cow's milk, is associated with increased risk. Milk consumption is also linked with various cancers. For example, nine separate studies have linked prostate cancer with high consumption of milk, including a 2010 study in the journal *Prostate*, showing more than a doubling of risk.[18] Cow's milk consumption has also been linked to multiple sclerosis.[19]

8. **Is it true that one glass of milk can contain 180 million white blood cells (pus cells) and still be considered safe to drink?** This is downright gross, but true. White blood cells (pus cells) are found naturally in dairy because they are important for the immune system development of the baby cows that are supposed to drink the milk. Humans aren't really supposed to drink cow's milk, and the white blood cells don't do anything to support human health or the human immune system.

9. **Is it true that many nonorganic dairy cows are given a hormone called bovine somatotropin (BST), also known as rBGH, to increase milk production?** Yes, and this hormone makes the cows sick and contributes to infections such as mastitis. The sick cows are then given antibiotics, which are then passed through into the milk.

10. **Is it true that the vast majority of dairy cows, including organically raised dairy cows, are fed a deviant diet of grain and are not free to pasture and graze the way nature intended?** Yes, and the health of the cow and the nutrients in her milk are directly affected by the foods she eats. Cows that don't eat the foods nature intended produce poor-quality milk, even if they are organic cows.

Our conclusion is that although there are nutrients found in milk that your body does need, such as calcium, vitamin D, magnesium, vitamin A, vitamin B12, potassium, and protein, milk is not exactly the cleanest source for these nutrients, and you definitely don't need to drink milk to get them! There are far better sources of *all of these nutrients* than dairy. Dairy foods are not a nutritional requirement. And if you are concerned about preventing osteoporosis, maintaining a healthy weight, and boosting your intake of bone-building nutrients such as vitamin K and calcium, one of the most important things you should do is swap the slogan Got Milk? for Got Greens? Instead of making an effort to consume three servings of dairy a day, try getting just one or two large servings of dark leafy greens each day. You will do your body, and your bones, a big favor!

WHY WE STILL EAT (A LITTLE) *REAL* CHEESE

WE EAT REAL cheese—very small amounts of it—only because, let's face it, cheese tastes good. We do not eat cheese because we think cheese is a nutrient-dense food choice. Because we know it is *not*. Instead, we look at cheese as a delicacy that should be consumed in extreme moderation. We think that if you eat healthfully 95 percent of the time then eating a little bit of splurge foods such as cheese is not going to be the end of the world. Now, if you can totally live without cheese more power to you! We haven't been able to give up real cheese completely just yet.

Dairy-Free Milk and Cream Substitutes That Actually Taste Good!

Once you become convinced that cow's milk is not the superfood the National Dairy Council would like you to believe, and once you decide to give it up, you are left with the issue of what to substitute it with. Soy milk and almond milk are not exactly the tastiest substitutes for dairy primarily because commercial soy milk can often have a distinctly nondairy funky taste that can be hard to get used to and commercial almond milk is simply too watered down to give you the creamy satisfaction you get from dairy. We've found the best-tasting substitutes for cow's milk are as follows:

- For cream we use homemade cashew cream (recipe on page 144) or hemp cream (recipe on page 306), both of which take less than 5 minutes to make. Cashew cream is particularly good in soups and cream-based recipes such as those you'll find in Part Four.

■ For convenience, for adding to cereal, or for baking, we use commercially bought hemp milk. Hemp milk has a favorable omega-3 fat to omega-6 fat profile and also has more fat and therefore a creamier texture than soy milk or almond milk. You can buy hemp milk at the supermarket in the nonrefrigerated section near the boxed soy milks, but you can make it at home (see page 130).

■ For smoothies we use nut milks made from raw nuts like macadamia nuts, almonds, and pecans. These are blended with water in our high-speed blender. Check out some of our smoothie recipes in Part Four. You can also try the following 1-minute recipe:

1-minute nut milk

Note: This recipe works best with "creamy" nuts such as macadamia nuts, pecans, and walnuts.

1 cup raw nuts (ideally, soaked for 1 hour or more)
3 cups water
2 or 3 pitted dates
1 teaspoon pure vanilla extract
Pinch of unrefined sea salt

Place all ingredients in a high-speed blender (such as a Vitamix) and blend until smooth and creamy. Store nut milk in a covered container in the fridge for 2 days. Shake well before using.

DR-COW TREE NUT CHEESES

IN ADDITION TO eating small amounts of real dairy cheese, we also indulge (guilt-free we might add) in Dr-Cow tree nut cheeses. Dr-Cow nut cheeses are made from—you guessed it—nuts! A 100 percent organic, living raw, vegan, and gourmet alternative to dairy cheese, Dr-Cow produces a wide variety of artisan fresh and aged nut cheeses that truly can hold their own against the very best gourmet dairy cheese. (Aged macadamia nut cheese is among our favorites.) Dr-Cow cheeses are made with absolutely no preservatives, stabilizers, artificial ingredients, or additives of any kind. They are a true treat indeed.

We hope this chapter has helped put protein in perspective. If you follow our nutrient-dense whole foods diet emphasizing plenty of fruits and vegetables along with whole grains, beans, nuts, and seeds plus some fish you will get all the protein you need (and all the other nutrients too!) to sustain your body day to day without overloading it. It is your choice whether you choose to eat protein-rich animal foods other than fish such as beef, chicken, and eggs. We consider ourselves fishy flexitarians because we eat mostly a vegan diet but we do eat fish and a bit of high-quality pastured beef, chicken, and eggs too. Sounds fishy, we know, but it works for us. We don't feel deprived. And we certainly aren't malnourished!

CLEAN CUISINE AND WINE
A Perfect Pairing?

Wine makes daily living easier, less hurried, with fewer tensions and more tolerance.

—BENJAMIN FRANKLIN

It is no surprise why many people the world over love the taste of wine. The two natural substances known to convey the flavor of food most effectively are fat and alcohol. We all know a salad with a drizzle of oil will taste immensely better than dry lettuce leaves. Anyone who cooks regularly, or enjoys eating, can tell you a little bit of fat goes *a very long way* to enhance the flavor of pretty much any food. Wine has the same effect. Wine enthusiasts will tell you wine with dinner simply makes the food taste better.

But beyond the taste-enhancing benefits of wine and beyond the obvious temporary relaxation benefits a glass of wine provides, does wine really have any intrinsic health-promoting properties? This is a question we get asked frequently by our Clean Cuisine readers. And we received a flurry of questions asking whether we drink wine regularly or just on special occasions after we posted photos on the Clean Cuisine Facebook page of us in Napa Valley sipping wine on our vacation. The truth is we do drink wine regularly and not just on vacation or special occasions. We drink wine in *moderation,* but we do drink it regularly.

Is Wine Healthful?

We don't make recommendations to avoid certain foods or beverages unless there is clear-cut scientific research to validate those recommendations. And there is absolutely *no* scientific rationale to support avoiding wine for the *average* person. Unless you have a specific reason to stay away from alcohol, such as medication conflicts, liver disease, or a history of alcohol abuse, we believe the scientific literature strongly supports that moderate consumption of wine is, in fact, healthful for most people. **Moderate consumption means one or two glasses daily if you are a man and one glass a day if you are a woman.** Also, most of the studies show that it's the first one or two drinks *per week* that are the most beneficial for heart health. A close look at the medical literature makes it is hard to ignore the fact that the occasional glass of wine is very likely to provide health benefits for many, many people, especially as you age.

One of the earliest scientific studies on the subject of wine and health was published in the *Journal of the American Medical Association* in 1904.[1] Since then, a flood of research has shown moderate drinkers tend to have better health and live longer than those who are either abstainers or heavy drinkers.[2] Researchers at Harvard studied more than 80,000 men aged 40 to 84 for nearly 11 years and found the risk of dying was 23 percent less for those who had two to four drinks per week and 22 percent less for those who had five or six drinks a week.[3] It is important to note the benefits of alcohol do *not* increase with more drinks. The take-home message here is *not* that more wine is better. It is a fact that excessive consumption of alcohol poses serious health risks. The only acceptable way to consume alcohol in any form is in *moderation*.

WINE IS THE HEALTHIEST ALCOHOLIC BEVERAGE

WHILE WE DO say a nice glass of wine can be the perfect pairing to a Clean Cuisine dinner, unfortunately we just can't say the same about a shot of vodka or a bottle of beer. This is because in comparison to hard liquor and beer, wine contains more antioxidants and is very low in sugar. Hard liquor is also low in sugar as long as you don't add sugary mixers, but hard liquor is also devoid of antioxidants; beer contains antioxidants yet most varieties also contain a good deal of empty-calorie sugars and starches. As for whether to drink red or white, the research is not clear-cut just yet. Both red and white wine contain antioxidants, but because red wine is fermented with the grape skins and rich in resveratrol it is believed to be the better choice. Climate also plays a role because wines produced in humid climates generally contain more resveratrol than wines produced in drier regions. And Pinot Noir is believed to contain twice as much resveratrol as either Cabernet Sauvignon or Merlot. In the grand scheme, however, whether you choose red or white really doesn't make so much difference as long as you choose wine over beer or hard liquor.

> **NOTE:** Low-carb beers do contain significantly less sugar than regular beer, but they also contain significantly less antioxidants.

Is Wine Healthy for Your Heart?

Moderate consumption of alcohol appears to increase good HDL cholesterol and reduce the formation of clots that block arteries. More than 100 studies suggest light to moderate drinkers have a lower risk of heart disease. Study after study has shown that men who drink moderately are 30 to 40 percent less likely to have a heart attack than men who don't drink at all. In fact, moderate alcohol consumption appears to be more effective than just about every other lifestyle modification factor used to lower the risk of heart disease and other diseases. Only cessation of smoking is proven more effective. Further, other medical research suggests that adding alcohol to a healthful diet is more effective than just following the diet alone.

Moderate wine consumption is also linked to a decreased risk of stroke. Stroke is the third leading cause of death in the United States. There are two types of stroke, and the most common (ischemic) has the same origin as heart disease. So it's not far-fetched to assume that if moderate consumption of wine decreases risk of heart disease it also decreases the risk of stroke. Sure enough, the medical literature supports this theory. In a 16-year study examining data from the Copenhagen City Heart Study, researchers found intake of wine (but not beer or hard liquor) on either a monthly, weekly, or daily basis was associated with a lower risk of stroke as compared with not consuming wine at all.[4] This decreased risk of stroke was confirmed in the United States in the Northern Manhattan Stroke

Study. Researchers examined alcohol consumption in more than 1,800 Manhattan men and women. They found a one third decrease in the risk of stroke for men and women who consumed up to two drinks per day.[5]

Does Drinking Wine Increase Risk of Breast Cancer?

As a surgeon who operates on breast cancer patients regularly, Andy can't ignore the fact that drinking alcohol of any sort has been linked to an increased risk of breast cancer. However, when you delve a little deeper into the research, the increased risk may not be as clear-cut as many scientists have thought. New Canadian research showed drinking didn't increase the chances of breast cancer at all in women at high genetic risk for the disease. And while it certainly *sounds* scary to read about alcohol increasing breast cancer risk, if you analyze the research you see the increased risk is not as great as you might think. For example, women who drink the most (15 drinks or more per week) appear to have a 2.6 percent risk of being diagnosed with breast cancer over 7 years, compared with a 2 percent risk for those who had two or fewer drinks per week, a mere 0.6 percent increase in risk. And then there's the multicenter study of nearly 14,000 women showing that among postmenopausal women, wine was not related to breast cancer, but hard liquor was.

Furthermore, a Clean Cuisine lifestyle, with its plant forward diet and regular exercise program, is *much more likely* to offer protection from breast cancer than simply avoiding alcohol altogether. It is interesting that several studies have shown that only women whose diets are low in green vegetables and thus consume less than 350 micrograms of folate per day see their risk of breast cancer increase with alcohol consumption; the same is not true for women eating lots of vegetables and a folate-rich diet.[6] The Clean Cuisine diet we recommend is *extremely* rich in vegetables and folate as well as many other cancer-protecting substances.

Also note that the Clean Cuisine diet will decrease your body fat, which will further reduce your risk of breast cancer because having a lower body fat level will lower estrogen levels. One reason alcohol is believed to increase the risk of breast cancer is because alcohol increases estrogen levels. Estrogen levels are also increased in persons who are overweight. But then again, despite the media hype on breast cancer, according to the American Heart Association, heart disease is still the number one killer in women. Breast cancer prevention should not guide a woman's overall approach to good health. Clean eating with an emphasis on unrefined whole plant foods and fewer animal foods, regular exercise, and maintaining a healthy body weight and body fat level will offer far more protection against breast cancer than avoiding wine. You really have to take the big picture and the entire lifestyle into consideration and try not to lose the forest for the trees.

Is Wine Healthful If You Have Diabetes?

Although you might think wine would be a bad thing for someone with diabetes, studies show moderate consumption of wine is not only okay for the diabetic patient but can actually be health promoting, especially because diabetes particularly increases the risk of arterial aging and heart disease. Solid research suggests people who already have diabetes are less likely to develop heart disease if they drink alcohol.[7] And, believe it or not, moderate wine consumption has also been associated with a reduced fasting insulin concentration, improved insulin sensitivity, and a reduced risk for developing type 2 diabetes in the first place! In the Nurses' Health Study, moderate drinkers were at significantly less risk for developing diabetes as compared to teetotalers.[8] Studies also show moderate drinkers have lower insulin levels compared with nondrinkers consuming the same number of calories.[9] Our conclusion? We see no reason to avoid drinking wine even if you have diabetes.

Does Wine Make You Fat?

We've read countless diet books where authors tell you wine inhibits your body's ability to burn fat and that drinking wine regularly will lead to weight gain. And we can't tell you how many times we've heard friends at dinner say they are going to skip the wine to save calories for the dessert. Well, we can tell you right now this is a big fat mistake. From a weight management standpoint, you'd actually be far better off having a glass of wine than a slice of cake. Before we delve into the studies, we can tell you this much: We both have wine with dinner every night (with the exception that Andy abstains on the nights he is on emergency room call). We've been doing this for as long as we have been married, over a decade now, and both of us have perfectly healthy weights. Neither one of us has changed a clothing size or gained weight. Okay, so a sample size of two is not exactly statistical proof, so let's delve deeper into the science.

Actually, the science is right in line with our personal experience. We have believed for years that wine calories are not equal to food calories. In fact, in our first book we wrote, "the calories in alcohol do not appear to be metabolized in the same manner as the calories from carbohydrates, fats and protein. There is no scientific rationale to abstain from drinking moderate amounts of alcohol in an effort to maintain a healthy waistline."[10] We didn't just randomly come to this conclusion because we like to drink wine; we based our conclusion on studies published in medical journals. In April 1997, the *Journal of the American College of Nutrition* reported a 12-week crossover study in which 14 men were given two glasses of wine to drink every day for 6 weeks and then they were asked to abstain for 6 weeks. The men did not gain weight while they were drinking, nor did they lose weight when they stopped.[11] Two glasses of wine contain about 200 calories. Over a 6-week period these men should have gained about 2½ pounds, yet they didn't gain an ounce. Researchers theorize the alcohol may enter a futile cycle where it is not metabolized in the same way as carbohydrates, fat, or protein. This is very similar to the way that plant calories seem to be less likely to cause weight gain than animal protein calories, as we discussed earlier in this book.

Recently on CNN.com, R. Curtis Ellison, M.D., the director of the Institute on Lifestyle and Health at the Boston University School of Medicine, said the strongest evidence to date that calories from food and alcohol are not created equal comes from the March 8, 2010, issue of the *Archives of Internal Medicine*.[12] This study involved 19,220 healthy, normal-weight women done at the Harvard School of Public Health and Brigham and Women's Hospital in Boston, Massachusetts.[13] Dr. Ellison was quoted as saying, "Many other studies that are not nearly as well done as this suggest that calories from alcohol are metabolized differently. The alcohol calories probably don't count as much as the calories from a Hershey's Bar." We couldn't agree more wholeheartedly.

One study actually showed that women who routinely drank *moderate* amounts of alcohol, totaling about one drink per day, carried almost 10 pounds less body fat than women who did not drink at all.[14] Before this, researchers at the Centers for Disease Control and Prevention showed that, over a 10-year period, drinking alcohol seemed to have very little effect on body weight. However, in that study, drinkers tended to gain less weight

189

when compared with people who abstained from alcohol.[15] In a similar 10-year study, drinkers actually displayed a slight tendency to *lose* weight.[16]

Pouring in a Little Common Sense: If You Don't Drink Should You Start?

If you don't drink, you might ask whether you should start. This is a tough question and has more to do with personal values than anything else. We are not saying you should start drinking wine if you have a specific reason not to or you just don't want to or you just don't like the taste. If you have personally had a problem with alcohol abuse or other substance abuse, you obviously shouldn't start to drink again as the risks *far outweigh* the benefits. And we certainly are not saying wine should be your new weight-loss weapon of choice either. What we are saying is that if you enjoy wine and if it helps you relax and enhances your enjoyment of the Clean Cuisine lifestyle, then you shouldn't avoid wine because of an inaccurate perception that wine adds empty calories. The research just doesn't support that.

PART 3

The Clean Cuisine 8-Week Program

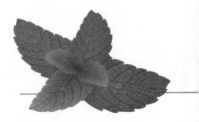

CLEAN CUISINE FULL FITNESS FUSION
The 30-Minute Solution

Take care of your body. It's the only place you have to live.
—JIM ROHN

Eating an anti-inflammatory clean diet alone is not enough to keep you healthy and slow aging. It doesn't matter how great your genes are or whether you need to lose a single pound, nobody can obtain optimal health without exercising. A *well-designed* fitness program that is done on a regular basis is an essential component of achieving optimal wellness and a key ingredient to any lifestyle prescription designed to help slow aging and help you look and feel your very best. We emphasize the importance of a well-designed fitness program because you simply can't take a haphazard approach to fitness. Walking around the park, weekend-warrior activities (tennis, golf anyone?), and darting around the gym while randomly hopping on an exercise device and simultaneously chatting on your cell phone is not the way to go about getting results. And if you don't get the results you are after, whatever they might be (anything from pain relief to fat loss to improved strength to more energy), then you will sooner or later call it quits and throw in the towel. Trust us, we get the issues and obstacles that keep people from exercising on a regular basis, so our *Clean Cuisine Full Fitness Fusion* 30-minute solution is created to deliver ma*ximum results in minimum time.*

What exactly is Full Fitness Fusion? It is a 30-minute *full* body workout

194

that is not only fully functional in nature but also fully transformational. Full Fitness Fusion will change your body. It will help you look and move as if you were 10 years younger. We focus on functional fitness and emphasize quality over quantity. And while you absolutely do need to work hard to get strong and fit, a workout should never cause pain or exhaustion. A good workout should feel fatiguing in an *exhilarating* way. And best of all, you don't need to spend hours at the gym to get in shape. Our fitness recommendations are realistic enough so that even the busiest of people can still get in shape—at home—without going to extremes.

Why Less Is Sometimes More

We are not going to suggest you start training for a marathon. For one, neither of us has run a marathon in our lives (we don't ever plan on doing so either) and two, we are not convinced excessive amounts of hardcore exercise such as marathon running are optimal for overall health, much less for slowing the aging process. We are absolutely positive a hardcore fitness program is not necessary for maintaining a healthy body weight and body fat percentage, reducing back pain, keeping your heart healthy, boosting mood, improving your cholesterol profile, reducing inflammation, and improving your metabolism either. You can certainly achieve all of these results and much more with our reasonable, doable, practical Full Fitness Fusion 30-minute solution..

Chemical reactions in your body that occur during and after extreme exercise regimens produce by-products and oxidative toxins that can damage DNA and accelerate aging. Eating a nutrient-, antioxidant- and phytonutrient-rich Clean Cuisine diet can help offset the oxidative damage created by exercise, but it cannot totally mitigate it. And by the way, because exercise increases oxidative damage, athletes and die-hard exercise enthusiasts actually need to pay *more* attention to what they eat than the average person who engages in light to moderate exercise. Most people think the more you exercise the more lenient you can be with your diet. Not true. The truth is, prolonged intense exercise dramatically increases the stress on your body and stress accelerates biological aging; if you don't adequately nourish your body, especially with antioxidants and phytonutrients (not more animal protein), during periods of intense training you will see and feel yourself getting older, not younger. If you happen to exercise 2 hours a day just because you love the endorphins, that still doesn't give you the green light to eat a Big Mac! We can't emphasize enough the more you exercise, the more attention you need to pay to eating Clean Cuisine and fueling your body with repairing antioxidants and phytonutrients.

Short, Intense Exercise + Clean Cuisine = A Strong, Healthy, and Youthful Body

The discussion connecting the dots between extreme fitness, poor nutrition, and accelerated aging is absolutely not intended to discourage you from exercising! Exercise is proven to promote longevity; plus the benefits you reap from a regular fitness program improve the overall quality of your life.[1] So the last thing we are encouraging is a bunch of couch potato Clean Cuisine acolytes. Instead, what we are saying is that *extreme fitness* most likely does not promote longevity and could negatively impact your quality of life (not to mention take up a lot of time), especially if you don't eat properly.

What we believe when it comes to exercise is that less is often more. In our opinions, the More Is Better mantra of fitness needs to be rethought. We are firm believers that short, *intense,* properly designed workouts that get your heart rate up and strengthen all of your major muscles are absolutely the fountain of youth when it comes to fitness regimens. Keep in mind, your cells are constantly regenerating and your muscle cells refresh every 90 days or so. On average, you renew about 1 percent of the cells in your body daily, and those new cells come in either stronger and younger or weaker and older. Your lifestyle and exercise habits play a tremendous role in cell regeneration, for better or worse. By exercising properly and refueling your body smartly, you can help your body grow younger and stronger. But to grow stronger you need to place a specific rather than haphazard demand on your muscles. That's where quality over quantity comes into play.

Quality over Quantity

As is the case with highly restrictive diets, fanatical exercise regimens that are physically draining or that require hours of your free time set the stage for failure. For those of you who, like us, do not enjoy exercising to extremes and also don't have the time to devote to fanatical fitness regimens, the good news is the properly designed and time-efficient Full Fitness Fusion workout that overloads your muscles, works your entire body, and takes just 30 minutes to complete can be far more effective than a lesser-quality workout lasting twice as long. Over and over, we see one of the main problems with a lot of workouts is that the focus is placed on the time spent working out rather than on the *intensity* and *quality* of the workout. Yet studies show you can reap significantly greater fat loss and significantly more metabolism-boosting muscle gain by performing short, high-intensity workouts as opposed to longer-duration, lower-intensity workouts. And you don't need to do traditional aerobic exercise (running, biking) to burn fat either. Hormonal changes occur with circuit-style resistance training exercises that create a fat-burning environment; specifically, resistance training can increase levels of triacylglycerol lipase activity, a measure of fat burning.[2]

In December 2006, Canadian researchers reported that seven sessions of high-intensity interval training over just 2 weeks increased women's fat-burning enzyme activity, boosting their ability to burn fat during exercise by 36 percent.[3] And it's not just what happens *during* the workout that matters either; intense circuit-style resistance training signals your body to burn a higher percentage of fat calories for many, many hours after your workout ends. The intensity of your workout is what increases the afterburn (also called excess postexercise oxygen consumption, or EPOC), and if your resistance training workout is intense enough you can burn almost double the amount of calories in the afterburn period than you would burn during the time spent doing moderate, steady-state cardio exercise such as jogging or biking. Fat oxidation is increased after resistance exercise, but not aerobic exercise, even 16 hours after the initial performance.[4] But, understand, the key to being able to reap the benefits of the afterburn is that the initial exercise must be intense.

Anyone who has ever exercised knows it is impossible to exercise for a long duration yet keep the intensity high. So ultimately, when it comes to exercise, you must choose between quality and quantity. We choose quality. Not only do quality workouts deliver better results but they are quicker! Science shows longer workouts don't burn more fat. What burns the most fat and gets you fitter, firmer, faster is intense full-body workouts, which by default must be short. The longer people exercise, the more they pace themselves and the less intense (and less effective) their overall workout becomes.

You Can Burn Fat with Zero Cardio Workouts

How many times have you heard the advice that to be in fat burning mode you should exercise slow and steady? Go for a long hike. Ride your bike for 40 miles at a moderate pace. Run a marathon. Swim a whole bunch of laps (just go slowly). Yet when the slow-and-steady exercise approach is put to the test it doesn't exactly yield the fat-burning results we've been promised. In fact, in a study published in the *International Journal of Obesity*, a group of women who performed 20 minutes of interval sprints on a stationary bike three days a week lost an average of 5½ pounds over 15 weeks compared to a similar group who performed slow-and-steady cycling for 40 minutes three days a week. These time-wasting women actually *gained* an average of 1 pound of fat over the same period, not the result most of them were seeking.[5] It's also important to keep in mind the more your body adapts to a workout, the fewer calories you burn; the body quickly adapts to steady-state aerobic exercise such as jogging, biking, walking, and the like, and you soon need to run longer or faster to get a real workout. A 12-month randomized study published in 2007 showed that subjects doing 6 hours of cardio-style exercise per week training 6 days a week for a full year lost an average of only 3 pounds.[6] That is a lot of exercise for not a lot of results. We are not impressed. Nor does that motivate us to start a 6-hour per week cardio-based exercise regimen! The truth is, you can burn fat with zero cardio workouts.

> NOTE: *A zero cardio workout does not mean you won't keep your heart rate elevated or won't condition your cardiovascular system while exercising; it just means you won't have to put in the typical 30 or 45 minutes of cardio time on the treadmill, bike, or elliptical trainer.*

We know from personal experience that zero cardio workouts do work for fat loss. Just as Ivy's MS diagnosis led us to the science behind the Clean Cuisine diet, we sort of stumbled on the science of exercise because of a congenital hip disorder she had called femoral retroversion (where her femur head was rotated 22 degrees off normal). Ivy's hip condition allowed her *extreme* flexibility in her gymnastics days, but as she got older and during a 25-pound pregnancy weight gain, the condition ultimately resulted in destruction of cartilage and a painful impingement in which her femoral head pressed against her hip socket (a condition made much worse by all the sitting she does to write the books!). It took over 10 years, *countless* alternative therapies, and a failed first hip surgery to get a proper diagnosis, and during that time her hip pain could be so severe that she was unable to do any form of cardio activity at all. Unwilling to give up being fit, Ivy used her fitness education background and spent a lot of time researching how to stay strong, lean, and fit without doing any cardio at all. Even though Ivy loved the high she could get from a quick jog or a dance workout, there have been months and months at a time where she was unable to even go for a fast fitness walk. Ironically, with her own body she noticed that during the hip flare-ups, which forced her to perform zero cardio workouts, her body fat would actually *go down*, not up.

The greatest test of this theory came after Ivy's major surgery performed to correct her congenital hip problem. This femoral derotational osteotomy involved intentionally breaking the longest bone in her body, the femur, totally derailing her fitness regimen. Her femur bone was broken in half and the shaft was rotated to put her femoral head in the normal position. After the surgery, Ivy was unable to walk for over 4 months; it took at least 7 months before she could walk without limping, and months after that to adjust to walking with her new anatomy. During the year it took to recover, she certainly couldn't do any form of cardio for more than a few minutes. (She could ride the stationary bike intensely for 1 or 2 minutes and use a hula hoop—more on that in a bit—while standing in place, but that was about it.) But she didn't just sit on the couch either. Even with a broken leg, with her zero cardio workouts she was able to maintain her fitness level. Not only did she not get fat with her zero cardio rehab, she actually *got leaner.*

The reason for this is that the steady-state jogging, biking, dancing, and so forth she loved to do as part of her old workout routines didn't put enough of a demand on her body to increase the afterburn, whereas the core training resistance exercises she subjected her healing body to did increase the afterburn. What is more, the cardio workouts she did in the past increased her appetite so she would eat more on the days she did cardio. After the surgery, Ivy lost considerable strength at first and a good 10 pounds, so she had to work hard to regain her strength, not just for appearance but so she could walk! She trained harder and more intensely that year than she ever has yet without doing any cardio work. As a result, she got stronger and had less body fat than before the surgery; the intense workouts she did tore muscle down and significantly boosted her metabolism postworkout as her body went into repair mode. Now that her hip is all fixed, she still enjoys dancing, the occasional jog, family bike rides, and beach walks, but she doesn't do those activities to get fit or lean. She does those activities for fun and for stress relief and because they no longer hurt.

Muscle Power and the Afterburn

If you are not convinced the afterburn is actually a bigger deal than the exercise itself, then let us more closely examine how your body burns calories with a pop quiz. Which of the following do you think accounts for the greatest percentage of calories you burn during the course of the day?

A. The calories you burn by exercising and moving.
B. The calories you burn by digesting breakfast, lunch, and dinner.
C. The calories you burn by supporting basic body functions such as pumping blood, tissue repair, thinking, and keeping warm.

Most people answer A, but C is the correct answer. The truth is about 70 percent of the calories you burn each day are burned solely to support basic bodily functions, including tissue repair. In other words, more than two thirds of your energy (calorie) intake is used solely to exist. Scientists call this type of metabolism your *basal metabolism*. Another 15 percent of the calories you burn are due to exercise and movement, and the remaining 15 percent of the calories your body burns are used to digest the food you eat.

Knowing these percentages, it should be obvious that the smartest, most time-efficient way to lose weight is to increase your basal metabolism. This is because a small change in 70 percent is a heck of a lot more significant than a small change in 15 percent! That's why our Full Fitness Fusion program is so different from most fitness programs. We don't focus on only the number of calories you burn while exercising; instead, we have created a complete fitness program designed to increase your basal metabolism and turn up the afterburn, so you burn calories long after the workout is over.

Keep in mind, intense exercise involving resistance strength training, which is what our Full Fitness Fusion workouts provide, causes your tissue to use more calories and increases your muscle mass, which in turn increases your total calorie expenditure. By increasing your muscle mass you increase the number of cells in your body that contain large numbers of calorie-burning mitochondria, and your body simply burns the food you eat faster. In essence, building lean muscles speeds up your metabolism. And as mentioned earlier, challenging your muscles in a way that forces your body to go into repair mode after your workout will not only lead to stronger, more metabolically active muscles but will also substantially increase the afterburn. And because our Full Fitness Fusion workouts are intense enough and varied enough to temporarily damage and constantly challenge your muscles, the afterburn effect can last for up to 48 hours after your workout. The results: you get fit *fast.*

OVERLOAD YOUR MUSCLES TO SEE RESULTS. LADIES, THIS INCLUDES YOU!

WITHOUT QUESTION, STRENGTH-TRAINING exercises have the greatest ability to transform your body. A properly designed resistance-training program can shape, tighten, and tone your muscles, lift any droopy areas, create symmetry, and incinerate unwanted fat by boosting your basal metabolism. But you are guaranteed to *not get results* if you fail to overload your muscles in your workout. This means if you are lifting soup cans and doing 50 reps of leg lifts, you shouldn't expect to see a visible change in your body shape or body composition anytime soon. If your workout strategy is to go for the burn by doing 100 arm circles, you should know that the burn you are feeling is lactic acid, but lactic acid buildup won't increase your metabolism or do a single thing to help change your body shape or help you lose a single pound.

You absolutely must work your muscles to fatigue to see a change in your body, there is just no way around it. This is a concept many men grasp onto in a heartbeat, yet women still fear. The concern is they will bulk up with a resistance-training program. Trust us; you won't bulk up, not if you do the functional-style full-body program that is built into our Clean Cuisine workouts. It is true that even women who isolate muscles (such as doing leg extension exercises on weight machines or biceps curls) while lifting very heavy weights can get big, bulky muscles, but we are not going to have you doing isolation bodybuilding strength-training routines. In comparison to a bodybuilder-style workout, our exercises work multiple muscle groups at once and will *not* bulk you up. Our workouts train your body in a multidirectional, multiplanar fashion, a system of training that defines functional fitness. You work every major muscle in your body in a balanced and functional way. You don't isolate muscles, and your heart rate stays elevated the entire workout. You don't spend hours on mind-numbing cardio machines. *And you get results incredibly fast.* Our Full Fitness Fusion workouts will sculpt, whittle, and tone your body from head to toe.

Oxygen In = Fat Out

One of the goals of our Full Fitness Fusion workouts is to force the body to consume a lot of oxygen. When you do intense resistance exercise, you force your body to breathe in a lot of oxygen, which enhances the ability of your mitochondria (the energy makers within your cells) to process oxygen, which in turn increases your body's ability to burn fat for energy. In simple terms, oxygen in equals fat out. The more oxygen you train your body to consume, the more calories and the more fat you will burn at rest. But you can't significantly boost oxygen consumption simply strolling around the park while chatting with a friend or riding the stationary bike at a steady-state while reading a magazine (if you can concentrate on reading a magazine while you exercise, you aren't working hard enough).

The only way to increase oxygen consumption is to work out at a high enough intensity that you have to breathe heavily (chatting should be a challenge). If you aren't breathing pretty heavily during your workout, you probably aren't going to be getting the results you want. By breathing heavily and getting more oxygen in you'll burn more fat. But again, it is a myth that the only way to increase your oxygen consumption is to do cardio-style exercises such as biking or jogging. Our Clean Cuisine workouts fuse the benefits of cardio training and strength training into one super-time-efficient and effective workout system that will increase oxygen consumption and your maximum oxygen uptake ($\dot{V}O_2max$). Full Fitness Fusion workouts increase your metabolism and improve your strength and muscle tone. And you don't have to jog a single lap.

NOTE: $\dot{V}O_2max$ is generally considered the best indicator of an athlete's cardiovascular fitness and is measured by the maximum amount of oxygen you can use during intense or maximal exercise.

So What Is Full Fitness Fusion?

Full Fitness Fusion is a 30-minute *full*-body workout that is not only fully functional in nature but also fully transformational. Our workouts are based on resistance circuit training, and each workout is designed to quickly fatigue your *whole body*. Each one works every major muscle and gets your heart pumping hard. The program fuses cardio and resistance training into one elegant workout system. But it goes beyond that. Recognizing your body will adapt to whatever stress you place on it, we have created a fusion approach to fitness that constantly challenges your muscles with a variety of different workout strategies to prevent plateauing and combat boredom.

In our 8-week program (Chapter 9) you'll notice we switch the workout program frequently to keep your body guessing. You'll also notice each workout works your *entire body,* and the exercises are functional in nature, meaning we don't isolate muscles but rather we work your muscles using compound movements to train your body to do real-world, functional, everyday activities as well as force your body to consume a lot of oxygen with each exercise. Full Fitness Fusion is all about total-body conditioning rather than the single-muscle, single-movement exercises you'll find in old-fashioned workouts and bodybuilder exercise programs. The dynamic combo movement exercises you'll see in our workouts target at least two major muscle groups (think quads and glutes) and train your body in different planes of motion (up and down, forward and back, side to side, diagonally, and with rotation), so they give you maximum bang for your movement buck. You'll breathe hard doing the exercises because the exercises use large muscle groups that require a lot of oxygen; you'll also keep your heart rate elevated because you won't stop to rest. Integrated into each workout are challenging core exercises that will flatten your stomach faster than any crunch-based traditional ab exercise routine. The core training component of the workout will also help alleviate and prevent low back and hip pain (part of the reason Ivy was able to tolerate her hip impingement for so long was because she had a very strong core).

The benefits to our Full Fitness Fusion approach are that it burns more calories (more muscles are used per exercise), strengthens the body more efficiently, and results in a more balanced physique. Functional training yields a balanced body that looks strong (and *is* strong) but not overdeveloped. Because you won't be isolating muscle groups like you would be doing with a traditional weight lifting program, you won't get bulky; instead you'll look sleek and firm.

Keep in mind, the goal of each workout is to put demands on your body it is not accustomed to; you want to go beyond your comfort zone and push your body. Pushing your body is how you get results. Obviously, you need to exercise some common sense here because you certainly don't want to push your body to injury! You absolutely have to listen to your body and stop if there is pain, especially in a joint. You should never do any exercises that strain your joints. But you can't lift only the least amount of weight either. You want to put stress on the muscles, not the joints. Those toning-style, soup-can workouts that are so popular in gyms and glamorous-looking workout videos simply don't get results. If you want to get fitter, firmer, faster you need to get your heart rate pumping during your workout, and you need to be breathing hard and working every major muscle hard. By working intensely, doing a variety of different functional exercises for large muscle groups, and moving quickly from one exercise to the next without resting you can achieve results quickly.

Short and Sweet 30-Minute Resistance Circuit Training Workouts

As mentioned earlier, the intensity of your workout matters a lot when it comes to getting results. It is not possible to exercise intensely for too long, so if you exercise for long stretches, your workout by default will not be intense and thus will not be as effective. Plus as a busy surgeon working over 70 hours a week, Andy has never really had the free time for anything more than a short workout. (We know for a fact from working with clients and patients over the years and hearing from our readers on CleanCuisine .com that other people relate to this time crunch too!) In addition, short workouts help keep your mind engaged. Believe it or not, making a mind–body connection and mentally engaging in your workout is every bit as essential as being physically engaged. Anybody can spend an hour putting his or her body through a series of mindless motions or walking around a park chatting up a storm with a friend, but to really push yourself physically—and to really see results— requires a strong mind, willpower, and focus. Our Full Fitness Fusion workouts require you to be present and to really mentally engage in each workout, but because each workout is just 30-minutes in length, you'll find it fairly easy to put forth the mental energy required to get results. Mentally disengaging and doing mindless exercise just won't deliver results.

Get Warm, Then Get on with It

The myth that stretching before a workout prevents injuries still prevails, so many fitness buffs continue to waste a lot of time stretching before they start exercising. After analyzing the results of six controlled studies, scientists at the Centers for Disease Control and Prevention could find no relationship between preexercise stretching and injury prevention. In fact, vigorous stretching *before exercise,* when muscles are cold and therefore less supple, produces less benefit and may even leave your tendons more susceptible to injury. We support stretching but believe it is most effective after your workout when your muscles are already warm.

The best, most efficient way to prevent injury is to increase blood flow to all of your major muscle groups gradually with semi-challenging dynamic movements that increase your heart rate and prepare your muscles for the more strenuous exercises to follow. Examples of time-efficient and effective warmup exercises include squats without weights, overhead reaches, lunging side to side with opposite elbow touching opposite knee, and alternating high knee raises with arm swings. The warmup should actually get your heart rate elevated. In fact, if you are not in particularly good shape the warmup might actually feel like a workout! But that's okay. You don't necessarily want your warmup to be easy. If you haven't elevated your heart rate and you aren't feeling warm then you are *not* warmed up and you are *not* ready to start the real workout. Before each of our Full Fitness Fusion workouts you'll take 10 minutes to do our Fusion Activation Warmup on page 210. Once you get your heart rate elevated and have warmed up, you'll want to get on with your workout and then stretch *at the end,* when it will do the most good.

S-t-r-e-t-c-h It out *After* You Work Out

The importance of stretching is something we admittedly have not emphasized enough in our own workouts over the years. Stretching is important
but best done after your workout. While studying for her American College of Sports Medicine certification, Ivy learned flexibility was one of the
five components of physical fitness (the other four are cardiovascular fitness, muscular strength, muscular endurance, and a healthy body mass),
but because Ivy had always been very flexible due to years of gymnastics,
dance, and cheerleading, she put stretching for flexibility way down on
her exercise to do list. It wasn't until rehabbing from her first hip surgery—
which included a lot of stretching—that we both really began to appreciate
stretching firsthand and really began to research the importance of a
properly designed stretching routine. Again, we emphasize *properly
designed* stretching routine because you can't just do a downward dog for
30 seconds, a quick quad stretch, and a few side bends and let that be that.
To get results with stretching you need to stretch properly. In fact, a properly designed stretching routine is so important to your overall fitness
program that if you don't make time to stretch you simply won't get optimal results with your 30-minute Full Fitness Fusion workouts.

The workouts we have outlined in this chapter are all designed to
increase muscle strength. However, one negative consequence to all
strength training programs is that they create short, tight muscles that
can draw bones closer together, and this can eventually result in poor joint
mobility, pain, and even misalignment, *unless* you balance your strength
training workouts with a stretching routine. Proper stretching helps bring
alignment to the joints of your shoulders, hips, knees, and ankles. And
when your body is properly aligned, inflammation of the joints is reduced,
and mobility is increased. If you have super tight muscles that are holding
your body in a restricted position, then your joints are going to become
less mobile and lose their natural lubrication, which results in pain and
stiffness. A consistent flexibility program can do wonders for improving
range of motion and relieving stiffness, thus improving how you feel and
even how you look. An astonishing 31 million Americans suffer from
chronic back, neck, and shoulder pain and many of these issues stem from
acute immobility, musculoskeletal dysfunction, and poor posture. Regular
stretching can prevent and reduce muscle imbalances, prevent injuries,

improve structural problems, and help you achieve beautiful posture and a healthy-looking and properly aligned body.

And yes, a flexible body will look better too. It shouldn't come as any surprise that a supple body is going to move and look a lot younger than a stiff one! Lengthening and elongating your muscles helps with postural alignment that in turn helps return your body to a more neutral (and youthful!) position. Even if you don't exercise, you still need to stretch. For example, if you sit at a computer for hours each day (does anyone in the modern world *not* do this?), you will be shortening your iliopsoas muscles (your hip flexors). Tight iliopsoas muscles will then draw your pelvis into a posterior tilt causing your rear to push back and your stomach to protrude. By stretching your iliopsoas muscles, you will allow your pelvis to sit in a more neutral position, which will not only alleviate pressure on the vertebrae in your low back but also help flatten your stomach. And a flat stomach is going to do wonders for improving appearance.

Another benefit of stretching after a workout is that it will assist your body in releasing lactic acid from the muscle cells faster and more efficiently so free radicals and other toxins can quickly be escorted from your body. You can almost think of stretching as a form of postexercise detox because it helps your body get rid of waste products faster. And, of course, stretching improves circulation and increases blood flow to your muscles, which speeds muscle recovery after exercise. You are much less likely to experience soreness if you stretch your muscles *after* a workout.

A big mistake most people make with stretching, and one of the reasons they don't get results, is rushing through their stretches and failing to devote the time it takes to really lengthen the muscles. To get results with stretching you really need to hold each stretch for a good 45 seconds to one minute, sometimes even more. It takes time to elongate a muscle safely, so don't rush your stretches. Also, you should never stretch to the point of pain; you should feel tension while stretching but *never* pain. The key to lengthening muscle groups is to keep the tension continuous, all the while slowly going deeper into the stretch, which can be accomplished by making subtle positional changes while holding the stretch. Just remember to not bounce; keep your stretching static and breathe deeply to relax your body and ease tension while you are stretching.

> NOTE: *If you have had an injury or you are particularly tight or tense in one area, you may find you need to hold certain stretches for 3 or more minutes to get the best results.*

We are confident once you start incorporating a stretching routine into your lifestyle on a regular basis you will see an improvement in how you look, how you move, and how you feel. We have created two full-body flexibility and range-of-motion stretching routines that can be accessed at www.CleanCuisineandMore.com/stretchroutines. Stretch routine 1 is a more Western-style stretching routine composed of traditional flexibility exercises that target large muscle groups. Stretch routine 2 is a more Eastern-style stretching routine that incorporates yoga. We recommend you trade off doing one routine one day and the other routine the next. You can stretch as many as 7 days a week if you like. Just listen to your body and do what feels best.

207

WHAT IF YOU WANT TO ADD MORE EXERCISE?

WE REALIZE SOME of you may love activities such as jogging, playing tennis, dancing, going for long bike rides, or doing other exercises that are low-intensity and aerobic in nature. There is absolutely nothing wrong with doing any of these exercises for fun, but we absolutely don't want you replacing one of the real Full Fitness Fusion workouts with a low-intensity aerobic-style workout. Going for a leisurely bike ride or a walk on the beach or a hike in the park can be a great way to get outside and get some fresh air and soak in some vitamin D, not to mention relieve stress, but don't kid yourself thinking these sorts of activities can replace one of your real workouts.

If jogging and tennis are not enough and you love the rush many of us get from true cardio-style workouts, try our optional Sizzle Cardio Interval Workout at the end of this chapter for something more intense, and more effective, than the standard steady-state cardio workouts your body quickly adapts to. If you are time crunched, and if fat loss is a goal for you, cardio interval workouts are much more effective than just going for a run.

The Full Fitness Fusion Workouts

Equipment

For more details and pictures of the equipment, please visit: www.Clean CuisineandMore.com/equipment

RECOMMENDED ITEMS

Dumbbells: 2, 3, 5, 8, 10, and 12 pounds
Medicine Ball: light (2 or 4 pounds), nonbouncing
Jump rope
Resistance tubing with handles
- Basic fitness level: light (level 1) and medium (level 3)
- Intermediate fitness level: light (level 1) and heavy (level 5)

Exercise resistance mini-bands: light, medium, and heavy
Stability ball: size depends on your height
- 55 centimeters for people 5 feet to 5 feet 6 inches tall
- 65 centimeters for people 5 feet 7 inches to 6 feet tall
- 75 centimeters for people 6 feet 1 inch to 6 feet 6 inches tall

Towel

OPTIONAL ITEMS

Step
Sports hula hoop
Gliding discs
Stopwatch
Stationary bike

FULL FITNESS FUSION WORKOUT DVDS

VISIT CLEANCUISINEANDMORE.COM/FULLFITNESSFUSION to view our DVD collection. The workouts in this book stand on their own and are perfect for our 8-week Clean Cuisine Program but our growing Full Fitness Fusion Workout DVD collection led by Ivy can add variety to your fitness routine and provide the visual coaching that will help you take your workout to the next level. The DVD's can be modified for the beginner and advanced exerciser. They include a brief 5-minute dynamic warm-up, 30-minute workout, and a bonus 10-minute stretch and firm yoga sequence.

In the following pages you will find the Fusion Activation Warmup, four Full Fitness Fusion workouts (Strength Workout, Slim Workout, Sculpt Workout, and Stretch Yoga Workout), and a Cool Down Post-Workout Stretch. During the Clean Cuisine 8-week program we will be rotating the four Full Fitness Fusion workouts, but the Fusion Activation Warmup should be done *before each workout* and the Cool Down Post-Workout Stretch should be done *after each workout*.

10-Minute Fusion Activation Warmup

MEDICINE BALL (2–4 POUNDS) CHOPS

  ■ **10 REPS**

Stand with your feet hip width apart, toes facing forward, and knees ever so slightly bent. Hold the medicine ball in your hands with your arms overhead. Chop down and stop when the ball is between your feet. Return to starting position and repeat.

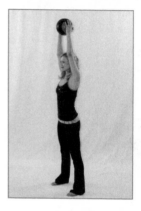 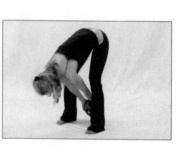

MEDICINE BALL (2–4 POUNDS) DIAGONAL CHOPS

  ■ **10 REPS LEFT / 10 REPS RIGHT**

Stand with your feet hip width apart, toes facing forward, and knees ever so slightly bent. Hold the medicine ball in your hands with your arms over your right shoulder. Twist your torso to the left, lifting your right heel off the ground, and pivoting your right toe inward, and chop down, aiming the ball toward your left toe. Return to starting position and repeat for 10 reps. Switch sides and repeat.

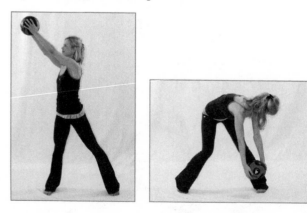

MEDICINE BALL (2–4 POUNDS)
ALTERNATING SIDE-TO-SIDE PIVOTS

■ 20 REPS

Stand with your feet hip width apart, toes facing forward, and knees ever so slightly bent. Hold the medicine ball in your hands with your arms directly in front of your body, elbows just slightly bent. Keeping the medicine ball in front of your body, twist your torso to the right while pivoting your left foot and lifting your left heel off the ground. Return to start position, and then twist to the left. Continue twisting back and forth for 20 reps.

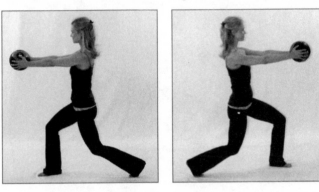

ALTERNATING REVERSE LUNGES WITH RAINBOW ARMS

■ 20 REPS

Stand up straight with your feet hip width apart. Step backward with your right leg, lowering your body to the ground. Reach your arms up and back as you twist your torso and arch over to the right ever so slightly. Press back to a standing position, and then repeat with your left leg. Alternate lunges for 20 reps.

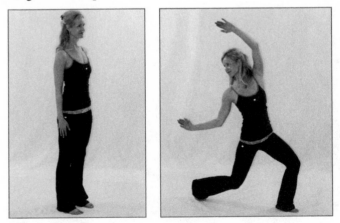

INCHWORM

■ **5 REPS**

Stand tall with your legs straight. Bend forward at the hips and place your hands on the floor. Keeping your legs straight, walk your hands forward as far as you can without letting your hips sag (keep your abdominal muscles pulled inward). Then take tiny steps to inch-walk your feet back to your hands. Then inch-walk your feet back to plank position. Inch-walk your hands back to your feet and stand up. That's 1 rep. Repeat 5 times.

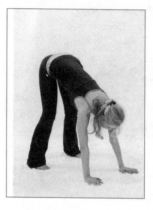 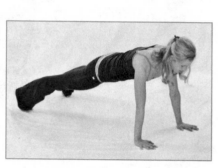

SINGLE LEG FORWARD AND BACKWARD HOPS

■ **10 REPS RIGHT LEG / 10 REPS LEFT LEG**

Stand on your right leg. Imagine there is a line drawn on the floor in front of you. Jump over the line with your right leg and land on your right foot. Then jump backward over the line to the starting position. Keep the jumps quick and small (you do not need to jump high!). Do 10 reps on your right leg and then switch sides.

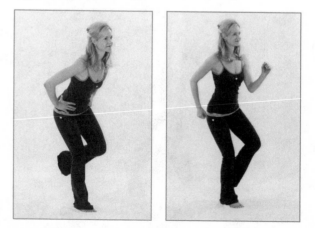

BEAR WALKS

■ **1 MINUTE**

Stand with your feet hip width apart, and bend over at your hips, placing 213 your hands on the ground in front of your feet. Distribute your weight equally between your hands and feet. Bring your right hand and left foot forward then bring your left hand and right foot forward. Continue walking on all fours for 1 full minute (to increase the intensity go faster).

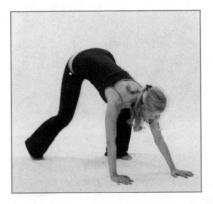

JUMPING JACKS (OR JOG IN PLACE)

■ **60 REPS**

Stand with your feet together and your hands at your sides. Simultaneously extend your arms above your head and jump up just enough to spread your feet out wide. Quickly reverse the movement.

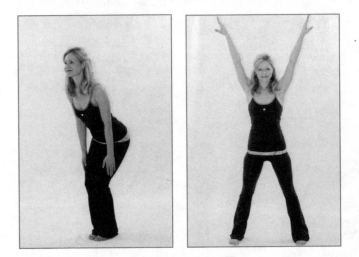

AROUND THE WORLDS

■ **5 REPS LEFT / 5 REPS RIGHT**

214

Stand with your feet a little wider than hip width apart and arms overhead. Keep your knees slightly soft. Bend over to the left and then down and over to the right and back up again, making a big circle with your arms. Repeat 5 times and then switch sides.

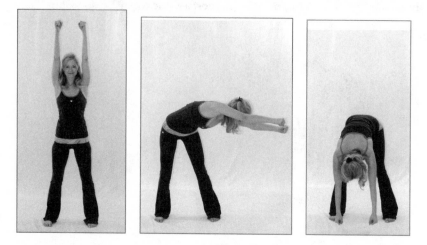

BRISK ALTERNATING OPPOSITE ELBOW–OPPOSITE KNEE

■ **60 REPS**

Stand with your feet hip width apart and arms down at your sides. Briskly bring your right knee up as you simultaneously bring your left elbow down to touch your knee. Repeat on the opposite side and continue alternating sides going at a brisk pace for 60 reps.

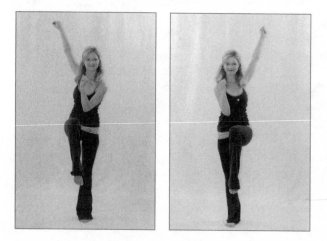

ALTERNATING SIDE-TO-SIDE LUNGES

■ **20 REPS**

Stand with your feet a few inches wider than shoulder width apart, toes 215
facing forward, and hands clasped with arms extended straight in front of
your body. Lunge to the left by bending your left knee and lowering your
hips toward the ground, keeping the weight in your left foot, and leaning
back slightly on your left heel. Be sure your left knee does not extend over
your left toe. Return to start position and lunge to the right. Continue
lunging side to side for 20 reps.

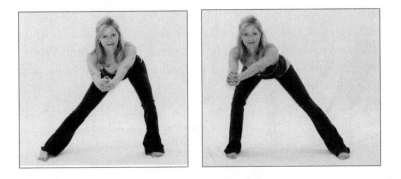

Workout 1: Strength Workout

216 The Strength Workout will create a foundation of full-body functional strength. You'll not only strengthen your muscles, you'll keep your heart rate elevated and strengthen your cardiovascular system too. Think of it as "cardio resistance training"—you are going to get a cardio workout burning calories and fat, but you'll also be simultaneously strengthening every major muscle in your body. You'll be doing what is called giant sets, during which you'll combine three or four exercises into a "station" and complete that station in a continuous fashion. No resting! When you've completed all the reps of each exercise in the station, you've finished one round of the giant set. Then you will repeat the station two more times through, again, without resting. The end result is an extremely time-efficient and effective full-body workout that will significantly boost your metabolism. But it's not easy.

▶ Start with the Fusion Activation Warmup (page 210).

Station 1 (Perform As a No Rest Circuit)

DUMBBELL SQUAT TO OVERHEAD PRESS

■ 8–12 POUNDS / 20 REPS

Stand with feet hip width apart and hands at your sides. Squat down, lowering your body as if you were sitting back into a chair, keeping your back in its natural alignment as you lower your legs. When your thighs are parallel to the floor, stand up and push your dumbbells straight overhead in one continuous movement. Lower the weights to the starting position and repeat.

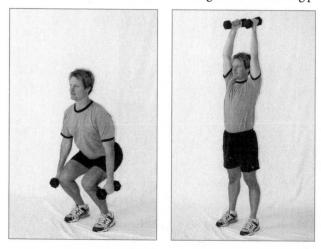

BACK ROW ON BOTH LEGS (STAGGER STANCE) WITH RESISTANCE TUBING

■ 10 REPS LEFT LEG / 10 REPS RIGHT LEG

Attach resistance tubing to the door, level with your chest, using the door attachment. Stand approximately 4 feet from the door with your feet in stagger stance with one foot slightly in front of the other (see photo), your toes forward, and your abdominal muscles contracted. Grasp the tube with your palms facing each other and pull your shoulders back. Pull the tube toward you. Return to start position and repeat.

> NOTE: *Be sure to stand upright the entire time; try not to lean forward or backward.*

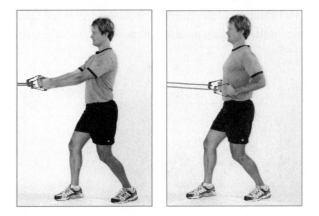

ON THE BALL BACK EXTENSION

■ 15 REPS

Lay facedown with your abs on the stability ball and your arms straight down. Place hands on the floor in front of the ball. Begin by lifting your arms straight to shoulder level so they look like a Y, palms facing each other, now slightly lift your chest up to bring your arms straight back with your thumbs facing up so that you create a straight line with your body. Return to the start position.

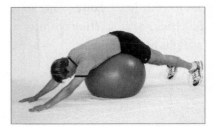
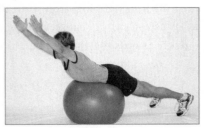

▶ Repeat station 1 a total of three times.

Station 2 (Perform As a No Rest Circuit)

OPPOSITE ARM / OPPOSITE LEG ROMANIAN DEADLIFT

▪ **10 REPS LEFT / 10 REPS RIGHT (NO WEIGHT FOR BEGINNERS; 8–10 POUNDS FOR ADVANCED)**

Stand on your left leg with your right arm reaching out toward the ground in front of you. Your right leg begins slightly off the ground. As you get stronger you can hold a dumbbell in your right hand. Stand with a neutral spine (don't let your back round). Bend at the hip, reaching for the floor with your right arm while pushing your right leg back to stretch your hamstrings. Go as low as you can while maintaining a neutral spine, and then contract and return to the starting position. Repeat on your other leg.

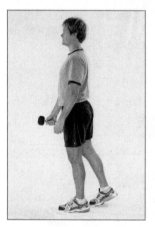
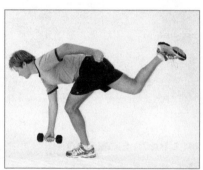

PUSHUPS WITH ONE HAND ON MEDICINE BALL

▪ **10 REPS EACH HAND**

Position a medicine ball on the floor. Place your left hand on the medicine ball and your right hand on the floor and assume a pushup position (advanced on your toes and beginners on your knees) with your body forming a straight line from your ankles to your head. Lower your body as far as you can go, pause, and then press back to the starting position as quickly as possible. Roll the ball to your right hand and repeat.

Beginner

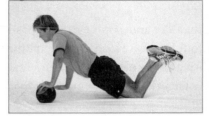
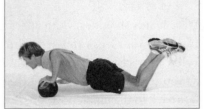

Advanced

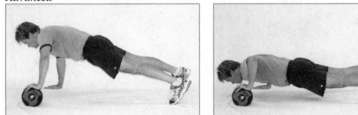

STATIC LUNGE (SINGLE-LEG LUNGE PRESS)

■ 10 REPS LEFT / 10 REPS RIGHT (NO WEIGHT FOR BEGINNERS; 8–10 POUNDS
FOR ADVANCED)

Stand in a split stance, with your front right heel about 3 feet in front of your left rear toe. Hold the dumbbells at your sides (if using). Both feet should face forward. Lower your body so your front knee is bent about 90 degrees and your rear knee nearly touches the floor. Keep your torso upright. Rise back up to the split position. Finish all reps on one leg and then switch sides.

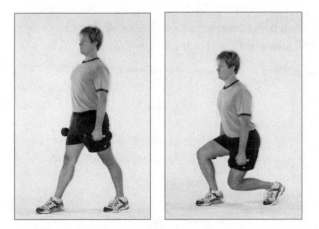

STABILITY BALL KNEE TUCKS

■ **10–15 REPS**

220 Place hands shoulder width apart on the floor and assume a plank position with your legs extended behind your body and shins resting on the ball. Contract your abdominals and bring your knees toward your chest as you round your back. Hold the position briefly and then return your legs back to the plank position.

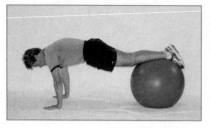 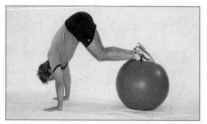

▶ Repeat station 2 a total of three times.

Station 3 (Perform As a No Rest Circuit)

TRAVELING SIDE STEP SQUATS WITH MINI-BAND

■ **10 SIDE STEPS LEFT / 10 SIDE STEPS RIGHT**

Place the mini-band around your ankles and stand with your feet hip width apart, putting slight tension on the band. Put your hands in prayer position, pressing your palms together (you should feel the muscles in your upper body working!). Step out to the right and squat, lowering your body as if you were sitting back into a chair, keeping your back in its natural alignment and your legs nearly perpendicular to the floor. When your thighs are parallel to the floor stand up and bring your left foot back close to your right foot. Travel to the right 10 times and then repeat going to the left.

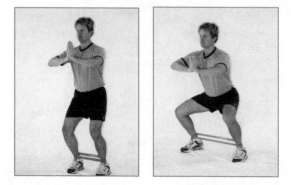

ALTERNATING ARCHER PULLS WITH RESISTANCE TUBING

■ **20 REPS TOTAL**

Attach the resistance tubing to the door, level with your chest, using the door
attachment. Stand approximately 4 feet from the door with your feet somewhat
more than hip width apart, your toes turned out and abdominals contracted.
Grasp the tube with your palms facing in and pull your shoulders back. Pull
your right hand toward your shoulder, keeping your elbow in line with your
shoulder, as you step back and rotate to the right. Return to start position and
repeat with the left hand. Alternate back and forth for 20 reps.

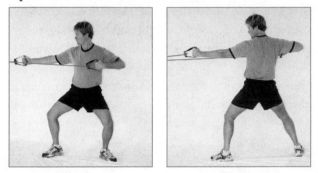

STANDING 2 O'CLOCK / 10 O'CLOCK ROTATIONS WITH RESISTANCE TUBING

■ **10 REPS LEFT / 10 REPS RIGHT**

Attach resistance tubing to the door, at waist height, using the door attachment. Stand approximately 4 feet from the door with your feet hip width
apart, your toes forward and abdominals contracted. Grasp the tube with both
hands and extend your arms in front of your chest, rotate your torso so that
your anchor point is at 2 o'clock. In one movement rotate your body to the left
and pull the band across your body so that your anchor point is at 10 o'clock.
Return to 2 o'clock position and repeat 10 times. Switch sides and repeat.

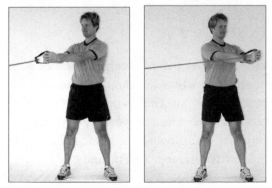

▶ Repeat station 3 a total of three times.

Cool Down BLTs on Stability Ball

Lie on floor with your calves or heels on the stability ball and your hands next to your hips on the floor. Do 10 reps of each of the following:

- B for bridges: hips lift up and down; engage your glutes by lifting your glutes and hips toward the ceiling
- L for leg curls: hips remain up and knees bend while you roll the ball toward your glutes; keep your abs tight and back straight as you engage your hamstring muscles by rolling the ball toward your glutes
- T for thrusts: adjust feet so just the soles of your feet are touching the ball and thrust hips up and down.

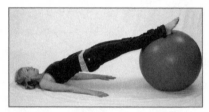
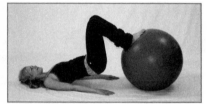
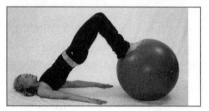

▶ Conclude with the Cool Down Post-Workout Stretch (page 255).

Workout 2: Slim Workout

The Slim Workout circuit fuses intense 1-minute cardio intervals with resistance exercises for a full-body functional workout that burns mega calories both during *and after* the workout. You'll work hard alternating between cardio bursts and resistance exercises, but you'll strip fat fast. It's a challenge for both mind and body! Think boot camp but friendlier, more fun, and with a more advanced, scientific approach behind it.

HOOPING CARDIO CORE INTERVALS

AS MENTIONED EARLIER, Ivy wasn't able to do any traditional cardio exercises for any length of time after her surgery, but she *was* able to hula hoop! Hooping for fitness is not something we invented; it is actually a relatively new workout trend that uses a giant 40-inch sports hoop such as the ones produced by Hoopnotica (see www .CleanCuisineandMore.com/equipment to learn more). Using a special sports hoop, hooping is a surprisingly easy exercise to learn (the sports hoop makes it much easier to learn compared to the hula hoop you might have used as a kid). Best of all, hooping really skyrockets your heart rate with zero impact on the joints. The faster you spin the hoop, the higher your heart rate climbs. In addition to getting your heart rate elevated, hooping effectively targets the notoriously neglected transverse abdominal muscles with the drawing in maneuver. By training the transverse abdominal muscles spinal stability is increased, abdominal muscles are pulled inward, posture is dramatically improved, and you are able to achieve the absolute flattest stomach possible. For the cardio interval component of the Slim Workout give hooping a try! You'll get fit, have fun, and feel like a kid again.

▶ First do the Fusion Activation Warmup (page 210).

Station 1 (Perform As a No Rest Circuit)

This station is a Quick Tempo Matrix made up of a series of seven exercises that you perform *quickly* 10 times without resting. Although you do not want to use momentum to do the movements, you do want to move quicker than you would normally move when lifting weights. Do not compromise form; it is better to lift a lighter weight and do the exercise properly with correct form than to use a heavier weight with poor form.

> NOTE: *If you are doing the Quick Tempo Matrix correctly and at the right tempo, it will increase your heart rate quickly.*

■ SUGGESTED WEIGHT: 2- TO 5-POUND DUMBBELLS FOR BEGINNER WOMEN, 8-POUND DUMBBELLS FOR BEGINNER MEN AND MORE ADVANCED WOMEN,

AND 10-POUND DUMBBELLS FOR MORE ADVANCED MEN

224   **MATRIX MOVE 1: ALTERNATING ROTATIONAL OVERHEAD PRESSES**

     ■ **10 REPS EACH SIDE**

Stand with your feet shoulder width apart and hold two dumbbells at your shoulders. Press your right hand dumbbell up overhead as you rotate your body to the left. Return to the starting position and repeat with the opposite side. Rotate back and forth, pressing one arm, then the other, overhead.

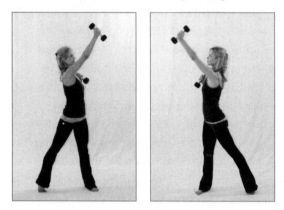

MATRIX MOVE 2: ALTERNATING OVERHEAD PRESSES

     ■ **10 REPS EACH SIDE**

Stand with your feet shoulder width apart and hold two dumbbells at your shoulders. Press one dumbbell overhead, keeping your palms facing inward. Return to start position and repeat with the opposite side. Alternate back and forth, pressing one arm, then the other, overhead.

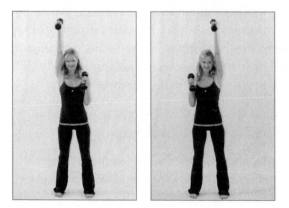

MATRIX MOVE 3: ALTERNATING HAMMER BICEPS CURLS

■ **10 REPS EACH SIDE**

Stand with your feet shoulder width apart and hold two dumbbells at your sides. Keeping your elbows in close to your waist, curl one dumbbell up to your shoulder, keeping your palms facing inward. Return to start position and repeat with the opposite side. Alternate back and forth, curling one arm, then the other.

225

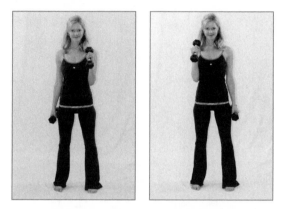

MATRIX MOVE 4: ALTERNATING BENT-OVER ROWS

■ **10 REPS EACH SIDE**

Stand with your feet shoulder width apart and bend over at the hips, keeping your back flat with your spine in a straight line, and your arms hanging down with your palms facing backward. Row one dumbbell up to your shoulder, keeping your elbow in line with your shoulder. Return to start position and repeat with the opposite side. Alternate back and forth, rowing one arm, then the other.

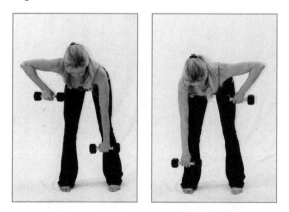

MATRIX MOVE 5: ALTERNATING LATERAL RAISES

■ 10 REPS EACH SIDE

226   Stand with your feet shoulder width apart and hold a dumbbell in each hand. Brace your abs and lift one arm straight out to the side, keeping your palm facing down and lifting the dumbbell straight out from the shoulder. Return to start position and repeat with the opposite side. Alternate back and forth, raising one arm, then the other.

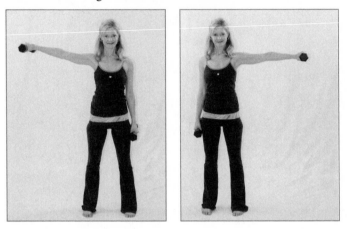

MATRIX MOVE 6: SIDE-STEP LUNGE WITH OVERHEAD PRESS

■ 10 REPS EACH SIDE

Stand with your feet shoulder width apart and hold a dumbbell in each hand. Step out to one side and bend that leg, lowering your hips while keeping most of your weight on the bent leg. Push off the bent leg while simultaneously driving both arms overhead as you stand up. Switch sides and repeat, alternating side steps with overhead press.

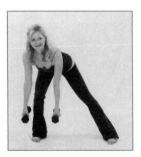
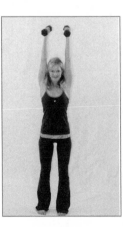
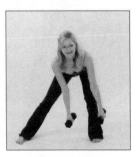

MATRIX MOVE 7: SQUATS WITH HAMMER BICEPS CURLS

■ **10 REPS**

Stand with your feet shoulder width apart and hold a dumbbell in each hand. Keeping your body upright, lower yourself into a squat position by bending at the knees and hips through a full range of motion, stopping once your hips are level with or below your knees. As you squat, be sure to maintain a tall posture; do not let your back round. As you stand up curl your dumbbells to your shoulders, keeping your palms facing inward. Repeat.

227

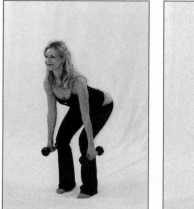
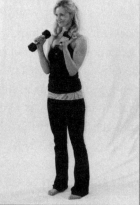

Station 2 (Perform As a No Rest Circuit)

Alternate between five strength stations and five 1-minute cardio stations for a total of 10 stations.

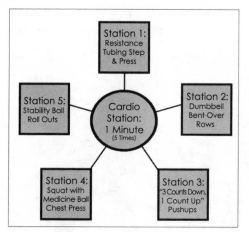

Strength Stations

STRENGTH STATION 1: RESISTANCE TUBING STEP AND PRESS (WITH ALTERNATING FEET)

■ **10 REPS LEFT / 10 REPS RIGHT**

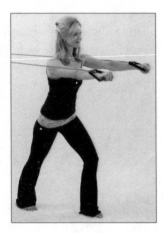

Attach the resistance tubing to the door, at shoulder height, using the door attachment. Stand approximately 4 feet away with your back to the door and feet shoulder width apart. Grasp the resistance tubing handles with your palms facing down. Step forward with one foot while pressing the resistance tubing forward, keeping your palms in line with your shoulders. Return to the start position. Switch sides and repeat, alternating forward steps with chest presses.

STRENGTH STATION 2: DUMBBELL BENT-OVER ROWS (WITH STAGGER STANCE)

■ **10 REPS LEFT / 10 REPS RIGHT**

Stand with one foot slightly in front of the other and bend forward at the hips, hold a dumbbell in each hand with arms straight in front of your body. Your back should be flat with your spine in a straight line. Squeeze your shoulder blades together as you row one dumbbell up to your side. Return to the start position and repeat, alternating rows back and forth with each arm for a total of 10 reps. Switch feet and repeat rows for 10 reps.

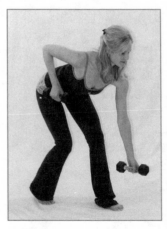
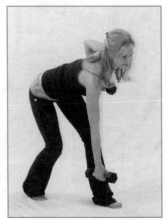

STRENGTH STATION 3: 3-COUNTS-DOWN / 1-COUNT-UP PUSHUPS

■ **10 REPS**

Get into pushup position (advanced on your toes and beginners on your knees), with your body forming a straight line from your ankles to your head. Lower your body to a count of 3, pause, and then press back to the starting position as quickly as possible. Repeat.

Beginner

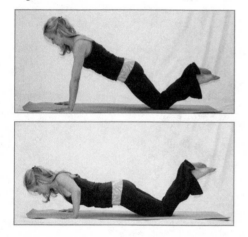

Advanced

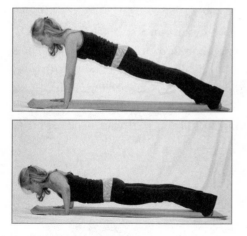

STRENGTH STATION 4: SQUAT WITH MEDICINE BALL CHEST PRESS

■ 15 REPS

Stand as tall as you can with your feet spread shoulder width apart and knees facing forward. Hold a medicine ball in front of your body with your arms extended straight. Lower your body as far as you can by pushing your hips back and bending at your knees. Bring the medicine ball in to your chest. Return to the start position as you simultaneously push the medicine ball in front of your body. Repeat.

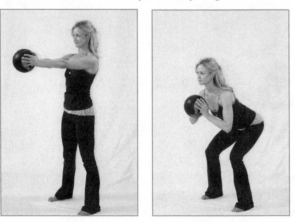

STRENGTH STATION 5: STABILITY BALL ROLL OUTS

■ 15 REPS

Kneel on the floor and place your forearms on a stability ball, drawing your abs in tight. Your upper arms should form 90-degree angles with your body. Roll the ball forward by pushing the ball forward with your elbows and forearms and letting your body lower toward the ground while maintaining a neutral spine and keeping your abs tight. Do not go beyond the point where you can maintain a stable back. If your back begins to arch, you've gone too far. Repeat.

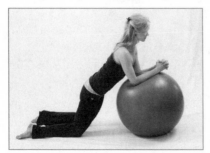
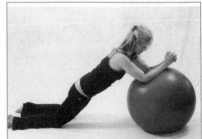

Cardio Stations

Choose *any* of the following cardio intervals to be performed for 1 minute at a time, alternating with the strength station intervals.

STATIONARY BIKE
Put the resistance on medium-high and peddle as fast as you can.

AIR BOXING
Stand with your right foot in front of your left and keep your knees slightly bent. Alternate jabs and upper cuts with both arms for 30 seconds. Do not extend your elbows straight when you punch; keep your elbows slightly bent. Switch legs and repeat for 30 seconds.

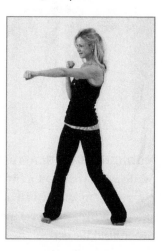

JUMPING JACKS
Standing with your feet together and your arms by your sides, jump and separate your legs slightly wider than shoulder width apart, simultaneously swinging your arms out to the side and up over your head. Jump back to starting position.

JUMPING ROPE
Stand with feet together and back straight. Hold the ends of the jump rope in your hands, with the rope behind your heels. Pass the rope over your head and, as it approaches your feet, *lightly bounce* them to the floor, springing from the balls of your feet. You do *not* need to jump high to get a good workout!

HULA HOOP WITH SPORTS HOOP
Stand up straight, keeping your feet slightly apart. Depending on your skill level, it may be helpful to place one of your feet faintly in front of the other. Hold the hula hoop with both hands and place it around your waist and against the small of your back. Lightly twirl the hula hoop in a counterclockwise motion with your hands and let go. To keep the hoop going, move your body forward and back with the hoop's rotation. If you

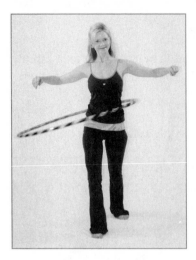

keep your swinging steady, the hula hoop should spin around just above your hips. It may take some practice to keep the hula hoop in rotation for long periods of time, but keep practicing and you will have it down soon! Don't laugh at the hula hoop! You'll be amazed how quickly your heart rate will soar while standing in place. If you haven't hula hooped since grade school visit Ivy at www.CleanCuisine andMore.com/hoop to learn how!

MEDICINE BALL SLAM

Stand with your feet a little more than shoulder width apart and hold a 4-pound medicine ball at your chest. Keep your core tight and in one smooth movement raise the ball overhead and forcefully slam the ball to the ground (be careful the ball doesn't come back and hit you in the face!). Catch the ball and repeat.

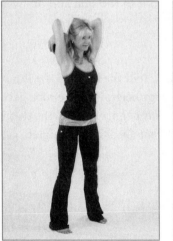
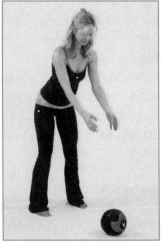

FOOTBALL SHUFFLES

Stand with your feet a little more than shoulder width apart and shuffle 4 times to the left and then 4 times to the right, keeping your feet low to the ground when you shuffle.

233

HIP-HOP TICK TOCK

Stand with feet together, arms down. Begin hops: jump onto left foot as you kick right leg to side, reaching left arm up and right arm down (as shown). On next hop, land on right foot, kick to left and switch arms, alternating sides.

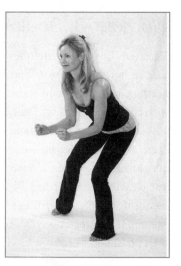

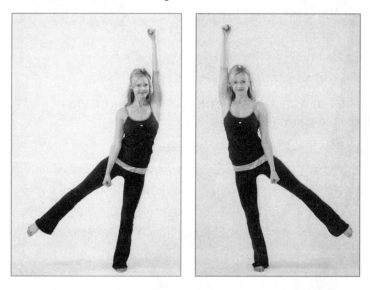

▶ Repeat the Station 1 "Matrix" moves and the Station 2 "Strength" and "Cardio" stations for a total of three times each.

▶ Next do the Cool Down BLTs on Stability Ball (page 222).

▶ Conclude with the Cool Down Post-Workout Stretch (page 255).

Workout 3: Sculpt Workout

234 The sculpt workout includes two challenging full-body super sets. The first set alternates lower body blast sculpting exercises with core conditioning, and the second set alternates upper body blast sculpting exercises with core conditioning. The core conditioning exercises target the muscles of your hips, back, glutes, and abdomen, but because there are no isolation exercises (no crunches, for example) the core exercises actually burn a lot of calories. The core exercises also work your deep transverse abdominal muscles, thus helping to pull your entire midsection inward. The result of combining calorie-burning core conditioning with upper and lower body exercises? Reduced body fat, sculpted arms and legs, and the flattest abdomen possible!

▶ First do the Fusion Activation Warmup (page 210).

Super Set 1: Lower Body Blast and Core Conditioning

LOWER BODY BLAST: ALTERNATING CURTSY LUNGE WITH STRAIGHT ARM DELTOID RAISES

■ **2–5 POUNDS / 20 TOTAL REPS**

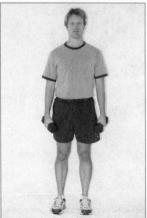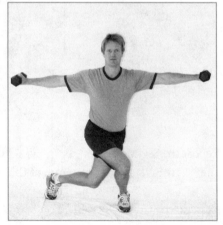

Start standing with your feet shoulder width apart, and dumbbells at your sides; then, keeping your weight on your right foot, take a big step back with your left leg, crossing it behind your right leg (as if about to do a curtsy) while raising your arms out to the sides, stopping at shoulder height. Slowly bend your knees and lower your body straight down until your front thigh is parallel to the floor, and both knees are bent at 90 degrees. Be sure to keep your abs drawn in and your back straight. As you lunge, keep your front knee directly over your ankle and don't let it roll in or out, your toes should point straight ahead. Alternate lunging side to side.

CORE CONDITIONING: SINGLE LEG BRIDGE WITH LEG EXTENSION

■ **6–8 REPS LEFT / 6–8 REPS RIGHT**

Lie on your back on the floor with your left leg bent 90 degrees, your left foot on the floor, and your right leg straight. Rest your arms on the floor, with your hands at your sides and palms pressing into the ground. Push off your left foot to lift your right leg, butt, and lower back off the floor as high as you can. *This is the starting position.* Keeping your pelvis lifted up high and stable, lower and lift your right leg. Your pelvis should not move at all while lowering and lifting your leg. Perform all reps on right side then switch sides.

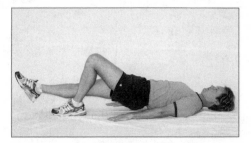

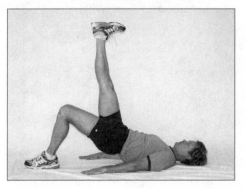

LOWER BODY BLAST: SLIDING SINGLE LEG REVERSE LUNGES WITH RESISTANCE TUBING ROWS

■ 10 REPS LEFT / 10 REPS RIGHT

Secure resistance tubing to a door, at waist level, using the door attachment. Hold the bands taut in front of you, one handle in each hand with palms facing inward. Stand with feet shoulder width apart and place a gliding disc (not shown) under each foot (athletic socks may work fine depending on the flooring). Slide your right foot back into a deep lunge. Draw your elbows back, bringing your hands to your rib cage. Stand back up. Repeat 10 reps on right leg then switch sides.

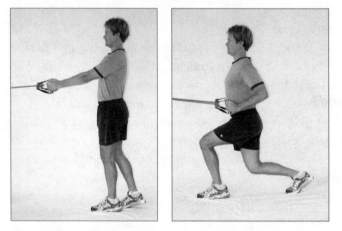

CORE CONDITIONING: OBLIQUE PLANK

■ 8 REPS LEFT / 8 REPS RIGHT

Lie on your right side with your knees straight. Prop your upper body up on your right elbow and forearm. Raise your hips so that your torso is higher than parallel to the floor. Pause, and then lower yourself back to starting position. Repeat all reps on left side and then switch to the right.

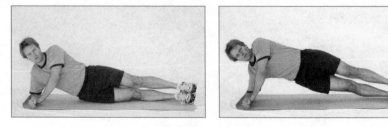

LOWER BODY BLAST: IN AND OUT PLYO SQUAT

■ **15 REPS**

Start standing with feet slightly wider than hip width. Bend your knees   237
and sit hips back into a low squat. Clasp your hands then jump straight
up, until both feet leave the ground (you don't need to jump high). Land
softly with your feet together, and sit back into a narrow squat position.
Repeat your jump again, landing with your feet wide next time. Alternate
landing your jumps in a narrow and wide squat, bringing feet in and then
out each time you lower. If you have a back or knee injury, you can omit the
jump and just squat up and down with your feet apart at shoulder width.

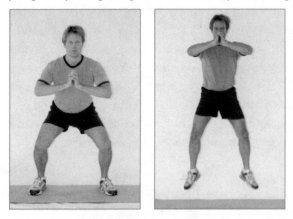

CORE CONDITIONING: ON THE BALL REVERSE HYPEREXTENSIONS

■ **15 REPS**

Lie on your stomach over the top of a stability ball with your hands and
forearms on the ground and your legs extended behind the ball, feet together
resting on the floor. Keeping your upper body stable, use your glutes to lift
your legs and create a straight diagonal line with your upper body. Keep
your shoulders back and down as you squeeze your glutes and inner thighs
together. Be sure to initiate the movement from your center, not your feet.

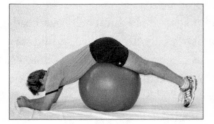 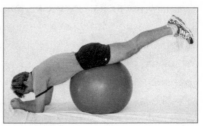

LOWER BODY BLAST: RUNNERS CROUCH TO REAR LEG LIFT
WITH STRAIGHT ARM TRICEPS SQUEEZES

▪ **12 REPS LEFT / 12 REPS RIGHT (2 POUNDS)**

Start standing with your feet together. Take a big step backward with your right leg. Reaching toward your left foot with both dumbbells, hinging slightly forward from your hips, bend both knees into a low lunge (be sure to keep your left knee directly over your left ankle at the bottom of your lunge; don't let your knee extend past your toes). Your right knee should be pointed straight down to the floor (like a sprinter about to start running). Next, press your body weight into your left leg and push down through your left foot as you stand up out of the lunge, lifting your right leg off the floor and straight up behind your hip. Your upper body should maintain the hinged forward position as you elevate with your back straight and abs tight and raise your arms straight behind you (you should feel your triceps muscles in the back of your arms working). Balance for one count and then lower back down into the lunge. If it's too hard to stand on one leg, try tapping your right foot lightly on the floor behind you as you stand up out of the lunge. Repeat 12 reps and then switch to the other side.

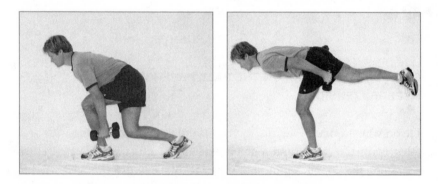

COMBO CORE CONDITIONING AND LOWER BODY BLAST:
SIDE STEP TO KNEE AND ARM RAISE

▪ **12–15 REPS LEFT / 12–15 REPS RIGHT (2 POUNDS)**

Start standing with your feet hip width apart, hold dumbbells overhead. Take a wide step to the side with your left foot (your right leg should stay extended), and bend your left knee, pushing your hips behind you. Keep your back flat, eyes looking straight ahead, touching the ground with your dumbbells. Push back to the start position and lift the dumbbells straight overhead. Complete 12 to 15 reps on each leg.

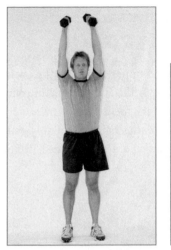
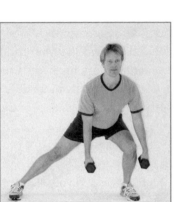

▶ Repeat Super Set 1 for a total of two times.

Super Set 2: Upper Body Blast and Core Conditioning

UPPER BODY BLAST: PLANK WITH PUSHUPS AND ALTERNATING ROWS

■ **10 TOTAL REPS (5–8 POUNDS)**

Holding dumbbells shoulder width apart on the floor, get into a bent-knee pushup position (balancing on your dumbbells and knees). Your shoulders should be directly over your hands, and your body should be in a straight line with abdominal muscles contracted. Row your left elbow behind your body, stopping at the middle of your back. Lower your arm to the floor as you lower into a pushup position. Push back up and repeat, alternating arms.

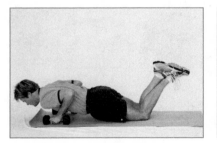
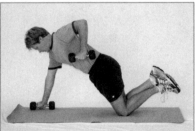

CORE CONDITIONING: SEATED RUSSIAN TWIST WITH MEDICINE BALL

■ **20 REPS**

Sit on the floor with your knees bent and your upper body leaning back slightly. Hold the medicine ball in your hands, extended out in front of your body. Keeping your torso completely still, rotate the medicine ball from side to side. To make the movement more difficult either increase the range of motion, the speed of your movements, or the weight of the medicine ball.

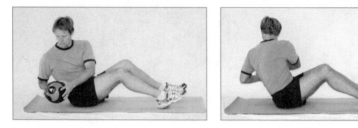

UPPER BODY BLAST: SPEEDY DUMBBELL BOXING

■ **100 ALTERNATING FAST PUNCHES IN FRONT OF BODY (2 POUNDS)**

Standing with your feet shoulder width apart, hold the dumbbells in front of your shoulders, making sure your palms are facing you. Turn your wrist over as you extend one arm in front of you, and then quickly bring it back to the starting point. Alternate arms so you have constant movement. Keep your core tight and do not lock your elbows when you punch out (keep your elbows slightly bent or soft when you extend your arms). Increase your speed to make this more challenging.

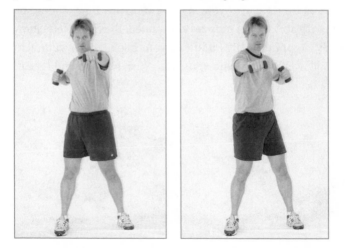

CORE CONDITIONING: RESISTANCE TUBING LIFTS (LOW TO HIGH)

■ **10 REPS LEFT / 10 REPS RIGHT**

Attach the resistance tubing to a stable object near your ankles. Clasp the band with both hands, and stand so that your right side faces the anchor. Keeping your arms fully extended and keeping both hands on the handle of the resistance tubing, rotate your arms up from slightly below your knees up to beyond shoulder height; the resistance increases as you elevate your arms. Pause, then return to the starting position. Complete all reps on one side, then switch sides and repeat.

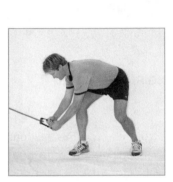 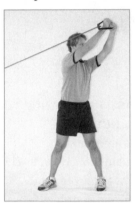

UPPER BODY BLAST: SUPER SLOW SINGLE ARM BENT OVER DUMBBELL ROW

■ **12 REPS LEFT / 12 REPS RIGHT (10–12 POUNDS)**

Bend over at the hips, holding one dumbbell straight down with one arm. Your back should be flat, with your spine in a straight line. Squeeze your shoulder blades together to row the dumbbell up very slowly (5 counts up) to your side, then lower the weight very slowly (5 counts down) to the starting position. Repeat all reps on one side and then switch sides.

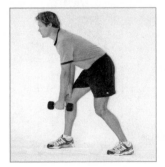 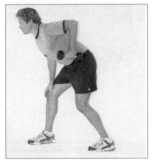

CORE CONDITIONING: PLANK WITH ALTERNATING KNEE PULLS

■ 16–20 REPS

Get in the basic plank position, with your hands under your shoulders and weight on the balls of your feet. Pull your abdominals in toward your spine and try to lengthen your body from your head to your feet. Keeping your abs strong, pull your left knee toward your left shoulder while rounding your back. Return to start position and repeat, alternating knees.

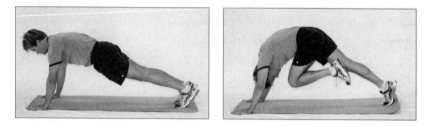

UPPER BODY BLAST: RESISTANCE TUBING REAR DELTOID FLY (STAGGER STANCE)

■ 10 REPS LEFT / 10 REPS RIGHT

Attach resistance tubing to a door, level with your chest, using the door attachment. Stand in a stagger stance, with one foot slightly in front of the other (see photo) and your toes forward and abdominal muscles contracted. Grasp the resistance tubing handles with your palms facing each other and shoulders back. Pull the tube out to both sides and then back with slightly bent arms. Return to start position and repeat. Do 10 reps with one leg forward and then switch legs.

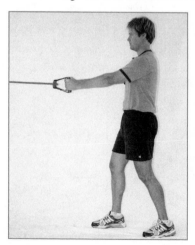
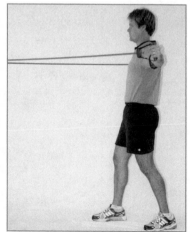

CORE CONDITIONING: STANDING ISOMETRIC TORSO TWISTS WITH TOWEL

■ **10 REPS LEFT / 10 REPS RIGHT**

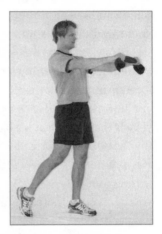

Stand with your feet hip width apart and hold onto the ends of a medium-size hand towel. Raise your arms in front of your chest and pull the towel taut (you should immediately feel the muscles in your upper body being activated; the harder you pull the towel the more intense the exercise). Keeping constant tension on the towel, quickly twist to the left about 12 inches, raising your right foot off the ground and rotating your right knee inward as you twist. Perform 10 quick twists on the left then switch sides to twist to the right 10 times.

UPPER BODY BLAST: ISOMETRIC FINGER LOCK CHEST PULL

■ **PERFORM TO FATIGUE**

Lock both middle fingers together. Pull hard and as doing so, slowly lift your hands from waist to above your head and back down again.

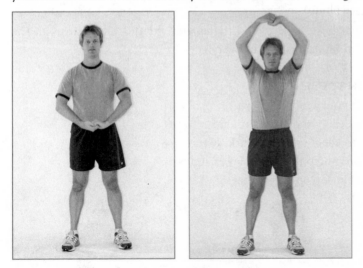

► Repeat Super Set 2 for a total of two times.
► Next, do the Cool Down BLTs on Stability Ball (page 222).
► Conclude with the Cool Down Post-Workout Stretch (page 255).

Workout 4: Stretch Yoga Workout

This yoga workout is much more than just a stretch routine; it's a full-body toning and strengthening workout that will help elongate your body, calm your mind, and take your fitness to a whole new level. Yoga will absolutely improve flexibility, but it also strengthens weaker muscle groups while simultaneously training stronger muscle groups. And it's not easy! Don't for a minute think that this workout is a rest day because we guarantee you'll work hard in each and every pose. One of the things we love about yoga is that it cultivates a balanced body and balanced strength by requiring the body to work as a whole. Yoga also calms your mind and helps you stay present. It's important to take deep long breaths through your nose throughout the entire workout; check in with yourself periodically, and if you find yourself breathing short and fast then guide your breath back to long and deep.

▶ You may skip the Fusion Activation Warmup because the yoga sequence effectively warms up your body.

Fat-Burning Sequence

Stay in each pose for 5 deep inhales and exhales. Flow through the sequence from one position to the next.

CHAIR (ON TOES)

Stand with your feet under your hips. Bend your knees deeply and extend your arms overhead. Try to keep a straight back by tucking your tailbone and pulling your lower abdominal muscles in. Go up on your toes if you can.

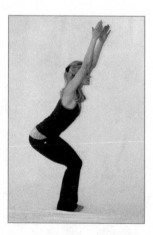

STANDING FORWARD BEND, CALF HOLD

Stand with your feet together. Bend your hips and knees deeply and carefully fold your torso over your legs, beginning with your belly and then your middle ribs. Grab your calves, bending your elbows slightly out to the sides. Straighten your legs as best you can.

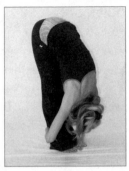

PLANK

Squat down with your hands by your feet. Jump back and straighten your legs so you are in one horizontal line, bringing your shoulder blades together. Make sure your hands are under your shoulders and your fingers spread wide. Keep your elbows straight, but do not lock your elbows; they should be slightly soft.

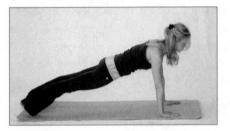

CHATURANGA

From plank pose, rock forward on toes so that your weight is more in the front of the body. Hands should be directly beneath your shoulders. Bend your elbows so they point straight back along your ribs and lower yourself to the floor. Pause when your upper arms are parallel to floor. Push up through your hands and transition to Upward Facing Dog pose by scooping forward and brushing your chest just above the floor. Keeping your palms pressed down, straighten your arms, roll your shoulders down and back, and press your chest forward. Keep your thighs and shins on the floor. This should be done as one smooth movement.

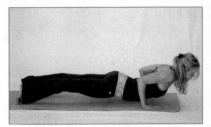
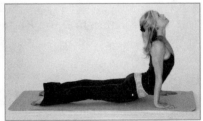

DOWN DOG

246

Spread your fingers wide on the mat, make sure your wrists are under your shoulders and your knees are under your hips. Walk or jump your feet back, lift your hips, and press your heels toward the floor. Relax your shoulders and head. Press your palms toward the floor.

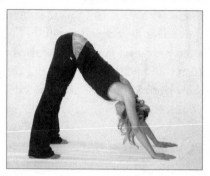

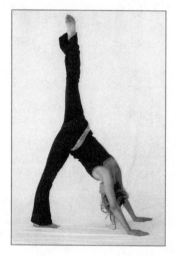

DOWN DOG SPLIT (RIGHT LEG)

From the Down Dog position lift your right leg up high behind you, pointing your toes. Keep your shoulders square to the floor, keep your fingers spread wide and press your palms to the floor.

KNEE TO FOREHEAD (RIGHT LEG)

Keeping your palms pressed to the ground, lift your hips and bring your right knee to your forehead, rounding your upper back.

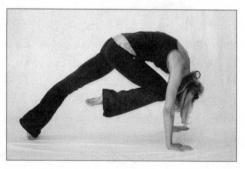

▶ Exhale, return to Down Dog Split, and repeat these two poses five more times.

KNEE TO CROSS LIFT (RIGHT LEG)

Keeping your palms pressed to the ground, slightly bend your elbows and bring your right knee across to the back of your left upper arm. Roll onto the inner edges of the toes of your left foot.

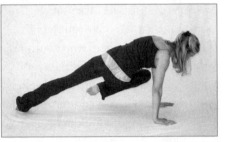

247

▶ Exhale, return to Down Dog Split, and repeat these two poses five more times.

RUNNERS LUNGE (RIGHT LEG)

Step forward with your right foot and extend your left leg straight behind you. Press your fingertips on the floor with one hand on each side of your right foot. Your right leg should be bent deeply and your left leg should be straight.

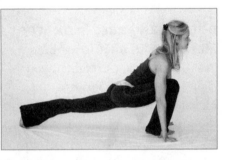

WARRIOR LUNGE PRESS (RIGHT LEG)

Bend your right knee over your right foot so your thigh is parallel to the floor. Extend your arms straight up over your ears. Put some weight onto your left foot, but keep your left heel off the ground. Sink your hips and relax your shoulders. Press up and down into a lunge position. Repeat for a total of six Warrior Lunge Presses. Note that the photo shows the up position.

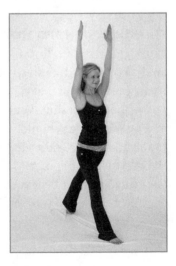

WARRIOR LUNGE PRESS AND TWIST (RIGHT LEG)

Moving on from the top position of Warrior Lunge Press, reach your left arm forward and your right arm back and open your torso to your right side as you sink your hips toward the ground. Make sure your shoulders are over your hips. Relax your shoulders and look back over your right hand. Press up from the lunge and return to the top of Warrior Lunge Press position. Continue pressing up and down into a lunge as you twist. Repeat for a total of six Warrior Lunge Press and Twists.

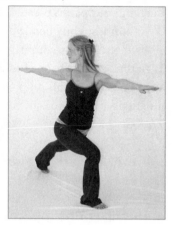

ROTATED TRIANGLE (RIGHT FOOT FORWARD)

Moving on from Warrior Lunge Press and Twist, straighten your right leg and hinge forward at the hips, lowering your right palm to the ground and placing it on the floor on the outside of your right foot (or on your shin). Extend your arms straight and open your shoulders. Look up to face your left hand.

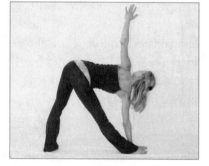

TRIANGLE (RIGHT FOOT FORWARD)

Moving on from Rotated Triangle, keep your legs straight and rotate your torso so that your chest faces right, extending your arms and opening your shoulders back toward the left side. Leading with the right side of your ribs, bring your shoulders out over your right leg, and either place your left hand

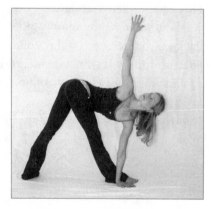

on your right shin or press your fingertips to the mat outside of your right foot. Open your torso and look up toward your right hand.

▶ Repeat the entire Fat Burning Sequence but change up your feet so that starting with Down Dog Split you are using your left leg. Go through the entire sequence a total of four times (two on the right and two on the left).

Lower Body Toning Sequence

Stay in each pose for five deep inhales and exhales. Flow through the sequence starting with your *right* leg.

WARRIOR 2 (RIGHT LEG)
Open your hips and shoulders to face your right side. Press through the outside edge of your left foot and lengthen your spine as you sink your hips low. Extend your right arm forward and your left arm back so they are parallel to the floor, reaching out evenly forward and back through your arms and fingertips. Focus your gaze over your right hand.

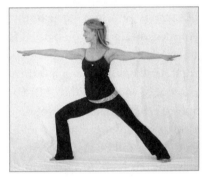

REVERSE WARRIOR (RIGHT LEG)
Keeping your hips low in Warrior 2, in one big movement cartwheel your arms back toward your left leg (touch the floor if you can). Extend your right arm straight up and square your hips. Look up toward your right hand.

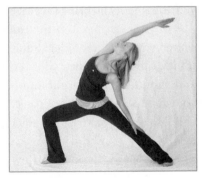

WARRIOR 3 WITH FINGERTIPS ON FLOOR (RIGHT LEG)

Moving on from Reverse Warrior in one big movement cartwheel your arms back over toward the right, shifting your weight into your right leg and straightening your leg, lifting your hips and raising your left leg until it is parallel to the floor. Flex your left foot, and press your fingertips against the floor a few inches in front of your right foot.

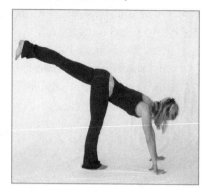

HALF MOON (STANDING ON RIGHT LEG)

Moving on from Warrior 3 with Fingertips on Floor keep both of your legs straight as you twist at the waist, placing the fingertips of your right hand on the floor a few inches in front of your right foot. Lift your left leg behind you, flexing your foot. Open your hips, torso, and shoulders to the left, and bring your left arm straight up. Look toward your left hand.

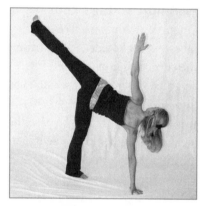

TWISTED HALF MOON (STANDING ON RIGHT LEG)

Moving on from Half Moon stay on your right foot and bring the fingertips of your left hand to the floor under your left shoulder. Square off your hips, then open your torso and shoulder to the right and lift your right arm straight up. You can check to see if your hips are square by dropping your head and making sure your left foot is pointing down.

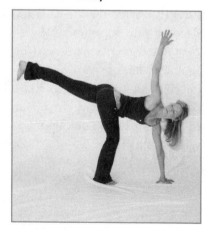

▶ Repeat the entire Lower Body Toning Sequence on your *left side.*
Go through this entire sequence a total of four times (two on the
right and two on the left).

Balance Sequence

Stay in each pose for five deep inhales and exhales.

TREE POSE WITH PRAYER PRESS
(STANDING ON LEFT LEG)

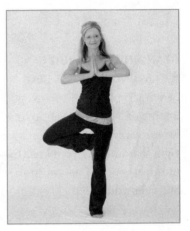

Balance on your left leg, pressing the
sole of your left foot into the ground.
Grab your right ankle with your right
hand. Place your right foot on the inside
of your left upper thigh, pressing the
soles of your right foot into your thigh.
When you feel steady, stand up straight
and press your palms together in prayer
position. Press your palms together as
hard as you can to activate the muscles
in your upper body.

STANDING TWISTED LEG EXTENSION
(STANDING ON LEFT LEG)

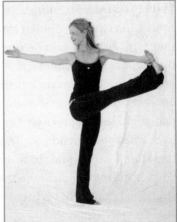

Moving on from Tree Pose with Prayer
Press, continue balancing on your left
leg, bend your right knee to your chest
and grab the outside of your right foot
with your left hand. Lengthen out of
your lower back and extend your right
leg forward. Open your torso toward
the right and extend your right arm
behind you, parallel to the floor. Look
toward your right hand.

AIRPLANE (STANDING ON LEFT LEG)

252

Moving on from Standing Twisted Leg Extension, continue balancing on your left leg and bring your right leg back, bending forward until your right leg and chest are parallel to ground (be sure to keep a flat back and concentrate on keeping your abs tight). Extend arms out to the side in airplane pose.

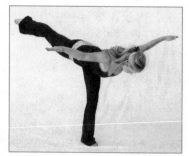

STANDING SHIN HUG
(STANDING ON LEFT LEG)

Moving on from Airplane, continue balancing on your left leg, moving your right leg forward, wrap your hands around your right shin and hug your knee to your chest. Stand up as tall as you possibly can to lengthen your back.

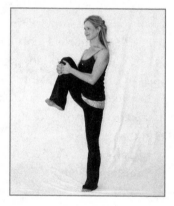

BIG TOE HOLD
(STANDING ON LEFT LEG)

Moving on from Standing Shin Hug, continue balancing on your left leg and bring the forefinger and middle finger of your right hand around your right big toe. Rest your left hand on your left hip for balance. Lengthen your back, and straighten your right leg. Do not sacrifice a straight back when you extend your leg; it is more important to keep your back straight and your standing leg straight than it is to straighten the leg that is lifted.

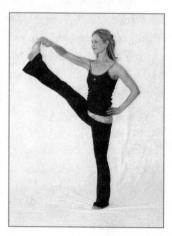

DANCER (STANDING ON LEFT LEG)

Moving on from Big Toe Hold, continue balancing on your left leg, come back to Standing Shin Hug, and grab the inside of your right shin (or ankle) with your right hand. Raise your right leg as high as you can behind you while continuing to hold your shin with your right hand. Reach your left arm up to counterbalance. Press your ankle or shin into your hand for additional stabilization.

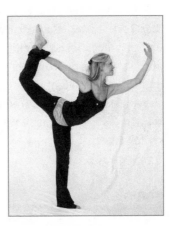

▶ Repeat the entire Balance Sequence standing on your *right leg*. Go through the entire sequence a total of four times (two on the right and two on the left).

On the Mat

CAT AND COW WITH LEG EXTENSION

■ **10 REPS RIGHT / 10 REPS LEFT**

Get on all fours with your hands shoulder width apart and your knees directly under your hips. Reach your right arm forward at shoulder height and reach your left leg behind you to hip height, keeping your toe and knee pointing downward. Bend your right arm and left knee toward your chest as your draw your abs in and round your spine, like a cat. Repeat 10 times and switch sides.

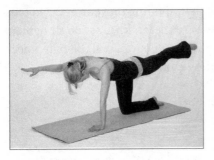
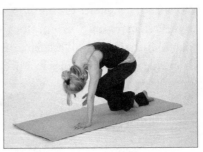

SIDE PLANK LIFTS ON FOREARM

Start on left side, left forearm and hip on floor, feet stacked. Lift hips to create a straight line from feet to head, and extend the right arm to sky (as shown). Hold for three counts then return to start. Repeat 10 times and switch sides.

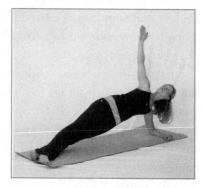

BRIDGE

Lie down on your back with your knees bent and feet flat on the floor. Place your hands on the floor next to your hips and gently lift your hips, pressing your arms into the floor. Lace your fingers together and press them toward your feet. Wiggle

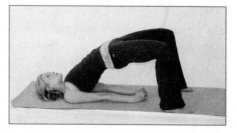

your shoulder blades together, and press your chest toward your chin. Keep your feet flat on the floor, and reach your hips up even farther. Hold for 5 deep inhales and exhales.

BICYCLES

■ **40–50 REPS**

Lie face up on your mat and place your hands behind your head lightly supporting it with your fingers. Bring your knees in to your chest and lift your shoulder blades off the floor without pulling on your neck. Rotate to the left, bringing the right elbow toward the left knee as you straighten the other leg. Switch sides, bringing the left elbow toward the right knee. Continue alternating sides in a pedaling motion for 40 to 50 reps.

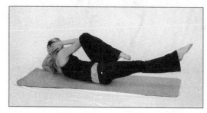
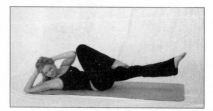

▶ The Cool Down BLTs on Stability Ball and Cool Down Post-Workout Stretch are not needed after the Stretch Yoga Workout.

Cool Down Post-Workout Stretch

The Cool Down Post-Workout Stretch routine targets all of your major muscles and will help speed recovery and reduce muscle imbalances. It is important not to rush through the stretches. **You want to hold each stretch for 30 to 60 seconds.** To relax your body, take big breaths in and out through your nose while you stretch.

FLOOR SPINAL TWIST (FOR UPPER AND LOWER BACK)

Sit on the floor with both legs extended straight in front of you. Cross your right leg over your left. Position your right foot near the outside of your left knee. Press your left arm against your right knee and thigh, pushing slightly, while rotating your shoulders, torso, and head to the right as far as you comfortably 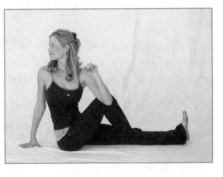 can. Hold the stretch for at least 30 seconds then switch sides and repeat.

LUNGING HIP STRETCH (FOR HIPS, QUADS, BUTT, BACK)

Position yourself on the floor, kneeling on both knees. Bring your right knee up and place your right foot in front of your body, keeping your right knee directly over your right ankle. Keep your back straight by placing both hands on your right thigh and pushing your upper torso backward. Hold the stretch for at least 30 seconds then switch sides and repeat.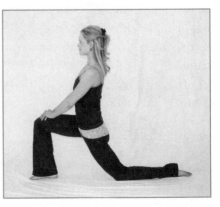

LYING TOWEL STRETCH COMBO (FOR HAMSTRINGS, CALVES, LOWER BACK, AND HIPS)

256 Lie on your back with your legs extended in front of your body. Wrap a towel around the middle of your left foot, and bring your straight or slightly bent leg up toward the ceiling while holding on to both ends of the towel until you feel the stretch in your hamstring. Apply continuous tension so your left leg gradually goes back farther throughout the stretch. Hold the stretch for at least 30 seconds and then repeat with the right leg.

Now, bring the towel around the top of your left foot and apply continuous tension so that your left calf gradually goes back farther throughout the stretch. This time you want to dorsiflex (pull) your foot forward toward your leg more so that you feel the stretch in your calf more than your hamstring. Hold the stretch for at least 30 seconds and then repeat with the right leg.

Drop the towel and lay your left leg across your body, keeping both shoulders flat on the floor, your left arm flat on the floor and your right elbow bent at a 90-degree angle. Hold the stretch for at least 30 seconds and then repeat with the right leg.

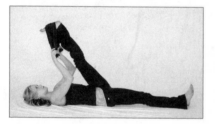 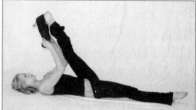

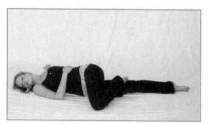

FIGURE FOUR STRETCH
(FOR GLUTES AND INNER THIGHS)

Hold on to a chair for support, cross your right ankle on top of your left thigh, and slightly bend your left leg. Gently press your hips back as if you were going to sit in a chair. Hold the stretch for at least 30 seconds and then switch sides and repeat.

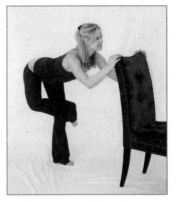

257

CHEST EXPANSION
(FOR SHOULDERS AND CHEST)

Stand with your feet hip width apart and legs slightly bent. Contract your abdominal muscles and keep your head, neck, and shoulders relaxed. Clasp your hands behind your back, and keeping your back straight, lift your arms behind you until you feel the stretch across your chest. Hold the stretch for at least 30 seconds.

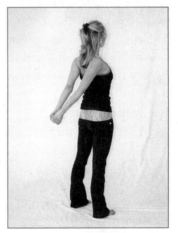

Sizzle Cardio Interval Workout (Optional)

Why is cardio interval training better than regular steady-state cardio? Cardio interval training challenges the body by continually surprising it with varying intensities. The problem with steady-state cardio is that your body gets better at it . . . quickly. Do a lot of steady-state cardio, and your body soon learns how to conserve fat and nutrients so that it can perform the activity in the most efficient way possible. But when fat loss is the goal, it's not efficiency we are looking for; we want to go for the biggest possible afterburn effect, which is exactly what cardio interval training delivers. Cardio interval training will help you shed fat super fast.

Perform this 15- to 20-minute workout one day per week either after your strength workout or on a different day.

Use any cardiovascular machine (bike, elliptical trainer, stair stepper, treadmill, and so on), and change it up frequently. Remember, the more variety the more you surprise your body!

THE ROUTINE

1. Warm up for 5 minutes at a light to moderate pace.
2. Perform 1 minute as fast as you can (at a level 8 or 9 intensity on a scale of 1 to 10), and then recover at a moderate pace for 1 minute (at a level 5 or 6 intensity). Repeat 7 to 10 times.
3. Cool down for 5 minutes at a light to moderate pace, at an intensity level less than 4.

The simple concept of cardio interval training can make your cardio efforts much more effective and rewarding. We do encourage cardio interval training as an optional challenge for those of you who love cardio workouts beginning in the third week of our 8-week Clean Cuisine Program (Chapter 9).

9

THE CLEAN CUISINE 8-WEEK PROGRAM
Putting It All Together to Change the Way You Age, Look, and Feel

Lots of people know what to do, but few people actually do what they know. Knowing is not enough! You must take action.
—ANTHONY ROBBINS

By now you should have a very clear understanding of the science behind Clean Cuisine. You should know just about everything you need to know to make the changes that will have a real impact on how you age, look, and feel. Now it's time to apply the science you've learned to everyday real life. And, by the way, we *so* hope you didn't just skip the science and jump ahead to this part! If you were a page skipper, we urge you to go back and read everything, otherwise you won't have a clear understanding as to why we make the recommendations we make.

Our recommendations are distinctly different from what you might find in other diet and nutrition books because we don't encourage you to count your food in the form of calories, points, fat grams, and so forth. Instead, we give you guidelines for choosing a balanced diet based on nutrient-dense, anti-inflammatory whole foods, and then let your appetite naturally regulate your intake. Also, instead of encouraging you to elimi-nate foods from the get-go, we start by asking you to focus on *increasing*

259

your intake of super good-for-you foods. By the end of 8 weeks you'll be so full and so well nourished you won't have room for, or cravings for, unhealthful foods. Studies show it's more psychologically sound to focus on positive changes. The incremental approach helps too. When people take our Health and Body Makeover Programs, they repeatedly tell us that by making small changes week by week they feel less overwhelmed so they actually stick to the program. By the end of the 8 weeks you will have learned, step by step, how to totally revamp your lifestyle and how to make Clean Cuisine living second nature. So without further chitchat let's jump right in to week 1.

CLEAN CUISINE CUSTOMIZED NUTRITION AND WELLNESS PROGRAM

WE REALIZE SOME people have special medical issues or food allergies that might require a customized program. Other people might simply want the support and accountability of a health coach to stay motivated and keep on track. Every great athlete or successful person will agree that to be successful you need some type of mentor or coach. The same is true when it comes to your health. We know that optimal health is a choice. Health is a result of the things we eat, the drinks we drink, the lifestyles we live, and the thoughts we think. Our Clean Cuisine Nutrition Coaches can assist you in helping to restore your body's true function and health with a thorough analysis of all the systems in the body. We work with cutting-edge testing and analysis to assess the areas of concern in your body and develop a customized care plan and program based on your evaluation and test results. By understanding your individual challenges, our coaches can help you take action and accomplish your health goals. To meet the needs of everyone, we have set up an online Clean Cuisine Customized Nutrition and Wellness Program. For more information visit www.CleanCuisineNutritionProgram.com.

Week 1

Focus

Got Phytonutrients?

3 Big Changes to Make This Week

- Start the day right. Eat a Clean Cuisine breakfast containing fruit every day. Check out our easy mix-and-match breakfasts and delicious recipe ideas starting on page 305.
- Redefine lunch. Eat a phytonutrient-rich Clean Cuisine lunch that includes a *huge* salad, or cooked vegetables, or vegetable soup every day. Our easy mix-and-match lunch suggestions and delicious recipes start on page 315.
- Go for a once-a-day phytonutrient-rich green pick-me-up. Drink a SuperGreen Smoothie at some point in the day, either first thing in the morning, in the midmorning, or in the midafternoon. Green smoothies can be made up to 24 hours in advance so long as they are mixed up a bit before serving. Our delicious smoothie creations, which can be made in less than 5 minutes, start on page 344.

  NOTE: SuperGreen Smoothies contain chia seeds for an omega-3 and fiber boost.

Nutritional Enhancement

Start taking a phytonutrient-rich supplement every day. Many greens supplements exist, but we like Juice Plus+ capsules for their convenience and the powdered phytonutrient boosters you can mix with water, such as Barlean's Greens, Green Vibrance, and New Chapter Berry Green.

NOTE: Mixing lemon juice with your phytonutrient booster can help cut the taste of the greens.

Challenge of the Week

Don't eat if you are not hungry. We can't emphasize the importance of this enough. Even if it is meal time, if you are not hungry, *don't eat*! Some people think they must eat first thing when they get up in order to ignite their metabolisms. This is absolutely not true. If you are not hungry first thing in the morning don't eat. Don't eat until you get hungry. If you don't happen to get hungry until 10:45 then 10:45 is breakfast time. This applies to the rest of the day as well. You will never experience optimal wellness or achieve your ideal body weight if you eat when you are not hungry.

Time-Saving Clean Cuisine Cooking Tip

We totally understand the challenges and constraints of day-to-day life, and we realize it isn't always easy to prepare a homespun meal every day of the week. We encourage you to plan ahead by getting in the habit of cooking big batches of super healthy foods that pay big leftover dividends. You cook once then eat twice, three times, or even more! Some of the foods we like to prepare in big batches are Sauces That Make the Meal (page 351), big pots of beans (page 336), cooked greens (page 400), slow-cooked meals and casseroles (page 369), and veggie soups (page 325). Having these sauces, healthy recipes, and tasty meals already prepared makes eating Clean Cuisine much more doable in the real world.

Sample Meal Plan for Week 1

▶ **BREAKFAST**

WEEKDAY BASIC BREAKFAST

- If you aren't particularly active or you tend not to be a big breakfast eater try a light No-Milk Shake breakfast made with fruit and nuts (page 310).
- If you are active or prefer a heartier breakfast try a Great Grains and Fruit Combo or a no-cook muesli (page 307), either drizzled with some hemp cream (page 306) or sprinkled with hemp seeds, flaxseeds, chia seeds, or finely chopped raw nuts. The fruit to grain ratio should be 2 to 1 (perhaps 1 cup fruit to ½ cup grains).
- If you are super hungry in the mornings try our basic recipe for Scrambled Eggs-N-Veggies (page 309), made with 2 pastured

organic eggs and ¾ cup of chopped vegetables. Eat your eggs with any fresh fruit.

WEEKDAY SUPER RUSH

- If you are super busy or on the go and want a ready-to-eat breakfast cereal, the following whole grain cereals are healthy options. Be sure to add fruit and keep your fruit to grain ratio 2 to 1. If you choose to add milk, use hemp milk, almond milk, or soy milk, but no cow's milk!

    Uncle Sam Original Cereal

    Post Shredded Wheat'n Bran

    Ezekiel 4:9 Sprouted Whole Grain Cereal (any variety)

LAID-BACK WEEKEND

- If you have the time, try making our Chia-Crusted French Toast with sprouted whole grain bread (page 308) or Gluten-Free Millet Pancakes (page 307). Be sure to also add fresh fruit!

WHAT TO DRINK WITH BREAKFAST

- Coffee with a little organic pastured cream or milk and green tea are both allowed. But no juice!

▶ LUNCH

WEEKDAY BASIC LUNCH

- Have a veggie soup or large salad along with ½ Loaded Baked Potato or 1 whole Sweet Potato Combo (page 323).
- Have a big bowl of beans or legumes (page 336), either by themselves or on top of cooked whole grains, such as brown rice, quinoa, millet, or amaranth. Our bean recipes include vegetables but be sure to add additional vegetables as a side dish too. A simple salad of dark greens like arugula, watercress, or spinach fills the bill. Or try a side of cooked greens (page 400).

WEEKDAY SUPER RUSH

- Make a 5-minute Clean Cuisine Super Salad. See our guide to creating super salads and our salad mix-and-match chart (page 322).

    NOTE: *If you have a big appetite add some sprouted whole grain bread (such as Food for Life brand) or a side of cooked whole grains.*

- If you want a more substantial salad try making it into a wrap! Wrap up your 5-minute Clean Cuisine Super Salad in a sprouted whole grain tortilla. Food for Life brand tortillas are a great choice.

LAID-BACK WEEKEND

If you have time to prepare something more elaborate, head on over to our recipe collection and check out recipe ideas in the Whole Grains and Earthy Sides section. Be sure to add a nice big salad for a complete meal. Or try one of our pasta recipes (page 369). Again, just be sure to add a big salad or some cooked greens. For a lighter lunch try a recipe from Vegilicious Sides (page 405) served along with some simple cooked whole grains or beans. Canned beans are fine, just look for a BPA-free brand such as Eden Organic.

WHAT TO DRINK WITH LUNCH

- Water, sparkling water, or green tea.

EARLY MORNING, MIDMORNING OR MIDAFTERNOON PICK-ME-UP

- Have a SuperGreen Smoothie (page 344) to further increase your phytonutrient intake.

▶ DINNER

We don't want to overwhelm you by giving you specific dinner guidelines. Instead, ask yourself the following questions:

- How can I add more vegetables and more greens to my dinner?
- Am I eating big portions of animal foods like chicken, beef, cheese, and pork? If so, how can I reduce my portion size of these foods?
- Am I keeping oil to a minimum?
- If I eat dessert can I add fruit? Better yet, can I make the fruit to dessert ratio more favorable, at least 3 parts fruit to 1 part dessert? Or how about a fruit-only dessert drizzled with our Spirited Chocolate Sauce (page 427).

WHAT TO DRINK WITH DINNER?

- Water, sparkling water, and/or a glass of wine.

NOTE: We won't have you start our Full Fitness Fusion workout program this week because we don't want to overwhelm you. When it comes to reducing inflammation and making the biggest dent in how you age, look, and feel, your food choices matter most. We would rather you focus your energy on cleaning up your diet before you start a formal exercise program.

Week 2

Focus

Continue with all of the changes you made in your lifestyle last week. The Full Fitness Fusion focus is strength this week.

3 BIG CHANGES TO MAKE THIS WEEK

- Begin the Strength Workout (page 216). This is to be performed on nonconsecutive days 3 days per week.
- Add in 1 cup of cooked greens (pages 400–404) or a large dark leafy green side salad (for example, arugula, watercress, spinach, Romaine, and mâche) with every one of your evening meals.
- Start consciously to reduce your consumption of animal foods like chicken, beef, and cheese. When you do eat animal foods, make sure they are of the absolute highest quality, as discussed in Chapter 6. Ideally you will not eat more than one animal food per day (with the exception of eggs); we encourage you to be ovo-vegetarians until dinnertime and to include fish or shellfish on your dinner menu at least three days a week. We also urge you to do meat-free Mondays (we've included some of our family's favorite dinners in Part Four).

Nutritional Enhancement

Take a broad-spectrum high-quality multivitamin, multimineral supplement every day, as recommended in a report published in the *Journal of the American Medical Association.*[1] Think of your multivitamin, multimineral supplement as a daily insurance policy. Everybody needs one, the problem is which one to choose? If you head to your natural foods store you'll be bombarded with a plethora of supplements lining the shelves, each one seemingly better than the next. You might just be tempted to buy the one that contains the most stuff. But when it comes to supplements, more is not always best. A multivitamin, multimineral supplement is designed to *complement* your anti-inflammatory Clean Cuisine diet but you don't want to go overboard. Getting an excess of certain nutrients such as iron, selenium, and copper can be toxic.

In addition to making sure you don't get too much of a good thing, it is equally important to seek out supplements containing the absolute very best ingredients. For example, you don't want a supplement that contains synthetic forms of vitamin E (DL-alpha-tocopherol). You don't even want one that contains just one of the natural forms of vitamin E (D-alpha tocopherol). Ideally, you want your supplement to reflect the way vitamin E is found in nature in real food, in the form of *mixed* tocopherols. When you hear about research linking vitamin E supplementation to negative health outcomes, it is important to note that in addition to other flaws, the research in those studies did not take into account the *type* of vitamin E that the subjects were taking. Supplementing with a reasonable dosage (not mega-dosing!) of natural vitamin E in the form of mixed tocopherols not only is safe but is an important strategy in reducing overall oxidative stress. The same thing for carotenoids; research has actually linked taking isolated beta-carotene to increased risk of lung cancer (in smokers anyway), but isolated beta-carotene is not something you would ever find in nature in your food. In food, you would obtain *mixed* carotenes. That's exactly what you want to look for in a supplement. You want to avoid supplements containing synthetic folic acid and instead look for one containing folate, which is the form naturally found in foods like green vegetables.

Balancing the fat-soluble vitamins A, D, and K is also critical. This is because when you take one fat-soluble vitamin you increase your body's need for the other fat-soluble vitamins. For example, one of the roles of vitamin D is to activate osteoblasts (bone-building cells) to increase bone density while one of the roles of vitamin A is to promote bone breakdown so that new bone can be laid down. Although these processes seem to oppose each other they are both necessary to maintain bone health. Vitamins A and D work closely together and if you take one you need to take the other. Also, taking vitamin D will increase your need for vitamin K2. There is an intimate relationship between fat-soluble vitamins, and they all play a vital role in optimizing health. Unfortunately, mainstream foods do not supply adequate amounts of vitamins A, D or K2, so supplementation is especially important.

And of course the bioavailability of the nutrients in your supplement is also important because if your body can't absorb and use what you ingest then why bother taking it? For example, minerals have a wide range of bioavailability, depending on the form they are in and what they are bonded to; chelated minerals are the absolute best because they are well absorbed by your body. As another example, if your supplement contains vitamin C, it also needs to contain bioflavonoids or you won't be able to fully absorb the vitamin C. Bioflavonoids also boost the activity of vitamin C once it has been absorbed.

If you are following our Clean Cuisine diet closely, the one potential drawback to eating less animal foods in your diet is that you could possibly shortchange yourself on vitamin B12. This will not be an issue for most people because Clean Cuisine is not a vegan diet. However, because some individuals need extra B12 and because some people do not effectively convert B12 supplements into the bioactive form their body can use, it is important to take a high-quality B12 supplement in the form of methylcobalamin.

> NOTE: *Vitamin B12 is water soluble so you don't need to worry about overdosing.*

Picking the perfect multivitamin/multimineral supplement is not exactly as easy as picking which flavor of bubble gum you like best. Here is a breakdown of approximately what you want to look for on a daily basis. We include these vitamins and minerals in our "Clean Cuisine Essentials" iron-free multi-vitamin multi-mineral supplement but you can also get these nutrients from a combination of other supplements on the market.

(Percent Daily Values (DV) are based on a 2000 calorie diet

VITAMIN/MINERAL	RECOMMENDED	DAILY VALUE
Vitamin A Palmitate	1,250 IU	25%
Natural Mixed Carotenes (alpha, beta, beta-cryptoxanthin, zeaxanthin & lutein)	7,500 IU	150%
Vitamin C (as calcium ascorbate & magnesium-potassium ascorbate complex)	600 mg	1000%
Vitamin D3 (as cholecalciferol)	1600 IU	400%

VITAMIN/MINERAL	RECOMMENDED	DAILY VALUE
Vitamin E (As D-alpha tocopherol succinate plus mixed tocopherols D-beta, D-delta, D-gamma)	200 IU	666%
Vitamin K (25% as vitamin K1 phytonadione and 75% as K2 menaquinone-7 from natto)	80 mcg	100%
Thiamine	50 mg	3333%
Vitamin B6	25 mg	1250%
Folate	400 mcg	100%
Vitamin B12	100 mcg	1666%
Biotin	150 mcg	50%
Pantothenic Acid	200 mg	2000%
Calcium	500 mg	50%
Iodine (from Kelp)	75 mcg	50%
Magnesium (75% as magnesium aspartate-ascorbate complex and 25% as magnesium glycinate chelate)	475 mg	94%
Zinc (as zinc glycinate chelate)	10 mg	67%
Selenium (as L-selenomethionine)	100 mcg	143%
Copper (as copper glycinate chelate)	1 mg	50%
Manganese (as manganese glycinate chelate)	1 mg	50%
Chromium (as chromium nicotinate glycinate chelate)	100 mcg	84%
Molybdenum (as molybdenum glycinate chelate)	75 mcg	100%
Potassium	50 mg	1.5%
Boron (as boron aspartate-citrate)	1 mg	N/A
Vanadium (as bisglycinato oxovanadium)	100 mcg	N/A
Choline (as choline bitartrate)	75 mg	N/A
Inositol	25 mg	N/A
Citrus Bioflavonoids	50 mg	N/A

Challenge of the Week

Rethink snacking and grazing. There is absolutely no proof that eating five or six times a day stokes or improves metabolism. If anything, in our experience working with people in our Health and Body Makeover Programs and in Andy's medical practice, snacking is one of the major diet habits that prevents people from losing weight and contributes substantially to the consumption of added empty calories. Unless it is an exercise day, the only real snack you should have on the Clean Cuisine program is your SuperGreen Smoothie. This isn't even really a snack because it is so very low in calories! If you get hungry try having some green tea instead. Not only is green tea loaded with antioxidants and anti-inflammatory agents, it also helps curb your appetite and even assists with weight loss.

Exercise is the one exception to our no snacking recommendations. We recognize some people (including Ivy) feel light-headed or get a low blood sugar sensation after exercising. If this applies to you, then we suggest having a small fruit and nut snack either before or after exercise. For the benefit of moderate exercisers, here are a few Clean Cuisine snack options that are loaded with nutrients and easy to digest. They are, therefore, just fine to eat before exercise as well:

> NOTE: *If you are particularly active and train hard or exercise competitively, you will want to consult with a holistic-minded sports nutritionist or one of our Clean Cuisine nutritionists (www.CleanCuisineNutritionProgram.com) because you will absolutely have increased energy demands.*

PRE- OR POST-EXERCISE SNACK IDEAS

- Good Greens bars are made with a proprietary blend of greens, vegetables, fruits, antioxidants, probiotics, and enzymes; these good-for-you bars pack a mighty nutrition punch. They come in a variety of tasty flavors, including chocolate raspberry, chocolate peanut butter (our favorite!!), chocolate coconut, and wildberry. For women, we suggest a half a Good Greens bar as a pre- or post-workout snack, and for active men we suggest a whole bar.
- Lärabars are available nationwide in natural foods stores and, unlike the vast majority of energy bars, they are made from the purest and simplest of ingredients—just fruit, nuts, and spices.

They taste amazing! There is a flavor for everyone too: key lime pie, apple pie, banana bread, blueberry muffin, carrot cake, chocolate coconut chew, ginger snap, to name just a few. For women, we suggest a half a Lärabar as a pre- or post-workout snack and for active men we suggest a whole bar.

- Small handful (about ⅓ cup) of homemade trail mix made with 1:1 ratio of dried organic fruit to raw nuts or seeds.
- Banana with 1 teaspoon raw almond butter.
- Apple slices with 1 teaspoon raw peanut butter.
- No-Milk Shakes (page 310): are rather filling so you may find you only need to drink a half a serving to refuel after a moderate workout.

Time-Saving Clean Cuisine Cooking Tip

Keep a big batch of cooked whole grains in your fridge at all times. See our chart on page 306 for how to easily cook whole grains using either the stovetop or a rice cooker. After they are cooked, whole grains will keep nicely in the fridge stored in a covered container for 3 days. Having whole grains ready-to-eat makes putting together Clean Cuisine meals super easy! For an incredibly delicious but easy-does-it dinner, try making one of our recipes from Sauces That Make the Meal (page 351). Serve the sauce with any cooked whole grain along with some beans (rinsed canned beans are fine) and lots of veggies. Frozen veggies such as chopped spinach and chopped kale are particularly good and can be thawed in the fridge overnight, heated in the microwave in no time, or stir-fried while still frozen with some extra-virgin olive oil or organic extra-virgin coconut oil and maybe some crushed garlic too.

Sample Meal Plan for Week 2

Because we are focusing on exercise, strength, convenience, and learning to love phytonutrients this week everything foodwise is the same as week 1, except we do ask you to add a 1 cup serving of cooked greens or a large dark leafy greens side salad (watercress, arugula, spinach, romaine, or mâche) to your dinner.

Week 3

Focus

The fat and oil change and the Clean Cuisine dinner, plus continue with all of the changes from last week. Full Fitness Fusion focus: continue performing the Strength Workout three times per week.

3 Big Changes to Make This Week

- Make a conscious effort to eat less oil in general and instead get the majority of your fat from healthy plant-based whole fats, such as raw nuts, raw seeds, avocado, olives, and coconut. Be sure to read the ingredients on all packaged foods you buy! Most packaged foods are made with too much oil,and most of the oils used are cheap, unhealthful, and highly processed oils.
- Cook with the right oils at the right temperature.
  - When you cook, use small amounts of the following heat-stable, antioxidant-rich oils: cold-pressed extra-virgin olive oil (over medium heat only; don't use high heat with olive oil), macadamia oil, and organic extra-virgin coconut oil.
  - When preparing no-heat recipes only use small amounts of the following omega-3-rich oils: cold-pressed flax oil, hemp oil, and walnut oil.

  NOTE: *Truffle oil and cold-pressed extra-virgin olive oil are not rich in omega-3s, but they can also be used in small amounts for no-heat recipes.*

- Start eating Clean Cuisine dinners.

Nutritional Enhancement

Supplement with an ultra-purified pharmaceutical-grade fish oil containing EPA and DHA. We recommend you supplement with at least 2,000 milligrams of *combined* EPA and DHA daily. If you have an inflammatory condition such as multiple sclerosis, asthma, or fibromyalgia, you should take 3,000 milligrams daily. Look for a pharmaceutical-grade fish oil that undergoes molecular distillation, ultra-filtration, and purity testing by an independent third-party testing organization. Freshness is a key factor in choosing a high-quality fish oil. Keep in mind, the omega-3 fats in fish can oxidize easily if not handled properly, and oxidized oils can potentially be very harmful. Any fishy taste is a tip-off that your fish oil supplement isn't up to snuff in the freshness department. If your fish oil supplement has a fishy taste you absolutely don't want to take it. For years now our family has taken and recommended both Barlean's and Nordic Naturals as manufacturers of superior-quality pharmaceutical-grade fish oil supplements. If you can't stomach pills, Barlean's produces an incredible genius of a product called Omega Swirl (look for the ultra-high potency one to get the most EPA and DHA), a smoothie-tasting omega-3 supplement that is to-die-for delicious.

> NOTE: *If you are taking our Clean Cuisine Essentials daily supplement packets (www.CleanCuisineandMore.com/supplements) you will be getting 2,320 milligrams of combined EPA and DHA daily.*

If you are a strict vegan you will want to supplement with an algae-based omega-3 supplement, but you'll need to read labels carefully because many algae supplements contain only DHA and often not nearly in the same quantity as you'll get from fish oil supplements. You will need to take more algae supplements than fish oil supplements to get the same dosage. Barlean's Total Omega Vegan Swirl is an incredibly delicious smoothie-like plant-based omega-3 supplement containing DHA from algae sources that you take by the spoonful (no capsules!), and it's a great product for vegans. This product is good for nonvegans too, and kids love it!

> NOTE: *Krill oil is not a good substitute for fish oil because krill oil contains only a fraction of the EPA and DHA that is found in fish oil.*

Challenge of the Week

Consider pumping up your workout routine by adding one 20-minute cardio interval per week (see the Sizzle Cardio Interval Workout on page 258) in addition to the three times per week Strength Workout.

Time-Saving Clean Cuisine Cooking Tip

Rinsed, canned beans (we like the BPA-free Eden Organic brand) are a   273
perfect convenience food to keep in the fridge at all times. Store the rinsed
beans in covered containers for up to 3 days. You can then easily toss in
salads, add to soups, put on top of whole grains, eat with a sauce, or mash
into a quick hummus. Pretty much every bean makes a great hummus by
the way, including thawed frozen edamame.

Sample Meal Plan for Week 3

Everything is still the same as weeks 1 and 2, but we're adding to the
program.

▶ **BREAKFAST**

■ Continue with the breakfast options from week 1 (page 262), or
  consider switching things up by having a bowl of veggie soup
  (recipes in Part Four); who says you can't have soup for breakfast?
  Have a slice of toasted sprouted flourless whole grain bread (such
  as Food for Life's Ezekiel 4:9 bread) to dunk.

  WHAT TO DRINK WITH BREAKFAST?

■ Coffee with a little organic pastured cream or milk and green tea
  are both allowed. But no juice!

▶ **LUNCH**

■ Continue with the options discussed in week 1.

▶ **DINNER**

■ You can build your own customized daily dinner meals by following our general guidelines and mixing and matching meal
  choices from our Clean Cuisine recipe collection. We find it easiest to stick to a basic weekly dinner plan outline, including meat-
  free Monday and fish on Friday dinners, but don't feel you
  absolutely must follow this guideline exactly. If you repeat Tuesday's dinner on Wednesday and Thursday it's absolutely not the
  end of the world! The dinner meal plans are provided with the
  intention of showing you how to create a tremendous variety of

Clean Cuisine dinners. Additional Clean Cuisine dinner recipes are available free on our website (CleanCuisine.com), and for even more convenience, we've created *30 Eat Clean Dinners*, an entire month's worth of dinner menus plus complete grocery shopping lists, photos, and meal prep guidelines for sale at CleanCuisine .com.

IVY'S DINNER TIP

YOU MIGHT FIND it to be the least overwhelming to start the Clean Cuisine Program by finding seven recipes that your family really likes and making those same recipes over and over each week for a month. Once you make a recipe several times it becomes like second nature. After you master seven Clean Cuisine recipes you can branch out and add a few more to your recipe repertoire each month.

MEAT-FREE MONDAYS

- Large green salad *or* 1 cup cooked greens (page 400)
- Choose a vegetarian entrée
  - Baked tofu or tempeh smothered in a sauce (see Sauces That Make the Meal on page 351) served with a whole grain or starchy veggie side (page 405)
  - Vegetable chili (page 338)
  - Meat-Free Monday Meals (page 382)
  - Rice and beans with roasted vegetables (peppers, onions, etc.) topped with salsa or pico de gallo
  - Bean and mixed veggie burrito (use a sprouted whole grain tortilla or corn tortilla, such as Food for Life brand)
  - Sprouted whole grain pasta and marinara (see Clean Cuisine marinara on page 371 or try a high-quality store bought brand such as Rao's or Amy's) topped with broccoli, cauliflower, or roasted vegetables
  - Veggie stir-fry (with or without tofu) over black rice (page 383)
  - Meat-free burgers (page 361 and 364) served on a sprouted flourless bun (such as Food for Life brand)

TUESDAY

- Large green Salad *or* 1 cup cooked greens (page 400)
- Choose 1 entrée   275
  - Fish
  - Eggs, such as a frittata (page 376) or veggie omelet (but do not have eggs for dinner if you had eggs for breakfast)
  - Tofu or tempeh (with a sauce from page 351)
  - Clean Cuisine burgers (page 360)
- Choose 1 nonstarchy vegetable such as bok choy, eggplant, fennel, onions, tomatoes, rutabaga, radishes, bell peppers, broccoli, cauliflower, onions, artichoke, asparagus, leeks, spaghetti squash, green beans, snow peas, zucchini, cucumber, or Brussels sprouts (see the recipes in Part Four, or try simply steaming, roasting, or pan-sautéing)
- Choose 1 carbohydrate
  - *Light appetite:* Simply prepared (steamed or roasted) starchy earthy vegetable like carrots, beets, peas, butternut squash, parsnips, potatoes, sweet potatoes, or corn (page 391)
  - *Bigger appetite:* Simply prepared cooked whole grains or potatoes (page 323)

WEDNESDAY AND THURSDAY

- Large green salad *or* 1 cup cooked greens (page 400)
- Entrée: from our One-Dish and Slow-Cooked Dinners recipes (page 369); cook once and eat twice!

FISH ON FRIDAY

- Large green salad *or* 1 cup cooked greens (page 400)
- Fish (page 390)
- Choose a nonstarchy vegetable such as bok choy, eggplant, fennel, onions, tomatoes, rutabaga, radishes, bell peppers, broccoli, cauliflower, onions, artichoke, asparagus, leeks, spaghetti squash, green beans, snow peas, zucchini, cucumber, or Brussels sprouts (see recipes in Part Four or try simply steaming, roasting, or pan-sautéing)
- Choose 1 carbohydrate
  - *Light appetite:* Simply prepared (steamed or roasted) starchy earthy vegetable like carrots, beets, peas, butternut squash, parsnips, sweet potatoes or corn

- *Bigger appetite:* Simply prepared cooked whole grains or potatoes (page 418)

SATURDAY AND SUNDAY

- Large green salad *or* 1 cup cooked greens (page 400)
- Choose 1 entrée
  - Small serving fish (page 390)
  - Eggs, such as a frittata (page 376) or veggie omelet (but do not have eggs for dinner if you had eggs for breakfast)
  - Small serving pastured chicken, beef, or lamb

  HINT: *Making kabobs is a great way to reduce your meat serving size without feeling deprived and a great idea for an outdoor weekend.*

  - Baked, grilled, or pan-seared tofu or tempeh (try topping with one of the sauces on page 351)
  - Clean Cuisine burgers (page 360)
- Choose a nonstarchy vegetable such as bok choy, eggplant, fennel, onions, tomatoes, rutabaga, radishes, bell peppers, broccoli, cauliflower, onions, artichoke, asparagus, leeks, spaghetti squash, green beans, snow peas, zucchini, cucumber, or Brussels sprouts (see recipes in Part Four or try simply steaming, roasting, or pan-sautéing)
- Choose 1 carbohydrate
  - *Light appetite:* Simply prepared (steamed or roasted) starchy earthy vegetable such as carrots, beets, peas, butternut squash, parsnips, sweet potatoes or corn
  - *Bigger appetite:* Simply prepared cooked whole grains or potatoes (page 418)

WHAT TO DRINK WITH DINNER

- Water, sparkling water, and/or a glass of wine

ADDITIONAL TWO-WEEK MENU MEAL PLAN

HUNGRY FOR MORE meal planning ideas? We've done all the thinking and planning for you! Check out www.CleanCuisineMealPlanner.com for a complimentary, printable Clean Cuisine meal plan for two weeks of breakfast, lunch, and dinner ideas. We've also included a complete one-week meal plan at the end of this chapter.

Week 4

Focus

Continue with the food program as described in week 3. Full Fitness Fusion focus: Slim Workout. We'll be modifying the workout program to combat boredom and the plateau effect.

3 BIG CHANGES TO MAKE THIS WEEK

- Begin the Slim Workout (page 222) to be performed on nonconsecutive days for 30 minutes at a time 3 days per week. If desired, continue doing the 20-minute Sizzle Cardio Interval Workout (page 258) one time per week.
- Go for flavor! The more flavor you can add to your food from garlic, fresh and dried herbs (dill, basil, oregano, thyme, rosemary), and spices (ginger, cardamom, turmeric, cumin, cinnamon) the more antioxidants and phytonutrients you'll get. Not to mention the better your food will taste!
- Start incorporating nondairy vegan fermented foods and beverages containing probiotics into your daily diet. Fermented foods and beverages improve digestion, help restore the balance of bacteria in your gut, and even boost your body's ability to absorb the nutrients from the foods you eat. Here are some of the foods and beverages you can try adding this week:
  - Fermented vegetables such as raw sauerkraut or kimchi are excellent examples. Please note, raw sauerkraut is *not* the stuff squatting unrefrigerated in the can on the supermarket shelf; you'll find raw sauerkraut (and kimchi) only in the *refrigerated section* of your natural foods or health foods

store. Fermented vegetables such as raw sauerkraut and kimchi are delicious Clean Cuisine condiments when eaten alone or paired with savory dishes.

- Pickled carrots, beets, and cucumbers are also rich in probiotics and very tasty too.
- Kombucha is a tart and tangy fizzy and detoxifying beverage made from fermented tea and a great vegan source of probiotics as well as antioxidants and B vitamins. We think it's a bit risky to make your own kombucha unless you really know what you are doing; our family likes GT's Synergy brand instead of home brews.
- Traditional miso served in Japanese restaurants is another excellent vegan source of probiotics made from fermented soybeans, barley, or rice. For the healthiest miso, look for a brand that is unpasteurized (we like Miso Master). It is easy to find unpasteurized miso in the refrigerated section of natural foods stores or in Asian markets. By the way, miso diluted in water makes a great substitute for vegetable broth in soup recipes.
- Nama shoyu is an unpasteurized soy sauce made from cultivated soybeans and wheat; it is aged for months or even years. Nama shoyu is free of preservatives and full of enzymes and probiotics. Look for it in the natural foods store.
- Tempeh is another vegan food rich in probiotics. Originating from Indonesia, tempeh is made from fermented soybeans. It has a nutty, slightly mushroomy taste and makes a good substitute for meat. It is particularly good when crumbled and used as a ground beef substitute to add into sauces and as a filler for a stuffed pepper.

NOTE: *Although dairy products such as yogurt and kefir are the most popular and well-publicized probiotics, they are not the best choice from a stability or bioavailability standpoint.*

Nutritional Enhancement

Add a probiotic supplement. Probiotics are living, friendly bacteria that stay alive in your intestine after being consumed. These microscopic organisms work hard to alter the overall intestinal environment to a favorable one by crowding out bad bacteria that might otherwise dominate and harm health. Even though they are bacteria, probiotics actually help protect your body from infection. Probiotics can work with your immune system to improve your health and prevent, or even treat, certain diseases. Regular consumption of probiotics will help your body properly digest, process, and use the food you eat. Probiotic consumption also increases the bioavailability of minerals, especially calcium. In addition, they have a cleansing effect on your body and have been shown to support liver function and detoxification. These friendly bacteria filter toxins in the gut before they get into the bloodstream. The presence of probiotics speeds up the transfer time of toxic waste in your colon, thus preventing toxins from staying in your body and being reabsorbed in your bloodstream.

When looking for a probiotic supplement it is important to realize not all probiotics are equal from a quality or bioavailability standpoint (meaning your body doesn't always absorb the probiotics that the label claims it has). Many mass-market probiotic supplements contain a limited number of good bacteria and are manufactured in such a way that the good bacteria cannot necessarily survive (such as being exposed to heat, moisture, and light) or contain fillers and added sugars that interfere with their bioavailability. It is also important to look for a brand that contains strains of bacteria that have been clinically documented for their effectiveness (such as *Lactobacillus*, *Bifidobacterium*, and *Saccharomyces*). We suggest you look for a dairy-free probiotic because cow's milk allergy is one of the most common allergies. And finally, it is important to look for a brand that is shipped refrigerated and sold refrigerated to maintain shelf-life because heat is an enemy of probiotic viability.

Our Clean Cuisine Probiotic Blend contains a high-potency 25-billion-plus CFU hypoallergenic blend of 12 certified probiotic species to offer the most complete spectrum of microorganisms available and is certified dairy free. The Clean Cuisine Probiotic Blend is a scientifically formulated unique combination of colonizing and transient strains providing broad coverage to support a healthy balance of microflora across the entire gastrointestinal tract. Another excellent dairy-free brand is Dr. Ohhira's

Probiotics premium broad-spectrum probiotic supplement containing 12 strains of friendly bacteria. This award-winning brand was developed by Japanese microbiologist Iichiroh Ohhira, Ph.D., and, to our knowledge, is the only brand that relies on a natural fermentation process based in ancient Japanese tradition.

> NOTE: *You can purchase Clean Cuisine Probiotic Blend online at www.cleancuisineandmore.com/supplements. Use the code GIFT to receive a 20 percent discount off your first order.*

Challenge of the Week

Think kaleidoscope colors! The more variety of colorful fruits and vegetables you eat the more complete your exposure to the full array of antiaging phytonutrients and antioxidants.

Time-Saving Clean Cuisine Cooking Tip

Start planning your meals and your grocery list once a week. Ivy likes to do this on Sunday. She writes out everything we are going to have for dinner the upcoming week and then writes down the ingredients on a grocery list organized into the following categories: eggs, breads, and grains; fresh fruits and veggies; frozen; fish; meat; tofu and tempeh; spices; beans and canned goods; and nuts and seeds. Andy isn't involved in the meal planning and grocery stuff so he wouldn't know how much help this really is, but it saves Ivy a tremendous amount of time! It also safeguards against impulsive supermarket choices that can sabotage your clean eating goals.

Sample Meal Plan for Week 4

Everything is still the same as week 3.

Week 5

Focus

Become a fishy flexitarian. Continue with the program from last week but make the following changes.

3 BIG CHANGES TO MAKE THIS WEEK:

- Eat two or three fish meals for dinner per week, including our fish on Friday Dinners (page 390). Do meat-free Mondays in earnest now, go vegan all day!
- Replace cow's milk with hemp milk or almond milk for all meals and all recipes. Replace dairy cream with cashew cream (page 144) or hemp cream.
- Switch up your workout routine by doing Strength Workout for 30 minutes, 2 days per week and the Slim Workout for 30 minutes 1 day per week. If desired, continue doing the 20-minute Sizzle Cardio Interval Workout once per week.

Nutritional Enhancement

Start drinking green tea. And drink a lot of it! The goal should be to drink *at least* 3 or 4 cups a day. The health benefits associated with drinking antioxidant-rich green tea have been touted for centuries. A study published in the *European Journal of Clinical Nutrition* demonstrated that tea is a healthier choice than almost any beverage, *including pure water,* because tea not only rehydrates as well as water but also provides a rich supply of polyphenols (antioxidants) that are protective against heart disease and many other diseases too![2] What is more, a Japanese study published in the *Journal of the American Medical Association* suggests that drinking green tea lowers risk of death due to all causes, including cardiovascular disease.[3]

In a 2011 study published in the *Journal of Nutrition,* green tea was shown to boost skin elasticity and hydration and help protect against ultraviolet light–induced skin damage.[4] People in China, India, Japan, and Thailand have consumed green tea and used it for medicinal purposes for centuries. Most of the research showing the health benefits of green tea is based on the amount of green tea typically consumed in Asian countries—about 3 cups per day. Green tea is rich in catechins, a special type of antioxidant that really should be ranked right up there along with the other well-known antioxidants like vitamins E and C. Catechins are potent free-radical scavengers, antiagers, and health promoters. Not only does green tea wash toxins out of the system through its liquid content but the catechins in green tea are known to improve liver function and augment weight loss by increasing the metabolism of fats by the liver (a thermogenic effect), inhibiting lipase (a fat absorption enzyme) in the digestive tract, and providing a feeling of satiety and fullness.[5] Researchers have also found the catechins in green tea help reduce body fat, lower systolic blood pressure, and decrease LDL cholesterol, all of which in turn contribute to a decrease in cardiovascular disease risk.

But, as with most things, not all green tea is created equal, in health benefits or in taste. Although plenty of high-quality green teas are out there, we particularly like Costco's Kirkland Signature Green Tea for taste and price. Kirkland tea is made from sencha green tea from Japan. In keeping with the Japanese tradition, Kirkland Signature Green Tea is gently steamed, rolled, and then dried. The minimal processing stops the oxidation and preserves the freshness, aroma, and color of the tea leaf. If you are not a member of Costco, Ito En teas offers a great online resource that enables you to choose from a wide variety of Japanese green teas. Teavana also offers an amazing Matcha Japanese green tea powder. Some retailers also carry Ito En teas. It's worth noting that by adding just a little squirt of vitamin C–rich freshly squeezed lemon or freshly squeezed orange juice you can significantly boost the amount of catechins your body absorbs, thus boosting the health, antioxidant, and detoxifying benefits of green tea.

Challenge of the Week

Take 3 minutes in the morning and 3 minutes in the evening to sit quietly, breathe deeply, and focus on your breath. By putting attention on your breath, you will change your state of consciousness, begin to relax, and detach from ordinary awareness. Many systems of meditation use focus on breath as the main technique.

Time-Saving Clean Cuisine Cooking Tip

Keep frozen fruit and frozen vegetables on hand at all times for fast food prep. Although many health enthusiasts shun frozen produce for fresh, the cold truth is frozen fruits and veggies can sometimes be even more nutritious than fresh! Frozen produce is picked at the peak of freshness then flash frozen so nutrients are preserved. Keep in mind that if your spinach (or carrots, grapes, or apples) sits on the supermarket shelves too long or spends too much time driving around the country or flying in planes in transit to the supermarket, its nutrient content declines. Ideally, we would all eat our produce picked fresh from our own gardens every single day, the ultimate in produce utopia but not exactly real world either! 283

As for taste and texture, we have found certain brands, and certain vegetables or fruits within brands, are better than others. Cascadian Farm organic berries (blueberries, raspberries, blackberries, mixed berries) are all very good and particularly delicious in smoothies or topped with our Spirited Chocolate Sauce (page 427). They can be heated quickly on the stovetop or in the microwave so that the berries sort of melt right in with the sauce, mmmmm.

Frozen strawberries can be a little tricky because they are actually much better than fresh strawberries in smoothies but we haven't found them to be good for much else. We do use a lot of frozen mango and pineapple (also in smoothies), and we absolutely love frozen wild blueberries when we can find them. Wild blueberries have considerably more antioxidants than standard blueberries. And we have great luck with pretty much any chopped frozen leafy green like kale, collards, turnips, and mustard greens. You can use frozen chopped leafy greens a million and one ways. Here are three ideas:

- Sauté crushed garlic in a large skillet with a little extra-virgin olive oil or coconut oil over medium heat for 30 seconds then add the frozen chopped greens to the skillet, and sauté until the greens are heated through.
- Put the chopped frozen veggies on a microwave-safe plate and heat directly in the microwave for 2 minutes, or until heated through, then top with any of our sauces from page 351.
- Add thawed frozen chopped greens to soups, casseroles, and chilis, you'd be surprised at how they blend right in and barely change the taste.

And by the way, whatever you do, you don't want to prepare your frozen vegetables in water, which for whatever reason is the exact thing most frozen vegetable packages will tell you to do. Instead, you want to steam, microwave, or sauté the vegetables in a little oil while still frozen. Cooking frozen vegetables in water will give you a terrible-tasting result.

Frozen petite peas, corn, and edamame are also standbys in our house and can be prepared simply by heating in the microwave for a minute or so or steamed in a steamer. Frozen whole broccoli (but not chopped) is also surprisingly good, often better than fresh. And you can't go wrong with frozen asparagus, haricot verts (thin green beans), snap peas, and snow peas either. Again, these can be steamed, pan seared, microwaved, or sautéed. Frozen butternut squash is ideal for making squash-based soups or any recipe that requires puréeing. Frozen artichoke hearts are divine when placed directly from the freezer on a baking sheet, drizzled with a little extra-virgin olive oil, and a sprinkling of salt—maybe a bit of chopped fresh rosemary too—then roasted at 400°F for about 25 minutes. If you aren't accustomed to cooking with frozen vegetables, it might take a little trial and error to figure out how to optimize the taste, but once you get the hang of it you'll be *amazed* at how much time can be saved. And trust us, if you keep plenty of frozen fruits and vegetables on hand at all times you are guaranteed to eat more produce! Here are a few of our favorite flavor combos for quickly jazzing up frozen vegetables.

- Lemon juice, cold-pressed extra-virgin olive oil or flax oil, crushed garlic, balsamic vinegar
- Lime juice, minced cilantro, red pepper flakes, crushed garlic, cold-pressed extra-virgin olive oil
- Cold-pressed extra-virgin olive oil, oregano, basil, thyme
- Organic extra-virgin coconut oil, cumin, turmeric, garlic, ginger
- Dijon mustard, raw honey, lemon juice, crushed garlic, cold-pressed extra-virgin olive oil
- Mashed avocado, cold-pressed extra-virgin olive oil, crushed garlic, lemon juice, finely chopped cilantro

These combos are also good on whole grains, beans, and legumes.

Sample Meal Plan for Week 5

Keep everything the same as week 4 but remember to eat fish at least twice a week and eliminate the dairy products, except for the occasional cheese in a recipe.

Week 6

Focus

Continue, of course, with all of the changes from last week. Full Fitness Fusion focus: Sculpt Workout.

3 BIG CHANGES TO MAKE THIS WEEK

- Begin the Sculpt Workout (page 234) to be performed on non-consecutive days for 30 minutes at a time, 3 days per week. If desired, continue doing the 20-minute Sizzle Cardio Interval Workout once a week.
- Make sure you are eating at least one serving of beans (½ cup) a day.
- Make sure you are eating at least one serving (¼ cup) of nuts or seeds a day. Take nut and seed nutrition to a whole new level by soaking your nuts and seeds in water (page 142).

Nutritional Enhancement

Supplement with Vitamin K2 and Vitamin D3 and get a little sunshine too! Very few foods naturally contain ample amounts of fat-soluble vitamins K2 or D, but both are extremely important and both work synergistically, along with fat-soluble vitamin A (which you should already be getting from your food and from your multivitamin) to optimize health. In addition to what typically comes in a multivitamin you will most likely need to supplement with extra K2 and D to get the optimal amounts your body needs. Vitamin K2 is not easy to come by in your everyday diet. It is found in small amounts in certain pastured animal foods (including egg yolks) and is especially bountiful in natto, a vegan stinky slimy fermented superfood popular in Japan. Unfortunately natto tastes so darn terrible we just can't bring ourselves to eat it regardless of how healthful we know it is. It's important to note that vitamin K2 is not the same substance as the vitamin K1 you get in abundance from eating green leafy vegetables; K1 is primarily responsible for blood clotting but K2 is responsible for driving calcium into bones and keeping calcium out of arteries, veins, and soft tissue where it can cause damage. Vitamin K2 is so important for heart health that the Rotterdam Study published in the *Journal of*

Nutrition found that this single vitamin reduced the risk of death from cardiovascular disease by an incredible 50 percent and was associated with a reduced risk of dying from all causes.[6] In this study vitamin K1 had no effect. Another study conducted in 2009 showed similar results.[7]

> NOTE: *Atherosclerosis is a buildup of calcium-laden plaque that clogs the coronary arteries, or any artery in the body for that matter.*

But, because K2 is found in so few foods, it is very likely to be missing from your diet. We actually learned about the importance of vitamin K2 for bone health when Ivy was recovering from her derotational osteotomy surgery (which involved breaking her femur bone) and we wanted to make sure she was getting all the bone-building nutrients necessary to recover from the surgery. Not only did we learn the importance of K2 for bone health, including osteoporosis prevention and heart health, we also learned it played a valuable role in keeping teeth strong, veins healthy, and promoting smooth and wrinkle-free skin too! We feel supplementation of 60 to 100 micrograms of vitamin K2 derived from natto in the form of MK-7 is an optimal amount so long as you also get adequate vitamin A and vitamin D. Remember, all three of these fat-soluble vitamins work together.

Like vitamin K2, vitamin D is also limited in the food supply and found in relatively few sources—fatty fish, egg yolks, and certain mushrooms are about the only natural sources. It is important to note that the current recommended intake for vitamin D is insufficient for optimal health[8] and that taking vitamin D will increase your need for vitamin K2, so it is important to supplement with both vitamin D and K2 and not just cherry pick one or the other. Although it is certainly true your skin cells can manufacture vitamin D when they are exposed directly to the sun, vitamin D deficiency is estimated to affect more than 70 percent of us. This is a big problem because vitamin D is a super vitamin that fights aging, reduces inflammation, and decreases risk of disease on many different levels. Knowing that vitamin D has important anti-inflammatory benefits, it's also not surprising that studies have shown higher intake of vitamin D can decrease the risk for developing multiple sclerosis.[9]

> NOTE: *Dairy foods do not naturally contain Vitamin D; they are artificially fortified.*

Vitamin D even helps fight pain, including back pain. Although vitamin D, as synthesized by the skin from sunlight or taken as a supplement, is indeed a nutrient, once it is in your bloodstream it is further activated by your kidneys into a potent hormone that then works throughout your body in many tissues and organs, including muscles, nerves, and even your brain. Vitamin D plays a crucial role in supporting a healthy immune system, building and maintaining strong bones, protecting against heart disease and cancer, and even providing protection against the common cold. And, although calcium often gets all the credit for building strong bones, your body must have vitamin D to absorb calcium from foods, and then you also need vitamin K2 to guide the calcium into your bones where it is needed and away from your arteries where you don't want it! Vitamin D is especially important for controlling the release of stress hormones, improving mood, and maintaining a positive mental outlook. Maybe that's why all those vitamin D–drenched surfers at the beach always seem so relaxed and happy!

Oh and did you also know having enough vitamin D circulating in your system is associated with increased fat burning? But there's a catch; the fat-burning effects of vitamin D are not as effective if you are overweight because fat cells lock up vitamin D and sort of hold the vitamin captive so it can't do its good work. This means if you are overweight, it is very likely you are actually vitamin D deficient. The higher your body fat percentage, the less circulating vitamin D you are likely to have; in fact, obese people can require significantly more vitamin D than lean people.

Ideally you would get a blood test to determine your vitamin D level, and ideally you want your levels to be above 60 nanograms per liter (this is consistent with studies of lifeguards and of farmers in equatorial regions who spend a great deal of time outdoors). However, if you don't know your level you can supplement with 20 International Units of vitamin D3 (the most bioavailable form) per pound of body weight. Your multivitamin may contain some vitamin D3, but you will most likely need to take more to meet your optimal levels.

NOTE: *If you take our Clean Cuisine Essentials complete supplement system you will be getting a total of 1,600 International Units vitamin D3 and 60 micrograms vitamin K2.*

Challenge of the Week

Make sure you are taking time to get adequate rest and relaxation each week. You cannot possibly improve the way you age, look, and feel if you don't get enough R&R! Everybody has different sleep requirements, but in general a solid 8 hours of sleep each night is what the average adult needs to function best. Be sure you are getting enough sleep!

Sample Meal Plan for Week 6

The meal plan remains the same as for week 5.

Week 7

Focus

Time for a carb tune-up. Continue with the program as it has been developed through week 6.

3 BIG CHANGES TO MAKE THIS WEEK

- Get out of a whole wheat rut! Wheat is ubiquitous so most of us eat far more wheat than any other whole grain, and this short-changes us on the nutrients found in other whole grains and could potentially lead to wheat sensitivity. Start making an effort to incorporate wheat-free whole grains, such as oatmeal, barley, millet, quinoa, and amaranth into your diet. Limit your consumption of whole wheat foods to 1 serving a day.
- Limit your consumption of flour. Even if it is whole wheat or another type of whole grain flour, you are still far better off from a health and weight-loss standpoint eating the whole grain in its original form rather than eating flour. Whole grains in their natural form are digested slower and do a much better job at keeping blood sugar levels stable in comparison to flour. Make the switch to flourless sprouted whole grain breads and pastas. Flourless breads and pastas are digested slower and are more nutritious too; sprouting releases all of the vital nutrients stored within the whole grain and takes whole grain nutrition to a whole new level.

NOTE: Our favorite line of nationally distributed sprouted whole grain breads and pastas is the Food for Life brand.

- Switch up your workout routine by doing the Strength Workout for 30 minutes 1 day per week, the Slim Workout for 30 minutes 1 day per week, and the Sculpt Workout for 30 minutes 1 day per week. Or, give our Full Fitness Fusion workout DVD a try instead (visit www.CleanCuisineandMore.com/fullfitnessfusion to view our DVD collection). As before, if desired, continue doing the 20-minute "Sizzle" Cardio Interval Workout once per week.

Nutritional Enhancement

Start eating garlic, lots and lots of garlic. If you have been using our Clean Cuisine recipes you have surely noticed we use far more garlic than what is typical, for good reason too! The "stinking rose" truly is a functional food because it does far more than boost the flavor of your meals; garlic has incredible detoxifying, antioxidant, and anti-inflammatory properties and has been proven to protect against heart disease. A special compound in garlic lowers blood pressure by dilating blood vessel walls, and can even help lower cholesterol.[10] What's more, garlic not only lowers cholesterol but also improves your cholesterol profile by lowering the bad LDL cholesterol level and preventing the LDL cholesterol in your blood from oxidizing. Remember, bad cholesterol becomes bad for your arteries upon oxidation. Garlic is so helpful against heart disease that in Germany garlic supplements are actually registered and prescribed as drugs.

Garlic also boosts your resistance to infection. In fact, at the first sign of a cold we immediately eat two or three crushed garlic cloves mixed with some extra-virgin olive oil and "roasted" for 1 minute in the microwave. Garlic even helps activate liver enzymes that filter out junk and detoxify your body, especially from heavy metals such as mercury and cadmium. The power of garlic is mainly attributed to a compound called allicin, a sulfur-rich compound that gives garlic its strong taste and aroma. Allicin can be released from garlic only when the cloves are crushed, chewed, or cut, so swallowing whole garlic cloves won't do the trick. If you really don't want to eat more garlic, you can try one of a few very high quality garlic supplements such as Kyolic Aged Garlic Extract but keep in mind supplements are more expensive than fresh garlic, and fresh garlic is still your best bet for getting the most therapeutic benefits. Check out our Clean Cuisine recipe collection for garlic-forward ideas.

Challenge of the Week

Clean out your pantry! If you haven't already tossed the junk, now is the time so you aren't tempted to backslide when the 8-week program ends. Here's what you want to toss:

- **Carbohydrate foods containing refined flour and sugar:** bagels, biscuits, crackers, boxed mixes for preparing baked goods, breads, breakfast bars, cereals, muffins, pizza crusts, waffles, pretzels, rolls, and white pasta
- **All processed vegetable oils and packaged foods containing those oils:** soybean oil, cottonseed oil, pure vegetable oil, canola oil, corn oil, sunflower oil, safflower oil, hydrogenated oils, and partially hydrogenated oils
- **Sugary drinks and all juices, even those made from 100 percent juice**
- **Fake foods:** low-fat, fat-free, and sugar-free remakes of real food
- **All foods containing high fructose corn syrup**
- **Milk**

Sample Meal Plan for Week 7

Everything is still the same as week 6, except we are now limiting wheat to once per day so that there are more opportunities to enjoy the goodness of a variety of grains. We are also eliminating any residual junk food cheats listed under this week's challenge.

Week 8

Focus

Continue with the program from week 7. Full Fitness Fusion focus: Stretch Yoga Workout.

2 BIG CHANGES (JUST 2) TO MAKE THIS WEEK:

- Introduce the Stretch Yoga Workout (page 244) to be performed once a week for 30 minutes, continue the Strength Workout for 30 minutes 1 day per week and do the Slim Workout for 30 minutes 1 day per week. As always, if desired, continue doing the 20-minute Sizzle Cardio Interval Workout for one day every week.

- Go back and reread weeks 1 through 7 to make sure you are following the Clean Cuisine Program.

Nutritional Enhancement

Supplement with gamma-linolenic acid (GLA) in the form of evening primrose oil. GLA is a special omega-6 fat that is also an effective anti-inflammatory agent that offers none of the negative side effects of anti-inflammatory drugs. GLA works differently from the anti-inflammatory omega-3 fats. It is routinely recommended by in-the-know doctors for supporting hormonal balance, offsetting the bothersome symptoms of PMS and menopause, and supporting a balanced mood in general. And because GLA decreases inflammation it is helpful for anyone with an inflammatory condition such as MS, arthritis, allergies, or fibromyalgia. Research even supports GLA as being beneficial for lowering bad LDL cholesterol and improving the cholesterol ratio.[11]

This omega-6 fat is also widely recognized for promoting beauty on the outside in the form of clear, smooth skin and strong nails and lustrous hair. It has even been shown to be particularly beneficial in treating serious inflammatory skin conditions, including eczema and psoriasis. Unfortunately GLA is very difficult to find naturally from whole foods so supplementation is the only reasonable way to get a good dose. The vast majority of whole foods rich in omega-6 fat such as sunflower seeds and sesame seeds contain omega-6 fat in the form of linoleic acid (LA). If all goes perfectly your body is capable of converting LA into GLA. But all does not always go perfectly, and the conversion process from LA into the usable good fat GLA is often thwarted by a number of different internal and external factors. For example, the older you are, the less efficient the enzymes your body uses to convert LA into GLA become. Chronic health conditions such as diabetes, infection, poor nutrition, and stress further reduce your body's ability to convert dietary LA into GLA.

While it is true that GLA is an omega-6 fat and it is true we have emphasized not to eat a high ratio of omega-6 to omega-3 fats, GLA is a special omega-6 fat that is indeed anti-inflammatory. Supplementation with GLA is simple and affordable. GLA is naturally prevalent in the oils derived from four plant seeds: borage oil, evening primrose oil, hemp oil, and black currant oil. Of these four oils, borage oil has the highest percentage of GLA. We recommend GLA supplementation from evening primrose oil because it is the most widely researched. We suggest taking about 2,000 to 4,000 milligrams of a high-quality evening primrose oil (such as Barlean's) daily, which will give you about 200 fo 400 milligrams of GLA. If you take our Clean Cuisine Essentials complete supplement system you will be getting this recommended amount included in our daily packets.

> NOTE: *Hemp seeds are one of the only food sources of GLA that we are aware of. Hemp seeds are often used as a base for Ivy's creamy salad dressing recipes.*

Challenge of the Week

We so wish we could tell you candy is dandy and that dessert should be a guiltless pleasure, but that would not be truthful. By definition, desserts are sweet and therefore contain sugar. If you are a sugar lover you'll need to learn how to satisfy your sweet tooth without sabotaging your Clean Cuisine lifestyle. Not everybody loves sweets; Andy would much rather have salty potato chips than a piece of pie, but Ivy would choose the pie every time. We know there are a lot of sugar-loving Ivy's out there and we also realize how difficult it can be to totally cut sugar out of your diet. The good news is, as long as the rest of your diet consists of nutrient-dense, clean foods there is no reason you can't have a small, all-natural serving of a sweet treat as part of the Clean Cuisine lifestyle. As mentioned in Chapter 4, our overall strategy for incorporating sweets into our own diets is to sneak in nutrition whenever and wherever possible (and we keep our dessert portions small too). Here are some of Ivy's best tips for cleaning up your favorite dessert recipes and some of the strategies she has used in developing our family's dessert recipe collection (see Part Four):

- Ditch the cow's milk and substitute hemp milk, cashew cream, coconut milk, or almond milk.

- Eliminate butter, margarine, and highly refined vegetable oils like corn oil and soybean oil. Instead use more healthful oils such as extra-virgin olive oil (which can add a surprisingly welcome savory addition to many baked dessert recipes), macadamia nut oil, or extra-virgin coconut oil (a perfect replacement for butter).
- For moisture and substance consider puréed tofu, white soybeans, applesauce, ground flaxseed, prune purée, or baby food puréed fruit in place of empty-calorie oils.
- Reduce the sugar in all recipes substantially. Replace it with fruit sugars from fresh or frozen fruits, dried fruits, or date sugar.

  NOTE: *Date sugar can be purchased at natural food stores and is an all-natural sugar made from dehydrated ground whole dates; it is a great replacement for brown sugar and even contains antioxidants and phtyonutrients!*

- Try replacing sugar with unpasteurized raw honey. While honey is still very calorie dense, it also contains antioxidants, essential minerals, seven vitamins of the B complex group, amino acids, enzymes, and an array of phytonutrients. Because honey is sweeter than sugar, you need to use less—½ to ¾ cup for each cup of sugar.

  NOTE: *For each cup of sugar replaced, you should also reduce the amount of liquid in the recipe by ¼ cup. In addition, reduce the cooking temperature by 25°F because honey causes foods to brown more easily.*

- Try agave nectar instead of sugar. Although it's called nectar, agave is really more like a light syrup with a pleasant neutral flavor. Agave is particularly delicious when frozen and comes out caramel-like. All-natural agave nectar is made from the agave plant and is sweeter than sugar. When substituting this sweetener in baking recipes, you'll want to reduce the liquid slightly, maybe by as much as one third. You'll also want to reduce your oven temperature by 25°F to avoid over-browning.
- Use spice for sugar. To enhance the perception of sweetness, many recipes benefit from spices such as cinnamon, nutmeg, cardamom, allspice, pumpkin pie spice, or cloves. Orange or lemon zest can also boost flavor when sugar is reduced. *Pure* vanilla, lemon,

and almond extracts are also excellent sugar-free flavor boosters that simultaneously add richness and depth to numerous desserts.

- Adding liqueurs or spirits is another great way to add richness to your desserts. Try amaretto, brandy, coffee liqueur, rum, and bourbon. It doesn't take much so this is a safe indulgence.

- Celebrate the natural sweetness of nutrient-rich and fiber-rich fruits. We always make a fruit-based dessert whenever possible. Instead of sugar, why not try flavorful orange juice concentrate as a natural sweetener?

- Add crunch and satisfaction with nuts and richness with nut creams. Process nuts with water in a high-speed blender to form decadent nut creams that can replace dairy cream.

- Fiber up the flour. Making your own baked goods allows you more freedom to try healthful substitutions. Use white whole wheat flour or whole wheat pastry flour instead of all-purpose flour or add ¼ cup of ground flaxseed in place of ¼ cup of flour. Try tossing in some wheat germ or oatmeal too. Coconut flour, almond flour, and amaranth flour are slightly sweet, nutrient-rich flours ideal for desserts and definitely worth experimenting with.

- Add instant espresso to chocolate recipes to intensify the rich flavor of cocoa.

- Use dried fruit in place of half the chocolate chips in a recipe.

- Use unsweetened cocoa powder in place of sweetened cocoa powder.

- Make shot glass desserts! We got the idea for these mini indulgences while dining out at one of our favorite restaurants. The idea is so simple but so genius. Because the satisfaction of dessert mostly comes from the first few bites you create a dessert that is perfectly portioned to be just a few bites but presented so beautifully that you don't feel deprived. You can create an incredible assortment of shot glass desserts (key lime pie, pecan pie, and chocolate velvet cake come to mind), and to make them even more decadent try pouring a little liqueur on top before serving.

Sample Meal Plan for Week 8

Everything is still the same as week 7, but we've decided to reward your
efforts with some just desserts. Remember, when you eat dessert make
sure it contains at least some fruit! Enjoy!

A Week of Clean Cuisine Menus

> NOTE: *For an additional complimentary two-week meal plan,*
> *visit CleanCuisineMealPlanner.com. For ideas, inspiration, and*
> *300 recipes, visit CleanCuisineandMore.com.*

Monday

▶ **BREAKFAST**
- Carrot Cake No-Milk Shake (page 310)
- Coffee with a little organic pastured milk or organic pastured
  cream or green tea

▶ **LUNCH**
- Loaded baked potato, stuffed with mashed avocado, steamed
  broccoli florets (frozen is fine), and chopped chives
- Watercress salad with Creamy Herb Dressing (page 321)
- Sparkling mineral water (we especially love San Pellegrino) or
  green tea (try iced green tea!)

SMOOTHIE AND SNACK
- Citrus Splashy SuperGreen Smoothie pick-me-up (page 344)
  either midmorning, midafternoon, or first thing in the morning
  if you prefer to eat a late breakfast
- Optional snack (If you are especially active or muscular or it is
  an exercise day, you might feel you need a snack; let your appetite
  guide you: half or whole Good Greens bar or Lärabar *or* a handful
  of raw nuts or seeds and fruit *or* half of a No-Milk Shake [page
  310])

▶ **DINNER**

- Spring Barley & Quinoa Risotto with Asparagus & Shiitake Mushrooms (page 386)
- Side of steamed kale drizzled with extra-virgin olive oil
- Glass of wine, water, or sparkling mineral water
- Fresh raspberries with a small scoop of coconut ice cream (we like Coconut Bliss)

Tuesday

▶ **BREAKFAST**

- ½ cup cooked whole grain (millet, quinoa, oatmeal, etc.)
- 1 cup fresh strawberries
- ½ cup fresh hemp cream (page 306)
- Coffee with a little organic pastured milk or organic pastured cream *or* green tea

▶ **LUNCH**

- Clean Cuisine Super Salad (see chart on page 322) made with baby spinach leaves, edamame, organic corn, red onions, lightly steamed broccoli, orange bell pepper, chopped parsley, dried apples, Clean Cuisine Garlic Herb Salad Booster (page 319), drizzle of flax oil (we like Barlean's)
- Sparkling mineral water (we especially love San Pellegrino) or green tea (try it iced)

SMOOTHIE AND SNACK

- Blueberry-Ginger Cocktail SuperGreen Smoothie pick-me-up (page 345) either midmorning, midafternoon, or first thing in the morning if you prefer to eat a late breakfast
- Optional snack (If you are especially active or muscular or it is an exercise day, you might feel you need a snack; let your appetite guide you: half or whole Good Greens bar or Lärabar *or* a handful of raw nuts or seeds and fruit *or* half of a No-Milk Shake [page 310])

▶ **DINNER**

- New Orleans-Style Shrimp in BBQ Sauce (page 393) served over steamed black rice or millet

- Steamed spinach with a drizzle of extra-virgin olive oil
- Glass of wine, water, or sparkling mineral water
- Sliced bananas with a drizzle of Spirited Chocolate Sauce (page 427)

297

Wednesday

▶ **BREAKFAST**

- Fresh whole orange juice made with 2 peeled oranges, 2 pitted dates, and 3 ice cubes (put the oranges, dates, and ice in a high-speed blender and blend until smooth and creamy)
- Perfect Scrambled Eggs-n-Veggies (page 309) with veggie addition of 1 cup chopped frozen artichokes (thawed) and shallots sautéed in ½ teaspoon extra-virgin olive oil
- Coffee with a little organic pastured milk or organic pastured cream *or* green tea

▶ **LUNCH**

- Tuscan Slow-Baked Cannellini Beans with Shallots, Garlic, & Sage (page 336) served over steamed short grain brown rice or quinoa
- Arugula salad with shredded carrots and sunflower seeds and drizzled with hemp or flax oil (we like Barlean's) and lemon juice
- Sparkling mineral water (we especially love San Pellegrino) or green tea (try it iced)

SMOOTHIE AND SNACK

- Mango Spice Cake SuperGreen Smoothie pick-me-up (page 345) either midmorning, midafternoon, or first thing in the morning if you prefer to eat a late breakfast
- Optional snack (If you are especially active or muscular or it is an exercise day, you might feel you need a snack; let your appetite guide you: half or whole Good Greens bar or Lärabar *or* a handful of raw nuts or seeds and fruit *or* half of a No-Milk Shake [page 310])

▶ **DINNER**

- Clean Cuisine–Style Spaghetti Pie (page 369)
- Sautéed broccoli raab

- Glass of wine, water, or sparkling mineral water
- Key Lime, Blueberry, & Coconut Cloud Custards (page 434)

Thursday

▶ BREAKFAST

- Chocolate Cherry Bomb No-Milk Shake (page 312)
- Coffee with a little organic pastured milk or organic pastured cream *or* green tea

▶ LUNCH

- Salad wrap made with sprouted whole grain tortilla (such as Food for Life) and filled with chopped salad of arugula, black beans, avocado, chopped red bell peppers, cherry tomatoes, slivered raw almonds, cilantro, and a drizzle of extra virgin olive oil or flax oil (we like Barlean's)
- Sparkling mineral water (we especially love San Pellegrino) or green tea (try it iced)

SMOOTHIE AND SNACK

- Thai-Style Pineapple-Cilantro SuperGreen Smoothie pick-me-up (page 346) either midmorning, midafternoon, or first thing in the morning if you prefer to eat a late breakfast
- Optional snack (If you are especially active or muscular or it is an exercise day, you might feel you need a snack; let your appetite guide you: half or whole Good Greens bar or Lärabar *or* a handful of raw nuts or seeds and fruit *or* half of a No-Milk Shake [page 310])

▶ DINNER

- Chicken and Mushroom Casserole (page 373)
- Spinach salad with Succulent Tomato Salad Booster (page 318) and a drizzle of extra-virgin olive oil
- Glass of wine, water, or sparkling mineral water
- Clean Cuisine Chia & Chocolate Cookies (page 433)

Friday

▶ **BREAKFAST**
- ½ cup No-Cook Swiss Morning Muesli (page 307)
- 1 chopped apple
- ½ cup fresh hemp cream (page 306)
- Coffee with a little organic pastured milk or organic pastured cream, *or* green tea

▶ **LUNCH**
- Creamy All Greens Soup (page 328)
- Loaded baked sweet potato stuffed with Poblano Chile and Pumpkin Seed Mole Sauce (page 355)
- Sparkling mineral water (we especially love San Pellegrino) or green tea (try it iced)

SMOOTHIE AND SNACK
- Parsley–Apple SuperGreen Smoothie pick-me-up (page 349) either midmorning, midafternoon, or first thing in the morning if you prefer to eat a late breakfast
- Optional snack (If you are especially active or muscular or it is an exercise day, you might feel you need a snack; let your appetite guide you: half or whole Good Greens bar or Lärabar *or* a handful of raw nuts or seeds and fruit *or* half of a No-Milk Shake ([page 310]))

▶ **DINNER**
- Baked wild Alaskan salmon with Smoky Tri-Color Pepper Sauce (page 355)
- Braised Escarole with Sun-Dried Tomatoes (page 401)
- Steamed cauliflower
- Organic corn on the cob
- Glass of wine, water, or sparkling mineral water
- Blueberries with small scoop coconut ice cream (we like Coconut Bliss)

Saturday

▶ **BREAKFAST**
- Chia-Crusted French Toast (page 308)
- Fresh Strawberries
- Coffee with a little organic pastured milk or organic pastured cream *or* green tea

▶ **LUNCH**
- Mom's Cleaned-Up Clean Cuisine Tuna Casserole (page 398)
- Steamed spinach with a drizzle of extra-virgin olive oil
- Sparkling mineral water (we especially love San Pellegrino) or green tea (try it iced)

SMOOTHIE AND SNACK
- It's Easy Being Green SuperGreen Smoothie pick-me-up (page 349) either midmorning, midafternoon, or first thing in the morning if you prefer to eat a late breakfast
- Optional snack (If you are especially active or muscular or it is an exercise day, you might feel you need a snack; let your appetite guide you: half or whole Good Greens bar or Lärabar *or* a handful of raw nuts or seeds and fruit *or* half of a No-Milk Shake [page 310])

▶ **DINNER**
- Szechuan Lettuce Wraps with Dipping Sauce (page 388)
- Steamed bok choy
- Steamed black rice
- Glass of wine, water, or sparkling mineral water
- Slice of Blueberry Upside-Down Cake (page 426)

Sunday

▶ **BREAKFAST**
- Gluten-Free Millet Pancakes (page 307)
- Sliced bananas
- Coffee with a little organic pastured milk or organic pastured cream *or* green tea

▶ **LUNCH**

- Baked Quinoa Spinach Cakes (page 419)
- Clean Cuisine Caesar salad made with chopped romaine lettuce, 301
  halved cherry tomatoes, and Ivy's Vegan Caesar Salad Dressing
  (page 320)
- Sparkling mineral water (we especially love San Pellegrino) or
  green tea (try it iced)

SMOOTHIE AND SNACK

- Better Than V-8 SuperGreen Smoothie pick-me-up (page 349)
  either midmorning, midafternoon, or first thing in the morning
  if you prefer to eat a late breakfast
- Optional snack (If you are especially active or muscular or it is
  an exercise day, you might feel you need a snack; let your appetite
  guide you: half or whole Good Greens bar or Lärabar *or* a handful
  of raw nuts or seeds and fruit *or* half of a No-Milk Shake [page
  310])

▶ **DINNER**

- Greek Lamb (or Beef) Bulgur Burgers (page 367) served on a
  toasted sprouted whole grain bun (such as Food for Life) with
  slices of tomato
- Arugula salad with red onions, shredded carrots and Honey
  Lemon Thyme Vinaigrette (page 321)
- Glass of wine, water, or sparkling mineral water
- Stovetop Apple & Cherry Crumble (page 430)

PART 4

Clean Cuisine
Recipe
Collection

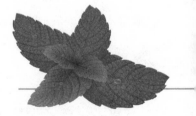

GO-TO BREAKFASTS
Great Grains With Fruit, Organic Pastured Eggs, And 5-Minute No-Milk Shakes

Great Grains with Fruit

- **Step 1:** Use the chart on page 306 to cook the whole grain of your choice.
- **Step 2:** Add any fruit (fresh or thawed frozen) of your choice to the cooked whole grains. Keep the fruit to grain ratio 2 to 1, meaning if you eat 1 cup of fruit then you want to have ½ cup of cooked whole grains.
- **Step 3:** Pour fresh hemp cream (page 306) on top of your whole grains or try sprinkling 1 or 2 tablespoons hemp seeds, ground flaxseeds, chia seeds, or raw nut crumbs (page 306) on top. You can also stir in a few teaspoons of raw nut or seed butter, such as almond butter or tahini.

OPTIONAL ADDITIONAL STEP
- **Step 4:** Boost flavor and antioxidants with a sprinkling of spice, such as cardamom, cinnamon, nutmeg, allspice, pumpkin pie spice (we like Simply Organic brand), or freshly grated ginger, lemon zest, or orange zest. If you want to add sweetness try just a drizzle of raw honey or 1 to 2 teaspoons date sugar.

	GRAIN in Cups	WATER in Cups	SALT (Opt.)	COOKING on Stovetop	COOKING in Rice Cooker
Steel Cut Oatmeal	1 Cup	4 Cups	Pinch	25–30 Minutes	20–25 Minutes
Millet	1 Cup	4 Cups	Pinch	20–30 Minutes	20–25 Minutes
Barley	1 Cup	4 Cups	Pinch	1 Hour	65–75 Minutes
Buckwheat	1 Cup	2 Cups	Pinch	20–30 Minutes	15–20 Minutes
Brown Rice (short grain)	1 Cup	2–2½ Cups	Pinch	50–60 Minutes	45–55 Minutes
Brown Rice (long grain)	1 Cup	2–2½ Cups	Pinch	45–50 Minutes	45–55 Minutes
Black Rice	1 Cup	1¾ Cups	Pinch	30 Minutes	30 Minutes
Wild Rice	1 Cup	3 Cups	Pinch	50–75 Minutes	50–60 Minutes
Quinoa	1 Cup	2 Cups	Pinch	20–30 Minutes	15–20 Minutes

NOTE: *We suggest you rotate your grains on a regular basis because each whole grain has its own unique vitamin, mineral, antioxidant, and phytonutrient profile. By rotating your grains you'll get exposed to a broad spectrum of nutrients.*

HOW TO MAKE NUT CRUMBS

TO MAKE NUT crumbs put any raw nut in a mini–food processor and pulse until crumblike. The nut crumbs will keep for up to a month stored in a self-sealing plastic bag in the freezer.

HOW TO MAKE FRESH HEMP CREAM

½ cup water
3 to 4 tablespoons hemp seeds
Pinch of unrefined sea salt

Place the water, hemp seeds, and salt in a high-speed blender (we like Vitamix) and blend until smooth and creamy. Hemp cream will keep for up to 3 days stored in a covered container in the fridge.

No-Cook Swiss Morning Muesli

SERVES 6

It really doesn't get much easier than this no-cook muesli, which keeps nicely for weeks if stored in a covered container or self-sealing plastic bag in the fridge. Sprinkle the muesli over chopped fresh fruit and drizzle some hemp cream on top. Yum!! P.S. Just a little bit of muesli trivia: the concept of muesli (which includes uncooked oats) was actually developed by a Swiss physician.

1 cup raw whole pecans

¼ cup ground chia seeds (such as Barlean's)

2 cups organic dried apricots

1 cup pitted dates

1 teaspoon ground cinnamon

1 teaspoon organic extra-virgin coconut oil (such as Barlean's)

1 cup old-fashioned oats

In a food processor, combine all the ingredients except the oats and pulse for about 2 minutes to combine. Transfer the mixture to a self-sealing plastic bag. Add the oats. Shake to combine. Serve.

Gluten-Free Millet Pancakes

SERVES 1

These are the pancakes Ivy and our son, Blake, invented when school was canceled for two days thanks to the threat of Hurricane Isaac. They are beyond delicious.

¼ cup, plus 1 tablespoon water

1 organic pastured egg

⅛ teaspoon pure vanilla extract

2 tablespoons hemp seeds

3 pitted dates

¼ cup, plus 1 tablespoon millet flour

½ teaspoon baking soda

⅛ teaspoon baking powder

Pinch of unrefined sea salt

⅛ teaspoon cinnamon

Organic extra-virgin coconut oil (such as Barlean's), for oiling the skillet

1. In a high-speed blender, combine all of the ingredients except for the coconut oil and blend until smooth and creamy.
2. Lightly oil the bottom of a skillet over medium heat. Once the skillet is hot, pour a small amount of batter in the pan. Cook until bubbles form on the surface, then flip the pancakes, and continue to cook until golden, 1 to 2 minutes. Repeat until the pancake batter is gone.
3. Serve warm with fresh fruit.

Chia-Crusted French Toast

SERVES 2

French toast is a classic favorite so it's good to know it can be incredibly health-ful too with just a few tweaks here and there. By using sprouted whole grain bread instead of regular bread made with empty-calorie white flour, by cooking with extra-virgin coconut oil instead of butter or highly refined vegetable oils, by using organic pastured eggs, and by dredging the bread in omega-3 and fi-ber-rich ground chia seeds, you'll get a super boost of nutrition in every yummy bite. It's so delicious you'll practically forget it's healthful too!

1 organic pastured egg, lightly beaten

2 tablespoons hemp milk (such as Pacific Naturals brand)

⅛ teaspoon ground cinnamon

2 slices sprouted whole grain bread (such as Ezekiel 4:9 Food for Life brand)

¼ cup ground chia seeds

Organic extra-virgin coconut oil (such as Barlean's)

Agave syrup or pure maple syrup to taste, optional

1. In a shallow bowl, whisk the egg, hemp milk, and cinnamon. Add the bread slices and turn them in the mixture to soak for 30 to 60 seconds.
2. Dredge both sides of the soaked bread slices in the ground chia seeds.
3. Lightly coat a large heavy skillet with coconut oil and heat over medium heat; when pan is hot add the bread slices and cook until golden brown, about 2 minutes. Flip and cook until golden brown, about 2 minutes. Drizzle with a smidgen of agave nectar or pure maple, if desired, and serve warm.

COOKWARE THAT MAKES FOODS TASTE BETTER

LOOKING FOR A simple to clean, nontoxic and green cookware that makes your food taste better? We recommend Xtrema—a 100 percent ceramic, non-scratch, nonreactive, and nontoxic cookware. Xtrema skillets, saucepans, woks, tea ware, and bakeware are manufactured with completely natural minerals, thus providing a much safer cooking alternative to traditional metal and nonstick coated cookware.

Foods cooked with Xtrema even taste better! That's because there are no heavy metals or toxins that can leach into the foods, which can distort the taste and nutritional value.

Xtrema also manufactures FridgeX, non-toxic, nonstick and stain-resistant silicone storage containers. Ivy loves a tidy kitchen and she especially loves that you can bake, serve, and store with FridgeX. The containers serve double-duty and go from freezer to oven without chipping or shattering. FridgeX is perfect for storing all of your Clean Cuisine leftovers too!

Learn more about Xtrema and FridgeX at www.Ceramcor.com. Clean Cuisine readers can enjoy a 10 percent savings by using coupon code: ccx10 at www.Ceramcor.com/clean.

Perfect Scrambled Organic Pastured Eggs-n-Veggies

SERVES 1

2 organic, pastured eggs

2 teaspoons water

Unrefined sea salt, to taste

Pinch of paprika

½ teaspoon organic extra-virgin coconut oil (such as Barlean's)

¾ cup finely chopped vegetables (onions, mushrooms, red or green bell peppers, carrots, zucchini, radishes, etc.)

1. Crack the eggs into a small bowl. Add the water, salt, and paprika. Use a fork to whisk the eggs vigorously (the more you whisk them, the fluffier they will be). Set whisked eggs aside.

2. Heat the oil in a small skillet over medium heat; add the vegetables and sauté until soft, 3 to 4 minutes. Pour the whisked eggs over the vegetables and scramble until the eggs are no longer runny (be careful not to overcook). Eat at once.

5-Minute No-Milk Shakes

As you now know from reading Chapter 6, we are not exactly big fans of cow's milk. Nut- and seed-based milks and no-milk shakes really do pack a far more powerful nutritional punch than cow's milk and with no nasty negatives either. Nut and seed milks are exactly what they imply—dairy-free (hormone and antibiotic free too) liquid nourishment made from ground nuts and seeds mixed with water. They are ultra-clean protein-rich vegan beverages supplying fiber, antioxidants, phytonutrients, vitamins, minerals, and essential fats. Milk and dairy just can't compete. Nut and seed milks also make the perfect neutral base for shakes because they blend so well with a wide array of fruits. You'll be blown away at how rich and creamy they taste. While you can absolutely buy almond milk or hemp milk ready made at the supermarket (and we regularly do so), nothing beats the taste or health benefits of fresh homemade raw nut and seed milk. And nothing could be easier to make either. All you need is a high-speed blender (we use a Vitamix), and you'll be good to go. We've included a few of our favorite shakes but once you get the hang of making them, you'll see you can put them together without a recipe. As we mentioned in Chapter 5, to boost nutrition and to make the nuts easier to grind you will want to soak them in water first. See page 142 for instructions.

Carrot Cake No-Milk Shake

SERVES 1

We thought up this shake for Andy's mom, Elaine, because her favorite dessert is carrot cake. This really does taste like carrot cake, we're not kidding! Feel free to substitute macadamia nuts for the pecans.

¼ cup raw whole pecans

1 carrot, peeled and cut into bite-size pieces

1 frozen banana, cut into bite-size pieces

½ cup frozen pineapple pieces

¼-inch segment ginger root (no need to peel)

¼ teaspoon ground cinnamon

1 cup coconut water (such as O.N.E.)

2 ice cubes

In a high-speed blender, combine all the ingredients except the ice cubes; blend until smooth and creamy. Add the ice cubes and blend again. Serve immediately.

BANANA FREEZE

FROZEN BANANAS ARE a staple food in our house because they make the richest, creamiest, sweetest, and most decadent smoothies on the planet. The best way to freeze bananas for use in smoothies is to remove the skins, then cut the banana into small chunks; place the banana chunks in individual self-sealing plastic bags and freeze. Bananas can be kept frozen for up to 4 weeks.

Eggnog No-Milk Shake

SERVES 2

This rich, velvety, sweet (but very low in sugar!) shake is dripping with yummy. Perfect for starting any holiday morning on a healthful note!

½ cup raw whole pecans

2 frozen bananas, cut into bite-size pieces

4 pitted dates

½ teaspoon ground cinnamon

½ teaspoon pure vanilla extract

¼ teaspoon ground nutmeg

2 teaspoons pure maple syrup (optional)

1½ cups ice cold water

2–3 ice cubes

In a high-speed blender, combine all the ingredients except the ice cubes; blend until smooth and creamy. Add the ice cubes and blend again. Serve immediately.

Blackberry-Almond No-Milk Shake

SERVES 1

1 tablespoon raw almond butter

¼ teaspoon pure almond extract

1 frozen banana, cut into bite-size pieces

¾ cup organic frozen blackberries

1 cup cold water

In a high-speed blender, combine all the ingredients; blend until smooth and creamy. Serve immediately.

Chocolate Cherry Bomb No-Milk Shake

SERVES 1

2 tablespoons raw cashews (about 16 cashews)

1 frozen banana, cut into bite-sized pieces

½ cup frozen cherries

1 tablespoon unsweetened high-quality cocoa powder (such as Ghirardelli or Green & Blacks)

⅛ teaspoon pure vanilla extract

¾ cup ice cold water

Pinch of unrefined sea salt

In a high-speed blender, combine all the ingredients; blend until smooth and creamy. Serve immediately.

Strawberry Banana Split No-Milk Shake

SERVES 1

2 tablespoons hemp seeds

1 frozen banana, cut into bite-size pieces

1 cup frozen organic strawberries

1½ cups very cold water

In a high-speed blender, combine all the ingredients; blend until smooth and creamy. Serve immediately.

313

Florida Sunshine No-Milk Shake

SERVES 1

> ¼ cup raw whole macadamia nuts (or 3 tablespoons hemp seeds)
>
> 1 orange, peeled and chopped
>
> ¾ cup frozen pineapple pieces
>
> 2 to 3 pitted dates (optional, if you want it a bit sweeter)
>
> 1 cup ice cold water or coconut water (such as O.N.E.)

In a high-speed blender, combine all the ingredients; blend until smooth and creamy. Serve immediately.

Georgia Peach Pie No-Milk Shake

SERVES 2

> ¼ cup chopped raw whole pecans
>
> 1 frozen banana, cut into bite-size pieces
>
> 1½ cup frozen peach pieces
>
> ¼ teaspoon ground cinnamon
>
> ¼ teaspoon pure vanilla extract
>
> 2 cups ice water

In a high-speed blender, combine all the ingredients; blend until smooth and creamy. Serve immediately.

Banana Açaí Superfood No-Milk Shake

SERVES 1

Containing two superfoods, açaí and hemp seeds, this is one of the easiest smoothies in the world to make. It's packed with antioxidants, omega fats, and phytonutrients and guaranteed to give you plenty of zip, pep, and go! It's mildly sweet made as is, but if you want it sweeter just add the dates.

1 tablespoon hemp seeds

1 frozen banana, cut into bite-size pieces

1 packet (100 grams) frozen unsweetened açaí smoothie packets (look for Sambazon brand)

¾ cup water

2 to 3 dates (optional, if you want it a bit sweeter)

In a high-speed blender, combine all the ingredients; blend until smooth and creamy. Serve immediately.

Ginger Blueberry & Mango Cobbler No Milk Shake

SERVES 1

½-inch piece fresh ginger, peeled

½ cup frozen blueberries

½ cup frozen mango pieces

¼ cup raw macadamia nuts

2 pitted dates

1 cup ice cold water

In a high-speed blender, combine all the ingredients; blend until smooth and creamy. Serve immediately.

Rise-n-Shine Green Goddess No-Milk Shake

SERVES 1

2 tablespoons hemp seeds

1 handful chopped kale

1 celery rib, chopped

3 pitted dates

½ cup frozen pineapple pieces

¾ cup frozen mango pieces

1-inch piece fresh ginger, peeled

¼ cup chopped parsley

Juice from 1 whole lime

1½ cups cold water

In a high-speed blender, combine all the ingredients; blend until smooth and creamy. Serve immediately.

REDEFINING LUNCH
Deliciously Nutritious Lunch Combos

Clean Cuisine Super Salads

Eating one gigantic raw salad each day is a great way to supercharge your Clean Cuisine lifestyle. But we know the obstacles to eating salad too, including the fact it's easy to get in a salad rut, especially if you are eating one every single day! We also recognize the idea of eating a salad day after day doesn't exactly sound super exciting. But honestly, the thing is salads can truly be incredibly tasty and super satisfying if you stick to just a few guidelines. Yes, really! You don't need to follow a strict "recipe" either; using creativity and imagination is part of the fun. Since learning how to make killer Clean Cuisine salads we truly look forward to our deliciously different salads. Here's a few of our best tips for building your own amazing four-star salad:

- **Mix up the lettuce leaves.** You want to combine soft lettuce (such as mâche, watercress, arugula, and spinach) with crunchy lettuce (such as radicchio, Belgian endive, and romaine) because the different textures provide important elements that elevate salad from ho-hum to *yum*!

315

NOTE: The darker the greens, the more nutrient bang for your buck. And the more greens you add the better!

- **Chop, chop, chop.** We learned about the culinary magic of a mezzaluna on a trip to New York City a few years ago. Our hotel was located right next to Fresh & Co, a casual quickie lunch spot that chopped up the most insanely delicious salads we had ever had. We were so hooked on the salads, we ate there for lunch every single day for our entire visit. And no matter which salad combination we tried, each one was over the top incredible. The secret was in the chopping. By using a mezzaluna (a half-moon shaped knife blade) the Fresh & Co salads were finely chopped in less than 2 minutes. The end result is chopped salad perfection... every single time. Do get a mezzaluna (you can get one for less than $30) and chop away. You'll be glad you did!

- **Add fresh herbs.** Not only do fresh herbs boost flavor but they boost the phytonutrient content of your salad, a lot. Experiment with a variety of fresh herbs. Our favorites in salad are parsley, cilantro, mint, basil, and tarragon.

- **Add zing with lemons, limes, or gourmet vinegar.** If you eat a salad every day, it really is worth it to experiment with gourmet vinegars. We particularly love the richness of balsamic vinegar (such as strawberry balsamic, blackberry ginger balsamic, and balsamic fig). For an extra-special treat that will greatly intensify the flavor of your balsamic vinegar (and your salad!) try reducing the vinegar in a skillet or saucepan over medium-high heat. Fresh lemons and limes are also delicious in salad, as are the zests.

- **Go for a drizzle of gourmet oils.** It's not a good idea to add tons of oil to your salad, but adding a little will no doubt boost the flavor. While you do want to avoid empty-calorie refined vegetable oils (such as soybean oil, pure vegetable oil, and corn oil) and bottled dressings made with those oils, you can absolutely drizzle small amounts of healthful omega-3-rich oils such as flax oil and walnut oil or monounsaturated oil such as cold-pressed extra-virgin olive oil. You can also experiment with high-quality gourmet oils that deliver big boosts of flavor in very small amounts. Some of our favorite gourmet oils for salad dressings are truffle oil (look for one in an extra-virgin olive oil base, such as Roland brand), avocado oil, pistachio oil, hazelnut oil, and lemon-infused extra-virgin olive oil. If you use one of our Salad Booster recipes you shouldn't need more than about 1 teaspoon of oil for your entire salad.

- **Supersize it.** Your salad is one dish where more is better! The bigger you can make your salad and the more dark greens and raw veggies you can add, the better. Your daily salad is a great way to get mega nutrition in one big tasty bowl. So think *big*!

317

- **Add dried fruit, raw nuts, and raw seeds.** Dried fruits, raw nuts, and raw seeds add tremendous flavor and satisfaction to your salad. There are so many different varieties of fruits, including exotic dried ones like goji berries and freeze dried pomegranates, plus tons of raw nuts and raw seeds (including hemp seeds!) to choose from. Mix and match and get creative. By far the tastiest way to eat dried fruit, raw nuts, and raw seeds on a salad is to use a food processor to process them into crumbs. By sprinkling on the dried fruit and nut crumbs you'll boost the flavor of your salad tremendously and need substantially less oil too. See our Salad Booster combinations for some great ideas.

- **Go for veggie variety!** There are so many different raw veggies to choose from that it's impossible to name them all. But think of creating your own salad bar. We like to store all sorts of raw veggies in various FridgeX (see page 309 for more information) containers in our fridge. That way, when it's time to make our salad we have them ready to go. Some of our favorite raw veggies are radishes, carrots, red and orange bell peppers, scallions, cherry tomatoes, red onions, and shredded beets. You can also add some kinds of thawed frozen vegetables, like organic corn and petite peas.

- **Beans beef up your salad.** Go ahead and add all kinds of beans, even thawed frozen organic edamame. These vegan foods help make your salad more nutritious, filling, and satisfying.

Clean Cuisine Salad Boosters

When it comes to boosting the flavor of *any* salad you need to add some fat. This is because fat is one of the most important conveyers of flavor that exist. It also means that if you make a fat-free salad, it just won't taste very good, and you probably won't be too enthused about eating it every day either. However, we recognize pouring excessive amounts of oil and dressings on top of your salad in the name of taste isn't exactly the best way to boost health either. Clean Cuisine Salad Boosters (www.CleanCui sineSaladBooster.com) are the tasty and nutritious alternatives to empty-calorie, processed bottled salad dressings and oily condiments.

Our Salad Boosters contain healthy whole fats from raw nuts and seeds. And because the raw nuts and seeds are ground into small crumbs they can be sprinkled over your salad so that you get a bit in every salad bite. If you simply add a few whole walnuts or almonds to your salad you might get the health benefits but you won't get the same taste satisfaction you get when the nuts are ground into crumbs. The Salad Boosters also include dried fruits that not only add a hint of sweetness but also a lot of moisture (because there is nothing worse than a dry salad).

Best of all the Salad Boosters are beyond easy to make yourself, and they keep for up to 2 months if stored in a self-sealing plastic bag in your freezer. Ivy likes to make a variety of Salad Booster batches in bulk quantity so we can grab and sprinkle on our salads anytime. We even like to travel with individual Salad Boosters in small plastic bags so we can enjoy tasty salads on the road. One of the greatest things about the Salad Boosters is that they are super versatile and *not* just for salads. You can sprinkle the boosters on top of just about any steamed vegetable, baked potato, whole grain, or bowl of beans for an effortless boost of flavor and nutrition.

Salad Boosters Master Directions

1. Put the first 3 ingredients in a high-speed blender or mini–food proces-sor and blend or process into crumbs.
2. Add the remaining ingredients and blend or process again until the mixture is crumbly and moist.
3. To use: Sprinkle a few tablespoons on top of your salad. Save the rest in a self-sealing plastic bag and store in the freezer.

NOTE: *All Salad Boosters are Vegan, Dairy Free, Gluten-Free*

SUCCULENT TOMATO SALAD BOOSTER

8 dried apricots

⅓ cup sun-dried tomatoes (preferably without salt), julienned or chopped

¼ cup plus 2 tablespoons pine nuts

1 garlic clove

2 pinches cayenne pepper

¼ cup hemp seeds

ALMOND-LIME SALAD BOOSTER

⅓ cup slivered almonds

5 pitted dates

½ teaspoon lime zest

1 teaspoon nutritional yeast (optional)

¼ teaspoon red pepper flakes (optional)

CURRY WALNUT SALAD BOOSTER

½ cup raw walnuts

3 tablespoons white raisins

¼ teaspoon ground turmeric

½ teaspoon curry powder

2 teaspoons freshly grated gingerroot

⅛ teaspoon unrefined sea salt

GARLIC-HERB SALAD BOOSTER

½ cup pine nuts or raw whole macadamia nuts

¼ cup white raisins

3 garlic cloves, chopped

½ teaspoon dried basil

½ teaspoon dried oregano

¼ teaspoon unrefined sea salt

READY-MADE GOURMET SUPERFOOD CLEAN CUISINE SALAD BOOSTERS

DON'T HAVE THE time to make your own Clean Cuisine Salad Booster? Check out our ready-made gourmet superfood Clean Cuisine Salad Boosters at www.CleanCuisineSaladBooster.com. We've included superfood ingredients such as goji berries, dried oyster mushrooms, nutritional yeast, hemp seeds, and green tea to supercharge your salad booster with omega-3s, fiber, phytonutrients, and antioxidants along with gourmet flavorings such as truffle salt for sensational taste. Our gourmet superfood Clean Cuisine Salad Booster blends are ideal for boosting the flavor (and nutritional profile) of so many different foods—including roasted vegetables, whole grains, potatoes, beans, whole grain crostinis, mushroom cap appetizers, and more! Check out the website for photos, inspiration, and ideas.

Clean Cuisine Salad Dressings

Dressings will keep in the refrigerator for 3 to 4 days if stored in a covered container.

Ivy's No Mayo, No Egg Caesar Salad Dressing

YIELDS APPROXIMATELY ½ CUP

This one is such a hit on our CleanCuisineandMore.com website that we had to include it in the book.

¼ cup hemp seeds

2 to 3 whole garlic cloves

¾ teaspoon Dijon mustard

1 teaspoon organic Worcestershire sauce (such as Annie's Naturals)

¼ cup cold-pressed extra-virgin olive oil

¼ cup freshly squeezed lemon juice

Unrefined sea salt, to taste

Freshly ground black pepper, to taste

½ teaspoon anchovy paste

Place all ingredients in a high-speed blender or food processor and blend or process until smooth and creamy.

Honey Lemon Thyme Vinaigrette

YIELDS APPROXIMATELY ½ CUP

3 garlic cloves

¼ of a whole lemon (including the rind), seeds removed

1 tablespoon fresh thyme leaves

3 teaspoons raw honey

⅓ cup flax oil (such as Barlean's)

¼ teaspoon unrefined sea salt

Pinch of freshly ground black pepper

Place all ingredients in a high-speed blender or food processor and blend or process until smooth and creamy.

Creamy Herb Dressing

YIELDS APPROXIMATELY ½ CUP

This rich and creamy dressing is actually a cross between the classic ranch and green goddess dressings, both of which are typically made with mayonnaise. Our cleaned-up mayo-free vegan version is so delish we promise you won't think twice about the missing mayo.

¼ cup plus 1 tablespoon hemp seeds

2 garlic cloves

1 teaspoon Dijon mustard

1 teaspoon organic Worcestershire (such as Annie's Naturals)

2 tablespoons chopped fresh chives

2 tablespoons chopped fresh parsley

¾ cup water

1 teaspoon raw honey

2 tablespoons cold-pressed extra-virgin olive oil

2 tablespoons lemon juice

Place all ingredients in a high speed blender or food processor and blend or process until smooth and creamy.

3-Step Clean Cuisine Salad Assembly

BUILD A CLEAN CUISINE 4-STAR SALAD

PICK 2 →   **GREENS**

(For Best Taste Mix Crunchy and Soft Lettuce Together)

- Mixed Greens
- Italian Blend
- Baby Spinach
- Radicchio
- Watercress
- Belgian Endive
- Mâche
- Romaine

PICK 1 →   **BEANS**

Drain and Rinse from BPA-Free Cans

- Black Beans
- Great Northern Beans
- Pinto Beans
- Cannellini Beans
- Kidney Beans
- Garbanzo Beans
- Legumes
- Split Peas
- Chick Peas
- Edamame Beans
- Petite Peas

PICK 2–3 → FRESH RAW OR LIGHTLY COOKED VEGGIES

- Radishes
- Carrots
- Red, Orange & Green Bell Peppers
- Scallions
- Tomatoes
- Red Onions
- Cucumbers
- Alfalfa Sprouts
- Corn
- Avocado
- Broccoli
- Green Beans
- Cauliflower
- Asparagus
- Mushrooms

PICK 1–2 → RAW NUTS, RAW SEEDS & DRIED FRUITS

- Raw Cashews
- Raw Almonds
- Raw Pine Nuts
- Raw Walnuts
- Raw Pecans
- Raw Peanuts
- Flax Seeds
- Raw Sunflower Seeds
- Hemp Seeds
- Dried Goji Berries
- Dried Pomegranates
- Dried Cranberries
- Raisins
- Prunes
- Dried Apricots
- Dried Peaches
- Dried Pears
- Dried Apples

PICK 1 →   **FRESH HERBS**

- Parsley
- Cilantro
- Mint
- Basil
- Tarragon
- Chives

PICK 1–2 →   **FINISHING TOUCHES**

- Squirt of Lime or Lemon
- Gourmet Vinegars
- Gourmet Oils (page 316)
- Salad Dressings (page 320)
- Salad Boosters (page 317)

1. In a large mixing bowl, combine the greens, beans, veggies, nuts, seeds, fruits and fresh herbs. Pour the mixture out onto a large chopping board. Use a mezzaluna (or knife) to finely chop all of the ingredients.

323

2. Sprinkle a Salad Booster (page 318) on top of the salad mixture and chop again. Season lightly with sea salt (we like Real Salt brand) and freshly ground black pepper, if desired.

3. Transfer the salad mixture back into the mixing bowl. Add the finishing touches. Gently toss to coat. Eat!

Perfect Loaded Baked Potato (Or Sweet Potato)

A perfect loaded baked potato (or sweet potato) starts, not surprisingly, with a perfectly baked potato. Sure you can microwave your spuds, but our favorite potatoes spend quality time in a real oven. Ovens transform potato skins into a crusty, thick, and full-flavored jacket, and the inside becomes soft, sweet, and fluffy. Microwaves just can't do a job like that!

SHOULD YOU EAT THE WHOLE POTATO?

THE SIZE OF your potato, your appetite, and your activity level should determine whether you eat an entire potato or just half. But whatever you do, be sure to eat the potato *with the skin* because the skins are loaded with fiber. Sweet potatoes are generally smaller and less filling than a white potato so you will most likely need to eat the entire sweet potato.

Perfect Baked Potato

SERVES 2

Although baked potatoes are always best straight from the oven, they are still very good eaten the next day, within 24 hours. If you want to store leftovers, just wrap your baked spud in plastic wrap or foil to keep it from drying out and store in the fridge.

2 Idaho or russet potatoes, scrubbed and dried

1 teaspoon cold-pressed extra-virgin olive oil

Unrefined sea salt, to taste

1. Preheat the oven to 400ºF.
2. Prick the potatoes all over with the tines of a fork. Rub the oil on the skins (to make them slightly crispy). Season the potatoes with salt to taste.
3. Place the potatoes on a rack in the oven and bake for about 1 hour, or until the insides feel soft when pricked with a fork. Eat warm.

Perfect Baked Sweet Potato

SERVES 2

Just like baked potatoes, baked sweet potatoes are best straight from the oven, yet they are still perfectly good to eat the next day too. If you want to store your leftover sweet potato just wrap it in plastic wrap or foil to keep it from drying out and store in the fridge.

2 medium sweet potatoes, unpeeled

1. Preheat the oven to 400ºF.
2. Prick the sweet potatoes several times with the tines of a fork.
3. Place the sweet potatoes on a rimmed baking sheet lined with foil. Bake 45 to 50 minutes, until tender. Eat warm.

LOADING YOUR PERFECT BAKED POTATO (OR SWEET POTATO)

ADD MOISTURE

- Hummus (look for one made with extra-virgin olive oil)
- Mashed avocado
- Parm-free pesto (look for a pesto made without Parmesan or make your own; page 354)
- Cashew Cream (page 144)
- Merlot Mushroom Gravy (page 351)
- Quick Romesco Sauce (page 352)
- Marinara sauce (page 371; or top-notch store bought sauce such as Rao's marinara)
- Poblano Chile and Pumpkin Seed Mole Sauce (page 355)
- Salsa
- Chopped olive tapenade

BOOST FLAVOR

- Garlic granules
- Roasted garlic
- Fresh chopped herbs (basil, chives, parsley, cilantro, oregano)
- Unrefined sea salt
- Freshly ground black pepper
- Salad Booster (www. CleanCuisineSaladBooster.com)

Vegetable Soups

Creamy Broccoli & Edamame Bisque

SERVES 4

This soup tastes so much like traditionally prepared cream of broccoli soup that you just won't believe it's dairy free. Our son Blake loves it as an after school snack. It is so good and goes so fast in our house that Ivy often makes a double batch (it freezes well too).

1 tablespoon cold-pressed extra-virgin olive oil

1 teaspoon organic extra-virgin coconut oil (such as Barlean's)

4 garlic cloves, minced

2 large shallots, chopped

1 leek, white and green parts, chopped

1 teaspoon ground coriander

Unrefined sea salt, to taste

6 cups organic vegetable broth

1 pound broccoli, trimmed, stems and florets chopped

1 cup organic shelled edamame

¼ cup short-grain brown rice

2 tablespoons freshly squeezed lemon juice

1. Heat the olive oil and coconut oil in a large saucepan over medium heat; add the garlic and shallots and sauté 3 to 4 minutes. Add the leek and sauté until very tender, about 10 minutes. Season with coriander and salt. Add ½ cup of the broth, scraping any brown bits from the bottom. Cook for 1 minute.

2. Add the remaining 5½ cups broth, the broccoli, edamame, and rice. Bring liquid to a boil. Reduce heat to low and simmer until the rice is soft and the broccoli is very tender, 15 minutes. Add the lemon juice.

3. Use an immersion blender to process the ingredients into a smooth and creamy bisque. Adjust seasoning. Serve warm or cold.

ALL SALT IS NOT CREATED EQUAL

DID YOU KNOW that all salt could technically be considered "sea salt"? Some salt is harvested from current oceans, some from dead seas, and some is mined from ancient sea beds, but the sea is ultimately the source of all salt. Sea water usually contains more than 60 essential trace minerals, but most salt producers today remove these high-profit minerals and sell them to vitamin manufacturers before selling the remaining cheap "table salt" to you. The problem is, when the trace minerals are removed you end up with a bitter flavor that many producers try to mask with chemicals or even sugar. Even worse, when you consume chemically treated or demineralized salt, your body's mineral balance doesn't respond optimally. "Table salt" is not healthy, but it's also not at all the same as "Real Salt" or Himalayan salt.

"REAL SALT" VS. HIMALAYAN SALT

"REAL SALT" (RealSalt.com) is a United States company that packages salt in its natural state without additives, chemicals, or heat processing of any kind. Real Salt's unique pinkish appearance and flecks of color come from more than 60 naturally occurring trace minerals.

Gluten-Free Soba Noodle Soup with Shiitakes, Carrots, Spinach, & Tofu

SERVES 4

This is really much more than just a soup side dish, in fact, we often eat it as a light meal. Look for soba noodles made entirely from buckwheat flour because they are more nutritious than soba made from whole wheat flour (100 percent buckwheat flour soba noodles are also gluten free.)

2 teaspoons extra-virgin coconut oil (such as Barlean's)

1 tablespoon minced gingerroot

6 garlic cloves, crushed

3 cups chopped carrots

1 tablespoon gluten-free soy sauce (such as San J)

1½ cups shiitake mushrooms, cut (use kitchen shears to cut the mushrooms)

4 scallions, chopped

¼ cup unpasteurized miso paste

8 cups hot water

8 ounces 100 percent buckwheat soba noodles, uncooked

3 tablespoons freshly squeezed lime juice

5 ounces baby spinach

7 to 10 ounces extra-firm organic tofu, drained and cut into small pieces

1. In a large saucepan, heat the oil over medium heat. Add the ginger and garlic; sauté 30 seconds. Add the carrots and sauté 4 to 5 minutes. Add the soy sauce and cook an additional minute. Add the mushrooms and scallions and sauté until tender, about 6 minutes.

2. Dissolve the miso paste in the hot water. Add the miso mixture to the saucepan with the vegetables; bring to a boil. Add the noodles and lime juice; reduce the heat to a simmer and cook 5 minutes. Add the spinach and cook until just wilted, about 1 minute. Taste the broth and add a bit of salt, if necessary.

3. Transfer soup to individual bowls and sprinkle with tofu. Drizzle soy sauce on top. Eat warm.

Mom's All-New Healing No-Chicken, No-Noodle Lemon-Turmeric Soup

SERVES 8

When Ivy was growing up, her mom made homemade chicken noodle soup every time her daughter was sick. There's nothing like slurping up Mom's homemade soup for extra comfort when you are under the weather. Although this soup is not exactly the way Ivy's mom made it, we picked the ingredients for their incredible healing, and flavor, properties. From a nutritional standpoint, this soup blows traditional chicken noodle soup out of the water. This is now the way Ivy's mom makes soup for all of us when we are feeling under the weather. Although we don't use noodles you can absolutely add cooked black rice if you want the soup to be a bit heartier (brown rice is also fine, but black rice has more antioxidants).

2 tablespoons organic extra-virgin coconut oil (such as Barlean's)

1 whole garlic bulb, minced

1 Spanish onion, finely chopped

3½ ounces shiitake mushrooms, cut into bite-size pieces (use kitchen shears for cutting)

3½ ounces maitake mushrooms, cut into bite-size pieces (use kitchen shears for cutting)

2 teaspoons ground turmeric

Freshly ground black pepper, to taste

Unrefined sea salt, to taste

1 medium-size leek, thinly sliced

3 cups chopped carrots

½ cup miso paste

10 cups very hot water

Juice from 1 whole lemon

2 teaspoons lemon zest

3 tablespoons chopped fresh tarragon

1 cup chopped fresh parsley

5 large handfuls chopped kale

1. Heat the oil in a large heavy saucepan over medium heat. Add the garlic and onions and sauté until soft, 3 to 4 minutes. Add the mushrooms and sauté until soft, 2 to 3 minutes.

2. Sprinkle the turmeric, pepper, and salt on the mushrooms. Add the leeks and carrots and sauté until soft, 3 to 4 minutes.
3. Dissolve the miso paste in 2 cups of the water and add the miso mixture to the saucepan with the vegetables. Add the remaining 8 cups of water and bring to a simmer.
4. Add the lemon juice, lemon zest, tarragon, parsley, and kale. Reduce the heat to medium-low and simmer until the greens are very wilted, for 10 minutes. Adjust seasoning. Serve warm.

SUPER TURMERIC

TURMERIC IS AN ultra-potent anti-inflammatory and healing spice. Pairing it with pepper increases the body's absorption by a whopping 2,000 percent!*

---

* G. Shoba, D. Joy, T. Joseph, et al., "Influence of Piperine on the Pharmacokinetics of Curcumin in Animals and Human Volunteers," *Planta Medica* 64, no. 4 (1998): 353–56.

Time-Saving Farmers' Market Vegetable Soup

SERVES 6

Okay, so we cheated a bit on this recipe by incorporating some frozen vegetables. We admit a real farmers' market soup would probably be made with only fresh veggies. But we have made this same soup using all fresh vegetables and not only does it take more time to make but we actually prefer this time-saving version. It might not be for veggie soup purists, but for the time-crunched among us, this one's a winner!

1½ pints cherry tomatoes, halved

3 tablespoons cold-pressed extra-virgin olive oil

Unrefined sea salt, to taste

Freshly ground black pepper, to taste

5 garlic cloves, chopped

1 large onion, finely chopped

4 carrots, finely chopped

4 celery ribs, finely chopped

1 tablespoon fresh thyme, chopped (or 1 teaspoon dried)

1 package (16 ounces) frozen cauliflower florets

1 box (9 ounces) frozen cut green beans

1 cup frozen organic corn kernels

4 cups baby organic spinach leaves

5 cups organic vegetable broth

2 tablespoons finely chopped parsley

¼ cup freshly squeezed lemon juice

1. Preheat the oven to 400°F. On a rimmed baking sheet, toss the tomatoes with 2 teaspoons of the olive oil and salt and pepper to taste. Roast for 15 minutes. Let cool, then mash with a potato masher.

2. Heat the remaining 1 tablespoon of olive oil in a large heavy saucepan over medium heat; add the garlic, onion, carrots, and celery and sauté until very soft, 10 minutes. Add the thyme and season with salt to taste. Stir in the cauliflower and green beans and sauté 4 to 5 minutes. Add the corn and sauté 1 minute. Add the spinach and cook until wilted, 1 minute. Add the mashed roasted tomatoes.

3. Add the vegetable broth. Increase the heat to high and bring to a boil; cook for 7 to 8 minutes. Remove the saucepan from heat and stir in the parsley and lemon juice. Adjust the seasoning. Let the soup sit for at least 15 minutes before serving. Serve warm.

Roasted Zucchini Soup with Tarragon & Lime

SERVES 6

When Ivy first made this soup she thought it would be an adult-only type of soup, but we were happily surprised when our son and his pal taste-tested it and asked for a bowl each. Not only do the kids like it but it also makes a mild-tasting and elegant dinner party soup (if serving to guests garnish with chopped chives). The soup will keep for 2 to 3 days if covered and stored in the fridge or for up to 1 month frozen.

5 zucchini, sliced into rounds

1 tablespoon cold-pressed extra-virgin olive oil

Unrefined sea salt, to taste

3 tablespoons freshly squeezed lime juice

3 tablespoons old-fashioned oats

⅓ cup pine nuts

1½ cups water

6 garlic cloves, crushed

2 shallots, chopped

2 cups organic vegetable broth

½ cup chopped fresh tarragon

⅛ teaspoon ground white pepper

1. Preheat the oven to 400°F.
2. Lightly oil the bottom of a cookie sheet or a large, heavy skillet. Place zucchini rounds in the prepared pan and drizzle 1 teaspoon of the oil on top. Toss the zucchini gently to coat with the oil and season lightly with salt. Roast for 30 to 35 minutes, or until soft. Remove the zucchini from the oven and set aside.
3. Place the lime juice, oats, pine nuts, and water in a high-speed blender or food processor. Blend or process until smooth and creamy. Set aside.
4. Heat the remaining 2 teaspoons of oil in a large saucepan over medium heat. Add the garlic and shallots and sauté until soft, 2 to 3 minutes. Pour in the pine nut mixture and vegetable broth. Bring the liquid to a simmer and cook for 5 minutes. Add the roasted zucchini and the tarragon and pepper.
5. Use an immersion blender to process the soup into a creamy consistency. Ladle the soup into bowls and serve warm.

Spiced Turmeric-Charged Creamy Cauliflower Soup

SERVES 6

With the anticancer, anti-inflammatory benefits of turmeric in the spotlight lately, Ivy gests a lot of requests from our online readers to create turmeric-charged recipes. She almost put this one on our website but decided to save it for the book instead.

1 tablespoon cold-pressed extra-virgin olive oil

½ onion, chopped

2 carrots, chopped

⅓ cup plus 1 tablespoon julienned sun-dried tomatoes, packed in oil, rinsed with water and patted dry

⅓ cup white raisins

½ teaspoon ground turmeric

¼ teaspoon red pepper flakes

Unrefined sea salt, to taste

1 head of cauliflower, trimmed of green leaves and coarsely chopped (about 6 cups)

6 cups organic vegetable broth

¼ cup pine nuts

1 tablespoon freshly squeezed lime juice

1. Heat the oil in a large heavy skillet over medium heat. Add the onion and carrots and sauté 2 to 3 minutes. Add the sun-dried tomatoes, raisins, turmeric, red pepper flakes, and salt; sauté until the onions and carrots are soft, 7 to 8 minutes. Add the cauliflower and toss to coat in the vegetable mixture. Cook for 3 to 4 minutes. Season with salt to taste.

2. Place 1 cup of the vegetable broth, the pine nuts, and lime juice in a high-speed blender or food processor; blend or process until smooth and creamy. Add the broth mixture to the saucepan. Pour the remaining 5 cups of broth into the saucepan. Increase the heat to high and bring to a boil. Reduce the heat and simmer until the cauliflower is tender, 20 minutes.

3. Use an immersion blender to process the soup into a creamy consistency. Adjust the seasoning, and add more broth or a bit of water if the soup is too thick. Serve warm.

Garlic and Carrot Soup

SERVES 6

We have to give credit to Samantha Gardner, our director of operations for CleanCuisine.com for helping Ivy develop this rich and creamy soup. It is just the thing to serve with lunch but it's also an elegant starter soup for entertaining. The secret to giving this soup (and just about any other soup) great depth is to layer the ingredients. To make it extra-special when serving to guests, Ivy sprinkles on Crunchy Garlicky Bread Crumb Topping (page 335) just before serving.

2 tablespoons cold-pressed extra-virgin olive oil

2 large shallots, finely chopped

1 cup chopped fennel stalks

1 whole garlic head, cloves separated and peeled (do *not* chop the garlic)

Unrefined sea salt, to taste

4 cups chopped carrots

¼ cup Chardonnay (look for a buttery flavored one, we especially love Kendall Jackson)

5 cups organic vegetable broth

¼ teaspoon white pepper

⅛ teaspoon ground cardamom

1. Heat the oil in a large heavy saucepan over medium heat. Add the shallots and fennel and sauté until the fennel starts to soften, 3 minutes. Add the whole garlic cloves and season with salt. Sauté until the garlic softens and the shallots and fennel become very soft, 5 to 6 minutes, being careful not to let the garlic burn.
2. Add the carrots and cook until they start to soften, 7 to 8 minutes.
3. Add the Chardonnay and cook until the liquid almost completely evaporates. Add the vegetable broth and simmer until carrots are very, very tender, 15 to 20 minutes. Add the pepper and cardamom.
4. Use an immersion blender and process until smooth and creamy. Adjust the seasoning. Serve warm.

CRUNCHY GARLICKY BREAD CRUMB TOPPING

5 garlic cloves

1 slice sprouted whole grain bread (such as Ezekiel 4:9 Food for Life brand), crusts removed

1 tablespoon cold-pressed extra-virgin olive oil

2 teaspoons chopped fresh thyme

1. Place the garlic and bread in a mini-food processor and process into fine crumbs. Set aside.
2. Heat the oil in a small heavy skillet over medium heat; add the bread crumb mixture and pan-fry until the bread crumbs start to turn golden, about 3 minutes. Add the thyme, and continue cooking for 30 seconds more.

Beans and Legumes

Tuscan Slow-Baked Cannellini Beans with Shallots, Garlic, & Sage

SERVES 4

In Italy foods such as minestrone, polenta, and risotto are often slow, slow cooked yielding a soft but deeply flavored dish, which is exactly what we've done here. Although the ingredients might sound rather simple the end result tastes anything but. Although we acknowledge cheese is not healthy, we have to admit that sprinkling a tablespoon or so of freshly grated cheese on top of the beans takes this dish over the top in taste.

1 tablespoon plus 1 teaspoon cold-pressed extra-virgin olive oil

2 large shallots, finely chopped

6 garlic cloves, crushed

Unrefined sea salt, to taste

2 tablespoons chopped fresh sage

5 ounces arugula

¼ cup white wine (look for a buttery flavored one, we especially love Kendall Jackson)

½ cup organic vegetable broth

2 cans (14.5 ounces) organic BPA-free cannellini beans, rinsed and drained

¼ cup raw walnut crumbs (page 306) and/or 4 tablespoons freshly grated Parmesan cheese (optional)

1. Preheat the oven to 325°F.
2. Heat 1 tablespoon of the oil over medium heat in a large heavy oven-proof skillet with tight-fitting lid; add the shallots and garlic and sauté until the shallots soften, 5–6 minutes.
3. Add the sage and sauté for 1 minute. Add the arugula and the remaining 1 teaspoon of oil and sauté until the arugula wilts, about 2 minutes. Add the wine and cook until it evaporates. Add the vegetable broth and beans and mix ingredients to combine well.
4. Cover the skillet and transfer to the oven; bake the beans for 50 minutes, or until the liquid evaporates and beans are soft and buttery. Serve with the walnut crumbs and cheese, if desired.

Smoky Pinto Beans with Oven-Roasted Tomatoes

SERVES 6 TO 8

Liquid smoke is the culinary secret to making healthful, smoky barbecue-flavored sensations with zero fuss. Ivy learned about liquid smoke from her mom, Gail, and once you start playing around with it in the kitchen you'll be amazed at how many dishes you can give that outdoor deliciousness with indoor ease. Look for all-natural Colgin brand liquid smoke in the condiment section at your supermarket (usually its right near the mustard). Colgin has several flavors too: natural hickory (which we use in this recipe), apple, mesquite, and pecan. This recipe really is beyond easy to make too. You can oven-roast the tomatoes anytime (up to 3 days in advance) with about only 5 minutes of hands-on time and then the rest of the recipe takes about 15 minutes or so. Easy peasy!

NOTE: Use an apple corer to core the tomatoes.

Oven-Roasted Tomatoes

Oven-roasted tomatoes can be prepared up to 3 days in advance.

2 pounds firm but ripe organic plum tomatoes, cored and halved lengthwise

2 teaspoons cold-pressed extra-virgin olive oil

Unrefined sea salt, to taste

Freshly ground black pepper, to taste

1. Preheat oven to 400°F and position the rack in the middle of the oven. Lightly oil a very large, rimmed baking sheet.
2. Arrange the tomatoes cut side up in the prepared pan. Make a tiny slit in each tomato and drizzle with the oil. Season with salt and pepper to taste.
3. Roast the tomatoes for about 1 hour, or until desired doneness. Remove the tomatoes from the oven and set aside to cool.

Smoky Pinto Beans

1 tablespoon plus 1 teaspoon cold-pressed extra-virgin olive oil

6 garlic cloves, minced

1 Spanish onion, finely chopped

Unrefined sea salt, to taste

2 cans (15 ounces) organic BPA-free pinto beans, rinsed and drained

1 recipe Oven-Roasted Tomatoes (page 337)

1 tablespoon natural hickory flavor liquid smoke

2 teaspoons Dijon mustard

1 tablespoon date sugar (or brown sugar)

1 teaspoon paprika

2 teaspoons ground cumin

1. Heat the oil in a large saucepan over medium heat; add the garlic and sauté 30 seconds. Add the onion, and sauté until soft, 4 to 5 minutes. Season with salt to taste. Stir in the pinto beans and tomatoes, lightly mashing the tomatoes with the back of a spatula.
2. Add the liquid smoke, Dijon mustard, sugar, paprika, and cumin. Reduce the heat to low and cook for 8 to 10 minutes, or until heated through. Serve warm.

VARIATION

This recipe is also delicious with a little organic grass-fed ground beef. If you want to use ground beef add 4 to 6 ounces along with the onions and cook until meat is no longer pink.

Smoky Tex-Mex Slow-Cooked Vegetarian Chili
SERVES 6 TO 8

We know chili lovers can take their chili pretty seriously (especially the ones who reside in Texas). Well we take our Clean Cuisine chilies serious too and so we've worked, tweaked, tasted, and revamped this one to perfection. The secret is the combo of liquid smoke (look for Colgin brand, available in the condiments section of any supermarket) and taco seasoning (we like Simply Organic brand). And sure, you could add a little ground pastured beef if you want, but once you taste this vegetarian dish, you'll see it doesn't need a thing . . . except a spoon.

NOTE: To make this gluten-free use vegetable broth instead of beer.

2 tablespoons cold-pressed extra-virgin olive oil

6 garlic cloves, minced

1 jalapeño pepper, seeds removed, finely chopped

1 small onion, finely chopped

3 carrots, chopped

2 medium zucchini, chopped

3 ears of organic corn, kernels removed

Unrefined sea salt, to taste

1 can (28 ounces) diced tomatoes

Juice from 1 whole lime

¼ cup beer or organic vegetable broth

2 tablespoons taco seasoning (we like Simply Organic)

2 tablespoons liquid smoke

1 tablespoon organic Worcestershire sauce (such as Annie's Naturals)

2 cans (15 ounces) BPA-free pinto beans, rinsed and drained

1 can (15 ounces) BPA-free kidney beans, rinsed and drained

1. Heat the oil in a large heavy skillet over medium heat; add the garlic and jalapeño and sauté 30 seconds. Add the onion and sauté until soft, 3 to 4 minutes. Add the carrots and sauté 2 to 3 minutes. Add the zucchini and corn kernels and sauté until soft, 3 to 4 minutes. Season with salt to taste. Transfer the vegetable mixture to a 5- or 6-quart slow cooker.

2. Add the tomatoes, lime juice, beer, taco seasoning, liquid smoke, Worcestershire sauce, and beans. Cook on low heat for 3 hours. Let sit 15 to 20 minutes before serving. Serve warm.

Fried Red Beans & Corn

SERVES 4

Ivy got the idea to make this rather unusual dish one day as an alternative to refried beans. It's delicious as is but we also like it as filler for our quesadillas (see "How to Make Clean Cuisine Quesadillas" on page 341 for tips).

1 can (15 ounces) BPA-free organic small red beans, rinsed and drained

1 cup frozen organic corn, thawed

1 tablespoon cold-pressed extra-virgin olive oil

6 garlic cloves, crushed

¾ cup finely chopped onion

Unrefined sea salt, to taste

1 chipotle chili in adobo sauce, seeds removed and finely chopped

2 tablespoons very finely chopped cilantro

1. Place the beans in a food processor and pulse 8 to 10 times, until coarsely chopped (do not purée). Remove the beans and set aside. Add the corn to the food processor and pulse 4 to 5 times, until coarsely chopped (take care not to overprocess). Remove the corn and set aside with the beans.

2. Heat the oil in a large heavy skillet over medium heat; add the garlic and onion and sauté until soft, 6 to 8 minutes. Season with salt to taste. Add the chipotle chili and sauté for 1 minute. Add the cilantro and sauté 30 seconds.

3. Add the chopped beans and corn to the skillet and mix well to blend. Sauté 2 to 3 minutes. Season with salt to taste.

HOW TO MAKE CLEAN CUISINE QUESADILLAS

QUESO **IS THE** Spanish word for "cheese." And a quesadilla is a toasted tortilla with melted cheese inside. So even though we aren't big cheese fans (for health reasons), we acknowledge that a quesadilla is not really a quesadilla if it's made without the cheese. But in addition to cheese, you can put practically anything in a quesadilla. And you don't necessarily need globs of cheese either. We don't recommend you use a rubber-eraser-tasting cheese alternative because you can get a lot of flavor for just a little real cheese; about 2 tablespoons of a shredded good-quality organic cheese (preferably one from grass-fed cows) is really all you need. And be sure to use a healthful tortilla too! We especially like sprouted corn tortillas from Food for Life brand.

To make a quesadilla the right way, you need to get the skillet pretty hot, so the best oil to use is heat-stable extra-virgin coconut oil. Don't worry, if you get a good-quality oil (such as Barlean's) your quesadilla will not taste like coconuts!

QUESADILLA

MAKES 1

Organic extra-virgin coconut oil (such as Barlean's)
2 sprouted corn tortillas (such as Food for Life)
⅓ cup Fried Red Beans & Corn (page 339) or ⅓ cup smashed
    red beans or pinto beans
2 tablespoons shredded organic cheese (such as Cheddar)

1. Lightly oil the bottom of a heavy skillet, and heat over medium-high heat.
2. Spread the bean mixure on one tortilla and sprinkle the cheese on top. Place the second tortilla on top of the cheese. Put the quesadilla in the hot skillet, and place a heavy object, such as a small saucepan, on top. Cook until tortillas are slightly browned but not burned, 2 to 3 minutes. Flip the tortilla and brown the other side. Serve hot.

Three-Bean Salad with Warm Balsamic-Shallot Reduction

SERVES 6

This is a gourmet, uptown version of the classic three-bean salad but it's still per-fect for family cookouts and casual entertaining. It also makes a nice fall side dish, and we've even seen it a time or two on our Thanksgiving dinner table.

¾ **pound fresh green beans, ends trimmed and cut into ½-inch segments**

1 **can (15 ounces) organic BPA-free black beans, rinsed and drained**

1 **can (15 ounces) BPA-free garbanzo beans, rinsed and drained**

1 **tablespoon plus 1 teaspoon cold-pressed extra-virgin olive oil**

4 **garlic cloves, minced**

2 **large shallots, finely chopped**

Unrefined sea salt, to taste

¼ **cup balsamic vinegar**

1 **teaspoon raw honey**

1 **teaspoon Dijon mustard**

1 **teaspoon organic Worcestershire sauce (such as Annie's Naturals)**

½ **cup fresh finely chopped parsley**

Freshly ground pepper, to taste

1. Prepare an ice bath.
2. Bring a large pot of salted water to a boil. Add the green beans and cook until fork-tender, about 7 minutes. Drain the beans in a colander and immediately plunge them into an ice bath to stop the cooking process and preserve the color. Drain and transfer the green beans to a medium-size serving bowl. Add the black beans and garbanzo beans. Set aside.
3. Heat the oil in a medium-size saucepan over medium heat; add the garlic and shallots and sauté until the shallots are very, very soft, 4 to 5 minutes. Season with salt.
4. Add the balsamic vinegar and cook until reduced by more than half, about 5 minutes. Stir in the honey, Dijon mustard, and Worcestershire sauce. Pour the balsamic-shallot mixture on top of the beans; toss the beans to coat. Add the parsley and toss again. Season with salt and pepper to taste. Let the beans sit at room temperature for at least 15 minutes to allow the flavors to fully develop. Serve at room temperature.

Southern Belle's Black-Eyed Pea Brunch Salad

SERVES 6   343

This is a simple but elegant salad, perfect for a brunch, with a Southern-style twist thanks to the black-eyed peas. If you want to give this dish a completely different flavor profile try substituting small white beans for the black-eyed peas, basil for the cilantro, and 1 teaspoon Italian seasoning for the cumin. To shave off a few extra minutes of prep time you can substitute 2 cups of thawed frozen organic corn for the fresh corn kernels.

1 tablespoon cold-pressed extra-virgin olive oil, plus more for lightly oiling skillet

3 ears of organic corn, kernels removed

Unrefined sea salt, to taste

1 can (15 ounces) BPA-free organic black-eyed peas, rinsed and drained

2 scallions, finely chopped

2 red bell peppers, finely chopped

⅔ cup very finely chopped cilantro

¼ of a whole lime

2 tablespoons hemp seeds

3 tablespoons water

3 garlic cloves

2 teaspoons ground cumin

1. Spread a very thin layer of oil on the bottom of a large heavy skillet. Heat the skillet over medium-high heat. Add the corn and pan-sear for 3 to 4 minutes. Season with salt and transfer to a medium-size serving bowl.

2. To the bowl, add the black-eyed peas, scallions, bell peppers, and cilantro; gently toss ingredients together. Set aside.

3. In a high-speed blender (such as a Vitamix) or food processor, add the lime, hemp seeds, water, garlic, cumin, and the remaining 1 tablespoon of oil; season with salt to taste. Process until creamy (the mixture should be a little thick and not totally smooth). Add the mixture to the corn and black-eyed peas. Gently toss to coat, adding more lime juice, if desired. Season with salt to taste. Let salad sit for at least 15 minutes before serving. Serve at room temperature.

GOT GREENS? SuperGreen Smoothies

Citrus Splashy SuperGreen Smoothie

SERVES 1

1 tablespoon chia seeds (such as Barlean's)

1 small handful arugula

1 whole orange, peeled

½ cup frozen pineapple pieces

2 pitted dates

1 tablespoon freshly squeezed lemon juice

1 cup ice cold water or coconut water (such as O.N.E.)

3 ice cubes

In a high-speed blender (such as a Vitamix), combine all the ingredients except the ice cubes; blend until smooth and creamy. Add the ice cubes and blend again. Drink cold.

Blueberry-Ginger Cocktail SuperGreen Smoothie

SERVES 1

1 tablespoon chia seeds (such as Barlean's)

2 handfuls chopped romaine lettuce

1 cup frozen blueberries

2 pitted dates

¼-inch piece gingerroot, peeled

1 cup ice cold water or coconut water (such as O.N.E.)

½ cup ice

In a high-speed blender (such as a Vitamix), combine all the ingredients except the ice; blend until smooth and creamy. Add the ice and blend again. Drink cold.

Mango Spice Cake SuperGreen Smoothie

SERVES 2

2 tablespoons chia seeds (such as Barlean's)

1 to 2 handfuls chopped kale

½ cup frozen pineapple pieces

1¼ cups frozen mango pieces

½-inch piece gingerroot, peeled

½ teaspoon ground cinnamon

¼ teaspoon ground nutmeg

2½ cups ice cold water or coconut water (such as O.N.E.)

In a high-speed blender (such as a Vitamix), combine all the ingredients; blend until smooth and creamy. Drink cold.

Thai-Style Pineapple-Cilantro SuperGreen Smoothie

SERVES 2

2 tablespoons chia seeds (such as Barlean's)

1 handful cilantro

1 handful parsley

1 cup frozen pineapple, pieces

1-inch piece gingerroot, peeled

3 cups ice cold water or coconut water (such as O.N.E.)

In a high-speed blender (such as a Vitamix), combine all the ingredients; blend until smooth and creamy. Drink cold.

Strawberry Mojito SuperGreen Smoothie

SERVES 1

1 tablespoon chia seeds (such as a Barlean's)

1 large handful chopped romaine

1 cup frozen strawberries

2 pitted dates

2 to 3 tablespoons chopped fresh mint

1 tablespoon lime juice

1 cup ice cold water or coconut water (such as O.N.E.)

¾ cup ice

In a high-speed blender (such as a Vitamix), combine all the ingredients except the ice; blend until smooth and creamy. Add the ice and blend again. Drink cold.

GREEN SMOOTHIE FAQ

ENJOYING A SUPERGREEN Smoothie every day is a key component of the Clean Cuisine lifestyle. Although drinking blended greens might seem a little odd at first, we promise you'll be hooked once you start. The vibrant energy and glow you'll get from your SuperGreen daily fix is just too good to give up. Plus SuperGreen Smoothies are incredibly refreshing and delicious. We get a lot of questions on our website about SuperGreen Smoothies so we thought we'd share our answers to the most frequently asked questions.

1. **Would juicing be better than drinking a smoothie?** No. Juices are not whole foods. Juice is a fractured food missing the fiber and its antioxidants, which are part of the whole fruit or vegetable. Keep in mind, fiber is also an essential component of detoxification and is crucial for helping rid your body of toxins. Once you reduce toxins, you'll absorb nutrients better. Fiber-rich foods also help stabilize blood sugar levels and keep you feeling full longer, but because juices are missing the fiber, they don't do a very good job at filling you up. You will undoubtedly end up being hungrier (and eating more!) if you drink juice instead of smoothies.

2. **Can't I just have an extra salad instead of a smoothie?** You could do this, but it's not optimal, especially if you have digestive issues. Your body assimilates considerably more vital nutrients from blended greens than from chewed greens because the blender breaks down the food into super teeny-tiny particles.

3. **Can I just drink the same SuperGreen Smoothie every day?** Yes and no. Sure, it would be better to drink the same Super-Green Smoothie every day than to have no SuperGreen Smoothie at all, but you'll be shortchanging your nutrition if you don't rotate your greens. Just like we suggest you eat a wide variety of whole grains, fruits, and vegetables, we also suggest you eat a wide variety of greens. This is because each and every green has its own unique nutrient, antioxidant, and phytonutrient profile. For optimal health, you want to switch up your greens and try different SuperGreen Smoothies every week.

4. How far in advance can I make my SuperGreen Smoothie? You can make SuperGreen Smoothies up to 24 hours in advance as long as you keep them cold in the refrigerator. Ivy often makes a double batch for us so we usually make a new one only every other day.

> *NOTE:* The chia seeds in the smoothies will thicken over time, so you may want to add more water if you don't drink your smoothie within 15 minutes after mixing. Another option is to put your smoothie back in the blender with 2 to 3 ice cubes for 30 seconds just before drinking to freshen it up.

5. How long does it take to make a SuperGreen Smoothie and clean up? No more than 5 minutes start to finish, considerably less time, effort, and mess than it takes to squeeze juice!

6. What if I don't like the taste? Add more fruit or dates for sweetness. Our SuperGreen Smoothie recipes do not have a particularly high fruit to greens ratio, but if you want to really mask the flavor of the greens simply add more fruit.

7. Why do you have chia seeds in every single SuperGreen Smoothie recipe? The chia seeds are not essential but we just add them for a fiber, omega-3, and antioxidant booster.

8. Why do you recommend coconut water as an alternative to water in every recipe? Coconut water adds a deliciously refreshing flavor to the green smoothies and it is an excellent source of potassium and other electrolytes.

9. What is the best blender to use? You really need a high-speed blender (1,000 watts or more) to fully break down the greens. We prefer Vitamix because we think it has more durability than the competition.*

---

* A Vitamix is not a cheap purchase, but if you really are serious about adopting the Clean Cuisine lifestyle you will want to invest in one. Learn more at Vitamix.com, and for free shipping use code 06-006758.

Parsley-Apple SuperGreen Smoothie

SERVES 2

    2 tablespoons chia seeds (such as a Barlean's)

    1 Granny Smith apple, cored and chopped (keep the skin on)

    1 cup frozen peach pieces

    2 handfuls parsley

    1 tablespoon freshly squeezed lemon juice

    2 cups ice cold water or coconut water (such as O.N.E.)

    3 ice cubes

In a high-speed blender (such as a Vitamix), combine all the ingredients except the ice cubes; blend until smooth and creamy. Add the ice cubes and blend again. Drink cold.

It's Easy Being Green SuperGreen Smoothie

SERVES 1

    1 tablespoon chia seeds (such as Barlean's)

    1 cup frozen peach pieces

    1 small handful arugula

    1 small handful parsley

    1 tablespoon freshly squeezed lemon juice

    1 cup ice cold water or coconut water (such as O.N.E.)

In a high-speed blender (such as a Vitamix), combine all the ingredients; blend until smooth and creamy. Drink cold.

Better Than V8 SuperGreen Smoothie

SERVES 1

    1 tablespoon chia seeds (such as Barlean's)

    1 tomato, chopped

    1 celery rib, chopped

    1 garlic clove

    1 handful parsley

1 teaspoon organic Worcestershire sauce (such as Annie's Naturals)

1 to 2 dashes Tabasco sauce (or other hot sauce)

¼ cup ice cold water

4 ice cubes

In a high-speed blender (such as a Vitamix), combine all the ingredients except the ice cubes; blend until smooth and creamy. Add the ice cubes and blend again. Drink cold.

NOTE: *Hungry for more Clean Cuisine recipes? Visit CleanCuisine.com for over 200 free recipes!!*

SAUCES THAT MAKE
THE MEAL

Merlot Mushroom Gravy

YIELDS APPROXIMATELY 1 CUP

*This stuff is just incredible. It's good to keep around too because you can
smother it on just about anything. Top off your cooked whole grains, baked
potato, or sweet potato; try it on baked butternut squash or spaghetti squash;
or dollop it on top of seared chicken breasts. We especially love smothering
our tofu steaks with it. The turnip in this recipe does wonders for adding body
and flavor to the gravy.*

1 tablespoon cold-pressed extra-virgin olive oil

6 cloves garlic, crushed

1 shallot, finely chopped

Unrefined sea salt, to taste

White pepper, to taste

¾ cup peeled, diced turnips

8 ounces gourmet mushroom blend (maitake, trumpet, shiitake, oyster)

2 tablespoons white whole wheat flour

¼ cup good quality merlot (don't use cooking wine!)

1 cup organic vegetable broth

1. Heat the oil in a medium-sized heavy skillet over medium heat; add the garlic and shallots and sauté 3 or 4 minutes, until shallots are tender. Season with salt and pepper to taste.
2. Add the turnips and sauté for 3 or 4 minutes, until soft. Add the mushrooms and sauté for 3 or 4 minutes, until soft. Season with salt and pepper to taste.
3. Sprinkle in the flour and stir to combine with the other ingredients. Add the merlot and cook for 1 or 2 minutes, until merlot evaporates. Add the broth and simmer for 5 to 8 minutes.
4. Remove skillet from heat and set aside. Use a hand-held stick blender to "cream" ingredients together. (*Note: you don't want a perfectly smooth gravy so don't overprocess!*)

For a sensational entrée, lightly salt extra-firm individual 4-ounce tofu steaks, spread the gravy on top, and bake at 400°F for about 20 minutes or until lightly golden. Mmmm!

Quick Romesco Sauce

YIELDS APPROXIMATELY 1 CUP

We first heard about romesco sauce from our dear friend Erin Lodeesen after she returned from a one-month trip to Spain (must be nice!). This sauce is a rich-tasting and savory condiment that adds the perfect spark to vegetables, beans, and seafood (Andy particularly likes it on plump seared scallops). And it is unspeakably delicious baked on top of tofu and finished with a squirt of lime. You can make a thinner and gluten-free sauce by omitting the toasted bread and nutritional yeast, but our family prefers the thicker version. Romesco sauce will keep for up to 3 days if stored in the fridge in a covered container. It can also be stored in the freezer for up to 1 month.

2 tablespoons cold-pressed extra-virgin olive oil
1 shallot, finely chopped
8 garlic cloves, crushed
3 tablespoons slivered almonds
2 tablespoons balsamic vinegar
1 can (14.5 ounces) BPA-free fire-roasted diced tomatoes
½ teaspoon red pepper flakes
1½ teaspoons paprika

¼ teaspoon unrefined sea salt

1 slice toasted, sprouted whole grain bread, broken into bite-size pieces (optional)

1 to 2 tablespoons nutritional yeast (optional)

1. Heat the oil in a large saucepan over medium heat; add the shallot and garlic and sauté until the shallot is soft, 3 to 4 minutes. Add the almonds and cook for 1 minute. Add the vinegar and cook until reduced by about half, about 2 minutes. Add the tomatoes, red pepper flakes, and paprika; simmer for 15 minutes. Add salt and season to taste and set the mixture aside to cool.

2. When cool, transfer the sauce to a high-speed blender or food processor and blend or process until smooth and creamy. Add toasted bread and nutritional yeast, if desired, and blend or process again. Serve warm or at room temperature.

WHY WE *LOVE* CLEAN CUISINE SAUCES

WE THINK ONE of the reasons people don't eat super healthful "Clean Cuisine" staple whole foods such as vegetables, whole grains, beans, lentils, fish, and tofu more often is because, let's face it, these healthful foods can taste bland and boring if served plain. This is where our homemade Sauces That Make the Meal step in to perk up even the most blah of foods. Our mole sauce will turn your corn on the cob into pure decadence and our Merlot Mushroom Gravy can transform tofu steaks into something you'd think should be served at a four-star restaurant. You'll be amazed at how a few tablespoons of a flavor-rich sauce will add a completely different flavor dimension to your entire meal. As much as we love sauces, we would never suggest you start pouring any old sauce on your food. Classically prepared sauces like hollandaise, béarnaise, and Alfredo certainly taste incredible, but dousing your healthful foods in these butter- and cream-laden sauces isn't exactly in the spirit of eating Clean Cuisine! Many times a sauce or the topping is a chef's secret, which makes restaurant food taste so good. If you know how to make a special sauce or topper you can eat gourmet restaurant-quality food from your own kitchen, every day. But unlike the butter, oil, and heavy cream sauces you'd likely get from a restaurant, ours are dairy free, guilt free, and loaded with nutrient-rich ingredients such as fresh herbs, nuts, seeds, olives, and citrus. Our sauces are so flavor forward that just a little bit goes a long, long way. Best of all, they are incredibly versatile and can be used to dress up just about any simply prepared whole food; try them on steamed vegetables, cooked whole grains, fish, beans, lentils, and tofu.

Indian Pesto

YIELDS APPROXIMATELY 1 CUP

We put this alternative-style pesto on everything from grilled fish (it's sensational on wild salmon), tofu steaks, grilled vegetable kabobs, black rice, and lentils. (Note: garam masala can be found in the spice section; it is a sweet, aromatic blend of spices, delivering warm and exotic flavors essential to traditional Indian cuisine.)

½ cup raw whole macadamia nuts

3 garlic cloves

½ cup fresh basil

½ cup fresh mint

½ cup cilantro

1 tablespoon freshly grated ginger

1 teaspoon garam masala

1 tablespoon freshly squeezed lime juice

⅛ teaspoon unrefined sea salt

2 tablespoons cold-pressed extra-virgin olive-oil

1 teaspoon raw honey

2 to 3 tablespoons water (to make a thinner pesto add more water as desired)

Place all ingredients in a food processor or high speed blender (such as a Vitamix) and process until smooth and creamy and well blended.

Smoky Tri-Color Pepper Sauce

YIELDS APPROXIMATELY 1 CUP

This very veggie sauce makes the perfect condiment for fish, chicken, tofu, tempeh, and even baked potatoes. Andy particularly likes it as a substitute for marinara on his sprouted whole grain pasta. The addition of hemp seeds adds a hint of creaminess along with lots of added nutrition.

2 tablespoons cold-pressed extra-virgin olive oil

2 shallots, chopped

1 red bell pepper, cored, seeded, and chopped

1 yellow bell pepper, cored, seeded, and chopped

1 orange bell pepper, cored, seeded, and chopped

5 garlic cloves, crushed

2 tablespoons hemp seeds

Unrefined sea salt, to taste

½ cup beer

2 tablespoons liquid smoke

¾ cup tomato purée

1 teaspoon dried oregano

1 teaspoon brown sugar or date sugar

1. Heat the oil in a large heavy skillet over medium heat. Add the shallots, bell peppers, garlic, hemp seeds, and salt; sauté, stirring frequently, for 8 to 10 minutes. Add the beer and cook for 3 minutes. Stir in the liquid smoke, tomato purée, oregano, and brown sugar. Reduce the heat and simmer until the sauce thickens, 15 to 20 minutes. Remove from the heat and set the sauce aside to cool.
2. Transfer the cooled sauce to a high-speed blender and process until smooth and creamy.

Poblano Chile & Pumpkin Seed Mole Sauce

YIELDS APPROXIMATELY 1 CUP

Mole sauce is to Mexican cuisine what béarnaise is to French cuisine; it's the sauce that ties the whole meal together. Mole sauce is a potent and intoxicating blend of spices and peppers with variations galore. Our Clean Cuisine version is super low in oil and gets its richness from superfood raw pumpkin seeds. Mole sauce is just the thing for serving with grilled or roasted corn, green peppers, tofu, fish, whole grains, pinto beans, and black beans. When you scan the ingredients, you'll think we made a mistake and that all those things couldn't possibly work together to create anything remotely edible, much less tasty. It takes a bit of blind faith to make, but trust us, it works and it is G.O.O.D.! Mole sauce will last 3 days stored in a covered container in the fridge.

2 poblano chilies

½ Spanish onion, quartered

3 teaspoons cold-pressed extra-virgin olive oil

½ cup raw pumpkin seeds

2 garlic cloves

1 teaspoon ground cumin

2 teaspoons ground cinnamon

1 teaspoon chili powder

⅛ teaspoon unrefined sea salt, plus more to taste

2 teaspoons unsweetened cocoa powder

½ cup fresh chopped cilantro

2 tablespoons freshly squeezed lime juice

⅓ cup organic vegetable broth

1. Preheat the oven to 375°F.
2. Place the chilies and onions in a large cast iron skillet or baking sheet and toss with 1 teaspoon of the oil. Roast for 30 to 35 minutes, or until the vegetables are very soft. Remove the vegetables from oven, transfer to a bowl, cover with plastic wrap, and let steam for about 10 minutes. Using paper towels, rub the skins off the chilies; then remove the stems, seeds, and ribs.
3. In a high-speed blender or food processor, add the roasted chilies and onions. Process for 30 seconds. Add the remaining 2 teaspoons of oil, the pumpkin seeds, garlic, cumin, cinnamon, chili powder, salt, cocoa powder, cilantro, lime juice, and vegetable broth. Blend or process until the ingredients are well blended, 1 minute. Serve warm.

Puttanesca Sauce

We love that this robust Napoletana sauce can virtually transport us to Italy with just a few basic pantry ingredients. It's divine over baked seafood of any sort, but we also love it mixed with a plate of whole grain spaghetti, spaghetti squash, cooked whole grains, beans, or chopped wilted greens. Heaven.

2 tablespoons cold-pressed extra-virgin olive oil

6 garlic cloves, crushed

2 small shallots, finely chopped

2 ounces anchovies, packed in olive oil, drained

2 pints grape tomatoes, halved

Pinch of brown sugar

1 cup chopped kalamata olives

2 tablespoons capers

2 tablespoons finely chopped parsley

½ teaspoon red pepper flakes

Heat the oil in a large saucepan over medium heat; add the garlic, shallots, and anchovies and sauté until the shallots soften, 3 to 4 minutes. Add the tomatoes and sugar; sauté until soft, 5 or 6 minutes. Stir in the olives, capers, parsley, and red pepper flakes; cook for 3 to 4 minutes. Remove from heat. If you prefer a chunkier sauce leave as is, otherwise use an immersion blender and pulse several times to purée slightly.

Almond Asian Sauce

YIELDS APPROXIMATELY 3/4 CUP

This is an exotic healthful raw twist on the classic peanut Asian sauce that is so popular. It's perfect as a dipping sauce for chicken, fish, or tofu and just the thing for sprucing up steamed veggies.

¼ cup raw almond butter

4 cloves garlic

2 tablespoons chopped scallions

3 tablespoons golden raisins

1 tablespoon freshly grated gingerroot

1 tablespoon freshly squeezed lime juice

3 teaspoons high-quality unpasteurized soy sauce

1 teaspoon rice wine vinegar

¼ cup plus 2 tablespoons water

Place all ingredients in a high-speed blender and blend until smooth and creamy.

So Easy Tomato & Caper Sauce

YIELDS APPROXIMATELY 1 CUP

We got the recipe for this delectable and very versatile sauce from our friend Jay Hatfield, a chef dedicated to making super-healthful, super-tasty Clean Cuisine as a personal chef (if you are lucky enough to live in the Palm Beach area check out www.eatrightnow4u.com and treat yourself to one of Jay's home cooked meals.) As Jay says, "The key to a successful meal and the secret to a healthy diet are the same: color, variety and texture." We admire Jay not only for his genius in the kitchen (just try this sauce and you'll see what we mean) but also for his passion for helping others improve their health through nutrition. Jay is a cancer survivor who was diagnosed with lung cancer at age 36, a diagnosis that changed his life, his eating habits, and his culinary career. Although he has cooked in kitchens across the country, from New York City to mountain lodges in Vermont, Jay now helps families at home learn to cook healthfully because he believes that is where his talent has the most impact. If you aren't lucky enough to live in Palm Beach County and have Chef Jay cook with you, you can at least make his sauce, which is just divine over baked fish, chicken, tofu, or rice and beans.

¼ cup white wine

3 garlic cloves, minced

1 medium yellow tomato, diced

1 medium tomato, diced

1 tablespoon cold-pressed extra-virgin olive oil

2 tablespoons finely chopped parsley

2 tablespoons finely chopped basil

1 tablespoon plus 2 teaspoons capers

Pour the wine into a medium sauce pan and bring the heat to high; reduce the wine by half. Add the tomatoes and garlic, and cook for 3 to 4 minutes on high heat. Reduce the heat to medium and add the olive oil, parsley, basil, and capers. Continue cooking for one additional minute. Serve warm.

NOT YOUR
MAMA'S BURGERS

Five-Star Portofino Portobello-Beef (or Buffalo) Burgers with Olive Tapenade

SERVES 5

Like most men, Andy loves a good burger. While not every single one of Ivy's not-all-beef burgers gets a five-star rating from Andy, this one did! Actually, Andy gave this one a two-thumbs-up, one thumb for taste and the other for moistness. Although we use pastured ground beef in this recipe it is also delicious made with pastured ground buffalo, which is leaner than beef.

½ cup pitted kalamata olives

¼ cup chopped parsley

5 ounces portobello mushrooms, gills removed (use a spoon to scoop the gills out) and coarsely chopped

¾ cup chopped onion

5 garlic cloves, chopped

1 tablespoon cold-pressed extra-virgin olive oil

Unrefined sea salt, to taste

Freshly ground black pepper, to taste

¾ pound pastured 95 percent (preferably organic) ground beef or ground buffalo

1. Place the olives and parsley in a mini–food processor and pulse several times until finely chopped. Set aside.
2. Put the mushrooms, onions, and garlic in a large food processor, and pulse until very finely chopped (be careful not to overprocess).
3. Heat the oil in a heavy skillet over medium heat; add the mushroom-onion mixture and season with salt and pepper to taste. Sauté, stirring occasionally, until vegetables begin to brown and the liquid has evaporated, 8 to 10 minutes. Add the olive-parsley mixture to the skillet and mix well to blend. Cook for 1 minute. Transfer to a bowl and cool, stirring occasionally.
4. Add the ground beef along with more salt and pepper to the mushroom-onion mixture. Use your hands to mix until well combined. Form into five 4-inch patties.
5. Lightly oil the bottom of the skillet and heat over medium-high heat; add the burgers and cook, turning once, about 8 minutes total for medium-rare. Serve warm.

Southern-Style Black-Eyed Pea Burgers

SERVES 6

Over the years Ivy has tried a number of different bean burger recipes, and time and again she has been disappointed. The burgers are either too dry when baked, too oily when fried, or just too blah. All we can say is that these bean burgers will not disappoint. The secret is to follow the directions exactly, and don't skip the food processor part! This is a great recipe for using leftover brown rice. Do be sure to use short-grain brown rice for this particular recipe though because it is stickier than long-grain and is therefore better for holding the burgers together.

1 celery rib, coarsely chopped

1 carrot, coarsely chopped

¼ cup fresh parsley

1 tablespoon cold-pressed extra-virgin olive oil

1 shallot, minced

5 garlic cloves, crushed

Unrefined sea salt, to taste plus ¼ teaspoon

¾ cup organic frozen corn, thawed

2 tablespoons stone-ground cornmeal (medium grind)

¼ cup julienned sun-dried tomatoes packed in extra-virgin olive oil, rinsed and patted dry

2 cups cooked short-grain brown rice

1 can (15 ounces) BPA-free organic black-eyed peas, rinsed and drained

1 pastured organic egg, lightly beaten

1 tablespoon organic Worcestershire sauce (such as Annie's Naturals)

1 to 2 dashes Tabasco or other hot sauce

1. Preheat the oven to 350°F. Line a large baking sheet with parchment paper.

2. Place the celery and carrot in a food processor and pulse several times until finely chopped. Remove celery and carrots from the food processor and set aside. Add the parsley to the food processor and pulse several times until very finely chopped. Remove the parsley and set aside (keep the parsley separate from the carrots and celery).

3. Heat the oil in a large heavy skillet over medium heat; add the shallots and garlic and sauté until soft, 3 to 4 minutes. Season with salt to taste. Add the celery and carrots and sauté until soft, 3 to 4 minutes. Add the corn and cook for 1 minute.

4. Transfer the sautéed vegetables to a large bowl. Add the parsley, cornmeal, tomatoes, brown rice, and black-eyed peas. Using your clean hands, mix thoroughly, mashing the black eyed peas ever so lightly. Add the egg, Worcestershire sauce, and Tabasco sauce and ¼ teaspoon salt. Continue mixing the ingredients until well blended but not mushy.

5. Divide the mixture in to six ½-cup portions and form into 6 patties, each about ½ inch thick. Place the patties in the prepared pan. Bake for 30 minutes, or until firm and lightly golden. Serve warm.

Cleaned-Up Sloppy Joes

SERVES 8

This classic all-American casual dinner entrée is one Andy's mom, Elaine, frequently made when Andy was growing up. Andy has always loved sloppy Joes so we decided to revamp the recipe. To health it up, we gave it a Clean Cuisine reduced-meat makeover by incorporating a medley of minced vegetables (they blend right into the tangy sauce) and a combo of crumbled pastured beef and tempeh (don't worry, the tempeh keeps a very low flavor profile and blends right in too). If you grew up eating and loving sloppy Joes you are going to fall in love all over again. Serve over toasted sprouted whole grain buns (such as Food for Life brand) with a large romaine side salad. Leftovers will keep for up to 4 days stored in a covered container in the fridge.

1 can (8 ounces) organic tomato sauce

1 tablespoon molasses

2 tablespoons organic Worcestershire sauce (such as Annie's Naturals)

1½ teaspoons Dijon mustard

1½ teaspoons ground cumin

1 teaspoon garlic granules

1 small onion, coarsely chopped

1 red bell pepper, coarsely chopped

2 celery ribs, coarsely chopped

¾ pound pastured (preferably organic) ground beef or buffalo

8 ounces tempeh

1 tablespoon cold-pressed extra-virgin olive oil

6 garlic cloves, minced

Unrefined sea salt, to taste

1. In a medium bowl mix together the tomato sauce, molasses, Worcestershire sauce, Dijon mustard, cumin, and garlic granules. Set aside.
2. Place the onions in a food processor and pulse to finely chop. Remove the onions and repeat with the bell pepper and celery. Take care not to overprocess the vegetables or they will become mushy. Set the vegetables aside.
3. Place the ground beef and tempeh in the food processor and pulse until well blended. Set the mixture aside.

4. Heat the oil in a large heavy skillet over medium heat. Add the garlic and onions and cook until the onions start to soften, 2 to 3 minutes. Season with salt to taste. Add the bell pepper and celery and cook until soft, 3 to 4 minutes. Season with salt to taste. Stir in the meat mixture, using a spatula to combine well. Cook until the meat is cooked through, 4 to 5 minutes. Pour in the sauce and simmer for 10 minutes. Serve warm.

Mexican Fiesta Pinto Bean Burgers

SERVES 6

Just like our Southern-Style Black-Eyed Pea Burgers (page 361), you need to follow the recipe for these Mexican burgers exactly for optimal results. The secret to making sensational bean burgers that are still healthful (and not fried in puddles of oil) is to finely chop the vegetables with a food processor, sauté them in a little oil, and take extra care you don't pulverize the beans into mush. If you overprocess the beans, the burgers end up tasting dry when baked (sure, you could fix that by frying them in oil but that sort of offsets all the good you are doing by eating a bean burger). If you follow the directions you'll be in south-of-the-border bean burger heaven in no time.

2 slices toasted sprouted whole grain bread, broken into bite-size pieces

2 carrots, coarsely chopped

¼ cup cilantro (or parsley)

1 can (15 ounces) BPA-free organic pinto beans, rinsed and drained

1 tablespoon cold-pressed extra-virgin olive oil

1 shallot, minced

5 garlic cloves, crushed

Unrefined sea salt, to taste plus ¼ teaspoon

2 tablespoons stone-ground cornmeal (medium grind)

1 can (4 ounces) chopped green chilies

1 organic pastured egg, lightly beaten

1 teaspoon ground cumin

Pinch of cayenne (optional)

1. Preheat the oven to 350°F. Line a large baking sheet with parchment paper.

2. Place the bread in a food processor and process into crumbs. Remove and set aside.

3. Place the carrots in the food processor and pulse several times until very finely chopped. Remove and set aside. Add the cilantro to the food processor and pulse until very finely chopped. Remove and set aside (keep the cilantro separate from the carrots).

4. Place the beans in the food processor and pulse until coarsely chopped, about 10 times. You do not want to process the beans into a smooth mixture.

5. Heat the oil in a large heavy skillet over medium heat; add the shallots and garlic and sauté until the shallots soften, 3 to 4 minutes. Season with salt to taste. Add the chopped carrots and sauté until soft, 3 to 4 minutes.

6. Transfer the shallot mixture to a large bowl. Add the cilantro, cornmeal, green chilies, bread crumbs, and beans. Using your hands, mix thoroughly, mashing the pinto beans in with the rest of the ingredients. Add the egg, cumin, and ¼ teaspoon salt. Add a pinch of cayenne if you like a spicy kick. Continue mixing the ingredients until well blended but not mushy.

7. Divide the mixture into five ½-cup portions and form into 5 patties, each about ½ inch thick. Place the patties in the prepared pan. Bake for 30 minutes, or until firm and lightly golden. Serve warm.

Baked Salmon Burgers with Chive Cream Sauce

SERVES 6

Ivy makes these salmon burgers a lot on weekend nights when our son has his friends over because the kids love them (usually the kids prefer ketchup to the chive cream sauce, but hey, at least they are eating fish). Our sister-in-law, Kim Larson, is especially fond of them. And, although he doesn't like to admit anything healthful tastes good, we've been told Andy's brother, Mike Larson, likes them too. The salmon cakes make the perfect meal nestled on top of a big bed of arugula and served with roasted radishes and corn on the cob (we often remove the kernels from the cob and sprinkle them on top of our salads).

Chive Cream Sauce

¼ cup pine nuts

¼ cup hemp seeds

2 garlic cloves

2 tablespoons chopped chives

2 tablespoons freshly squeezed lemon juice

¼ teaspoon unrefined sea salt

3 to 4 tablespoons water (use 3 tablespoons if you want a thicker sauce and 4 tablespoons if you want a thinner sauce)

Place all the ingredients in a high-speed blender (such as a Vitamix) or mini food processor; blend or process until smooth and creamy. Set aside.

Baked Salmon Burgers

2 slices toasted sprouted whole grain bread, broken into bite-size pieces

4 garlic cloves

1 tablespoon cold-pressed extra-virgin olive oil

2 shallots, minced

2 celery ribs, minced

2 tablespoons finely chopped parsley

1 can (15 ounces) wild sockeye salmon, drained

2 organic pastured eggs, lightly beaten

1 teaspoon Dijon mustard

2 teaspoons organic Worcestershire sauce (such as Annie's Naturals)

1 teaspoon Old Bay seasoning

Stone-ground cornmeal, for dusting (medium-grind)

1. Place the bread and garlic in a food processor and pulse into bread crumbs. Set aside.
2. Heat the oil in a large heavy skillet over medium heat; add the shallots and celery and sauté until soft, about 8 minutes. Stir in the parsley. Transfer the mixture to a large mixing bowl.
3. To the vegetable mixture, add the salmon (flaking the fish apart with a fork), eggs, Dijon mustard, Worcestershire sauce, and Old Bay seasoning. Using your hands, combine the ingredients to mix well.

4. Divide the mixture into six ½-cup portions and form into 6 patties, pressing each together with your hands. Sprinkle both sides of each patty with cornmeal. Transfer the patties to a large platter and place in the freezer for 10 minutes.

5. Preheat the oven to 400° F.

6. Remove the patties from the freezer and heat a thin layer of oil in a large heavy ovenproof skillet (such as Xtrema); when the skillet is hot carefully add 3 patties and cook for about 1½ minutes per side, or until they have a light golden crust. Repeat with the remaining patties. Transfer the patties to the oven and bake for 15 minutes. Serve warm with chive cream sauce.

Greek Lamb (or Beef) Bulgur Burgers

SERVES 4

You will not believe us until you try them, but we promise these burgers taste better than an all-beef patty. When Andy's brother, Mike, the ultimate burger connoisseur, exclaimed "This is really, really good—surprisingly good!," we knew we'd struck burger gold! We then had our good friend Cherie Fromson test them on her burger-loving husband, Abe, and he agreed. You'll just have to try them for yourself.

⅔ cup organic vegetable broth

⅓ cup coarse or medium-grind bulgur

¾ pound pastured (preferably organic) ground lamb or ground beef

¼ cup finely chopped mint

¼ cup plus 2 tablespoons finely chopped parsley

¼ cup minced onion

5 garlic cloves, crushed

½ teaspoon unrefined sea salt

¾ teaspoon ground cinnamon

2 teaspoons ground cumin

1. Bring the vegetable broth to a boil in a small saucepan. Stir in the bulgur, cover, and reduce the heat. Simmer until all of the water is absorbed, about 10 minutes. Remove from the heat and fluff with a fork. Transfer the bulgur to a medium mixing bowl and set aside to cool.

2. When the bulgur is cool enough to handle, add the remaining ingredients to the bowl and use your hands to mix thoroughly. Form the mixture into 4 equal patties, about ½ inch thick.

3. Lightly oil the bottom of a large heavy skillet and heat over medium-high heat; add the burgers and cook, turning once, about 8 minutes total for medium-rare. Serve warm.

ONE-DISH WONDERS AND SLOW-COOKED DINNERS

Clean Cuisine–Style Spaghetti Pie

SERVES: 6 TO 8

From what we've been told spaghetti pie is a big thing with Midwesterners. After receiving more than a few requests for a Clean Cuisine spaghetti pie on our website, Ivy decided to dig up a few recipes and see exactly what went into making this classic comfort food favorite. Turns out it's made from tons of cheese, beef, and sour cream and not very many vegetables. And certainly not sprouted whole grain pasta! Undeterred she came up with a Clean Cuisine version that we tested on Andy's parents, Ken and Elaine. They loved it so much that we had to include it in the book. You'll still get that comfy-cozy feeling from eating it, but not in a sofa-bound, food-slump sort of way. Spaghetti squash is our secret ingredient; it blends right in with the pasta and keeps a very low profile.

2 teaspoons cold-pressed extra-virgin olive oil

6 garlic cloves, crushed

10 ounces frozen chopped spinach, thawed and patted very, very dry with paper towels

Unrefined sea salt, to taste

369

½ cup finely chopped basil

4 cups cooked spaghetti squash (below)

4 cups cooked sprouted whole grain spaghetti or quinoa spaghetti

2 cups marinara sauce, store bought (such as Rao's) or homemade (try Clean Cuisine Marinara page 371)

1 organic pastured egg, lightly beaten

1 cup raw whole walnuts

1. Preheat oven to 350°F. Lightly oil the bottom of a 9 by 13-inch casserole.
2. Heat the oil in a large skillet over medium heat; add the garlic and sauté 30 seconds. Add the spinach and sauté 2 to 3 minutes. Season with salt to taste. Stir in the basil and the spaghetti squash flesh and gently toss the ingredients together. Add the cooked spaghetti and gently toss the ingredients once more. Remove skillet from heat and set aside.
3. In a medium bowl whisk together the marinara sauce and the egg. Stir the sauce into spaghetti mixture and gently toss to coat. Transfer the spaghetti squash mixture to the prepared casserole.
4. Place the walnuts in a food processor and pulse into crumbs. Sprinkle the nuts evenly over the top of the spaghetti mixture. Bake, uncovered, for 20 to 25 minutes, or until firm. Remove from the oven and allow to cool 10 minutes before serving. Serve warm.

HOW TO COOK SPAGHETTI SQUASH

BELIEVE IT OR not, spaghetti squash contains anti-inflammatory omega-3 fatty acids in the form of alpha-linolenic acid (ALA); in fact, 1 cup of spaghetti squash contains around 350 milligrams of ALA. We love spaghetti squash and frequently eat it with a bit of marinara or pesto on top. So good! And it's beyond easy to make. Whether you use it in the spaghetti pie or not you'll want to learn how to cook spaghetti squash. Here's how you do it.

1 spaghetti squash, 8 to 12 inches long
Cold-pressed extra-virgin olive oil or organic extra-virgin coconut oil
Unrefined sea salt, to taste

1. Preheat oven to 400°F.

2. Cut the squash in half lengthwise. Remove the seeds and pulp (just like cleaning out the inside of a pumpkin at Halloween).
3. Place the squash in a baking sheet cut side up. Brush with the oil and sprinkle with salt. Bake for 30 to 40 minutes, until the outer skin is soft and the flesh is very tender. Remove from the oven and let cool for at least 10 minutes. Pull a fork lengthwise through the flesh to separate it into long strands. It comes out easily and looks like thin spaghetti.

CLEAN CUISINE MARINARA

We'll be honest, Ivy doesn't often make marinara from scratch only because there are so many amazing prepared marinara sauces on the market (for the record, our absolute favorite is Rao's marinara). However, if you have a little bit of extra time to spare nothing beats homemade. Here's our standby recipe for versatile Clean Cuisine Marinara that can be served chunky style or smooth and creamy. Note that the quality of the tomatoes you use matters a lot; we prefer off-the-vine fresh-tasting, BPA-free Pomì brand boxed tomatoes (look for Pomì in boxes, not cans).

3 tablespoons cold-pressed extra-virgin olive oil

1 medium onion, finely chopped

8 garlic cloves, minced

Unrefined sea salt, to taste

2 carrots, peeled and finely chopped

2 celery ribs, finely chopped

Freshly ground black pepper, to taste

½ teaspoon dried oregano

1 box (24.46 ounces) BPA-free chopped tomatoes or canned BPA-free organic diced tomatoes

3 tablespoons dry white wine

1 teaspoon brown sugar

¼ cup chopped fresh basil

1. In a heavy saucepan, heat the oil to medium heat. Add the onion and garlic and sauté until the onion is translucent, 5 to 6 minutes. Season with salt to taste. Add the carrots and celery and season with salt and

pepper; sauté until all vegetables are soft, about 10 minutes. Add the oregano, tomatoes, wine, and sugar. Simmer, uncovered, stirring occasionally, for 40 to 45 minutes.

2. Remove from the heat. Season the sauce with additional salt and pepper to taste. Stir in the basil. If you want a chunky marinara leave as is, but if you want a smoother sauce use an immersion blender and process until smooth and creamy. The sauce can be made ahead and either frozen up to one month or stored in the refrigerator in a covered container for up to 4 days.

Italian-Style One-Dish Chicken Dinner

SERVES 6

This is a very veggie-forward clean spin on the classic Italian chicken cacciatora. You can stretch the recipe by serving it on top of cooked quinoa or brown rice. It's also delicious mixed with cannellini or garbanzo beans. Oh, and leftovers make the perfect sandwich combined with steamed spinach and nestled between slices of toasted sprouted whole grain bread.

1½ pounds skinless, boneless pastured chicken breasts, cut into 2-inch pieces

1 teaspoon unrefined sea salt

1 teaspoon freshly ground black pepper

Paprika, to taste

½ cup white whole wheat flour, for dredging

1 tablespoon organic extra-virgin coconut oil

1 tablespoon plus 1 teaspoon cold-pressed extra-virgin olive oil

1 large red bell pepper, chopped

1 onion, chopped

3 garlic cloves, finely chopped

8 ounces baby Portobello mushrooms, sliced

¾ cup dry red wine

1 can (28 ounces) crushed tomatoes, with juice

1 can (14.5 ounces) petite diced tomatoes with juice

¾ cup organic chicken broth

2 teaspoons garlic powder

Crushed red pepper flakes, to taste

1 teaspoon dried oregano

½ cup coarsely chopped parsley

1. Sprinkle the chicken pieces with 1 teaspoon each of salt and pepper. Liberally sprinkle the chicken with paprika. Dredge the chicken pieces in the flour to coat lightly. In a large heavy sauté pan heat the coconut oil over medium-high heat. Add the chicken pieces and sauté until just brown, about 5 minutes per side. (If all the chicken does not fit in the pan, sauté it in two batches.) Transfer the chicken to a plate and set aside.

2. Add the olive oil to the pan and heat over medium heat. Add the bell pepper, onion, and garlic; sauté over medium heat until the onion is tender, about 5 minutes. Season with salt and pepper. Add the mushrooms and cook 3 to 4 minutes. Add the wine and simmer until reduced by half, about 3 minutes.

3. Add the crushed and diced tomatoes, broth, garlic powder, crushed red pepper flakes, and oregano. Return the chicken pieces to the pan and turn them to coat in the sauce. Bring the sauce to a simmer. Continue simmering over medium-low heat until the chicken is just cooked through, about 30 minutes. Sprinkle chicken with parsley and serve.

Chicken and Mushroom Casserole

SERVES 6

This savory casserole is ideal for family dinners but can also be served to guests. Add a side of steamed spinach, and dinner is done.

⅓ cup raw cashews

4 garlic cloves

¾ cup water

1 pound skinless, boneless, pastured chicken breast halves, pounded thin with a mallet

Unrefined sea salt, to taste

Freshly ground black pepper, to taste

3 tablespoons cold-pressed extra-virgin olive oil

½ cup chopped onion

1 celery rib, finely chopped

1 shallot, finely chopped

10 ounces cremini mushrooms, halved

1 cup finely chopped carrots

3 tablespoons white whole wheat flour

3 tablespoons dry sherry or marsala

2¼ cups organic chicken broth

1 cup organic frozen petite peas, thawed

8 slices sprouted whole grain bread (such as Food for Life), trimmed of crusts and cut into triangles

2 tablespoons coarsely chopped parsley

⅓ cup freshly grated Parmesan

1. Place the cashews, garlic, and water in a high-speed blender; blend until smooth and creamy. Set the cashew cream aside.

2. Preheat the oven to 375ºF.

3. Pat the chicken dry with paper towels and then season on both sides with salt and pepper to taste. In a medium sauté pan, lightly spread 1 tablespoon of the olive oil over the bottom surface with a paper towel and heat over medium heat until the oil is shimmering. Add the chicken and sauté until golden brown on the bottom, 3 to 4 minutes. Turn over the chicken, reduce the heat to medium, and cook until opaque throughout, about 10 minutes. Use tongs to transfer the chicken to a plate.

4. Add the remaining 2 tablespoons of olive oil to the pan and heat. Add the onion, celery, shallot, mushrooms, carrots, and a pinch of salt. Cook, stirring occasionally, until the vegetables are soft and tender, 8 to 10 minutes. (Reduce the heat if the vegetables brown too quickly.) Stir in the flour and cook, stirring often, 2 minutes. Add sherry, chicken broth, and cashew cream; cook, scraping up the browned bits from the bottom with a wooden spoon, until the sauce has thickened, about 5 minutes. Season with salt and pepper. Stir in the peas.

5. Arrange the bread on the bottom of a shallow 2-quart baking dish, overlapping the slices slightly. Spoon half of the vegetables and sauce over the bread. Slice the chicken crosswise, ½-inch thick, and arrange on the vegetables. Top with any accumulated juices from the chicken. Spread the remaining vegetables and sauce over chicken; sprinkle evenly with parsley and Parmesan. Bake 25 to 30 minutes, until golden brown and bubbling. Let stand 15 minutes before serving.

Slow Cooker Taco Stew

SERVES 6

Andy grew up eating a taco stew that tasted very similar to this one. Although this version uses considerably less beef, sneaks in tempeh, and gets its cheesy goodness from nutritional yeast (not cheese) it doesn't taste one bit like "health food." And that's a good thing.

1 tablespoon cold-pressed extra-virgin olive oil

1 Spanish onion, finely chopped

5 garlic cloves, crushed

½ pound ground pastured (preferably organic) beef or buffalo

1 package (8 ounces) tempeh, crumbled

Unrefined sea salt, to taste

1 can (15 ounces) BPA-free chili beans, rinsed and drained

1 can (15 ounces) BPA-free kidney beans, rinsed and drained

1½ cups frozen organic corn kernels, thawed

1 can (8 ounces) BPA-free tomato sauce

1½ cups organic vegetable broth

1 can (28 ounces) crushed tomatoes

¼ cup nutritional yeast

1 can (4 ounces) chopped green chilies

1 package (1.13 ounces) all-natural taco seasoning mix (such as Simply Organic Southwest Taco Seasoning Mix)

1. Heat the oil in a large heavy skillet over medium heat. Add the onion and garlic and sauté until the onion softens, 5 minutes. Add the ground beef and tempeh, season with salt, and sauté until the meat is cooked through, about 4 minutes. Transfer the beef mixture to a 5- or 6-quart slow cooker.

2. To the slow cooker, add the chili beans, kidney beans, corn, tomato sauce, vegetable broth, crushed tomatoes, nutritional yeast, green chilies, and taco seasoning. Mix to blend the ingredients well. Cover and cook on low heat for 6 hours. Serve warm.

Mexican Frittata Ranchera with Black Beans

SERVES 6

We love frittata for dinner because they are the perfect make-ahead meal. You can prepare a frittata in the morning, refrigerate, and then quickly re-heat for dinner. And for the cook, frittatas are pretty much foolproof. In sharp comparison to the omelet, which must be folded over just so, the frittata is neither delicate nor fussy. Making a frittata doesn't require the fine art of folding a sheet of egg paper over an assortment of fillings and instead can be prepared without stress, worry, or any particular skill. We like that!

7 organic, pastured eggs

¼ cup finely chopped cilantro

¼ teaspoon unrefined sea salt, plus more to taste

¼ teaspoon freshly ground black pepper, plus more to taste

1 tablespoon cold-pressed extra-virgin olive oil

½ cup finely chopped onion

1 jalapeño pepper, seeds removed, finely chopped

1 orange bell pepper, finely chopped

1 pint grape tomatoes, halved

1 can (15 ounces) BPA-free organic black beans, rinsed and drained

1. Preheat the broiler, with rack 4 inches from the heat source.
2. In a large bowl, whisk together the eggs and cilantro; season with ¼ teaspoon salt and ¼ teaspoon pepper.
3. Heat the oil in a 9- or 10-inch ovenproof skillet (such as Xtrema) over medium heat. Add the onions, jalapeño, bell pepper, and tomatoes; cook, stirring occasionally, until the onion softens, about 6 minutes. Sprinkle the black beans on top. Pour the egg mixture on top of the black beans. Cover, reduce the heat to low, and cook until the eggs are almost set, 5 to 7 minutes.
4. Uncover the skillet and place the frittata under the broiler. Broil 3 to 4 minutes, or until the top is set and just beginning to brown.
5. Run a flexible spatula around the edge of the frittata to loosen it from the pan; cut into wedges and serve.

Slow Cooker Clean Cuisine Chili

SERVES 6 TO 8

Like most men, Andy appreciates a good, hearty, stick-to-your-ribs (but not your waist) chili. This is one of his favorites!

2 tablespoons cold-pressed extra-virgin olive oil

1 Spanish onion, finely chopped

3 carrots, chopped

2 tablespoons minced garlic

3 celery ribs, chopped

1 red or orange bell pepper, chopped

2 tablespoons minced canned chipotle chilies in adobo sauce, plus 1 to 2 teaspoons adobo sauce

Unrefined sea salt, to taste

3 tablespoons nutritional yeast

2 cans (15 ounces each) BPA-free organic small red beans, rinsed and drained

1 can (14.5 ounces) BPA-free diced tomatoes

2½ cups organic vegetable broth

2 teaspoons ground cumin

2 teaspoons chili powder

2 packages (8 ounces each) tempeh (such as Lightlife)

6 ounces beer

1 tablespoon raw honey

1. Heat 1 tablespoon of the oil in a large heavy pot over medium heat. Add the onion, carrots, and 1 tablespoon of the garlic; sauté until the onion is soft, 4 to 5 minutes. Add the celery, bell pepper, chipotle chilies, and adobo sauce; sauté until the bell pepper is crisp-tender, 4 to 5 minutes. Season with salt to taste.

2. Transfer the vegetable mixture to a 5- or 6-quart slow cooker. Add the nutritional yeast, beans, tomatoes, broth, cumin, and chili powder. Use a wooden spoon to stir the ingredients together.

3. Grate the tempeh. Pour the remaining 1 tablespoon of oil into the skillet used to sauté the vegetables; heat the oil over medium heat. Add the remaining 1 tablespoon of garlic and the grated tempeh and sauté until golden brown, about 8 minutes. Season with salt to taste. Add the beer

and honey and stir to scrape up any bits from the bottom of the pan. Let the beer reduce by half.

378   **4.** Transfer the tempeh mixture to the slow cooker and stir to combine. Cover and cook on low heat for 2 hours. Let chili sit for at least 20 minutes before eating. Serve warm.

Skillet Enchilada Black Beans, Chicken, & Rice

SERVES 4 TO 6

A delicious family-friendly dish, this skillet entrée can be transformed to a vegan dinner simply by substituting extra-firm tofu cubes for the chicken. You can also use it as a filling for enchiladas made with sprouted corn tortillas (such as Food for Life brand).

¾ pound skinless, boneless pastured chicken breasts, cut into bite-size pieces

Unrefined sea salt, to taste

¼ cup stone-ground cornmeal (medium grind)

2 teaspoons organic extra-virgin coconut oil (such as Barlean's)

1 tablespoon cold-pressed extra-virgin olive oil

1 Spanish onion, chopped

1 cup chopped celery

6 garlic cloves, minced

1 can (14.5 ounces) BPA-free fire-roasted diced tomatoes, drained

1 cup organic vegetable broth

1 can (4.5 ounces) chopped green chilies

2 tablespoons plus more to taste, all-natural taco seasoning (such as *Simply Organic* brand)

2 cans (15 ounces each) BPA-free organic black beans

1 cup chopped green Spanish olives (also known as Manzanilla olives)

2 cups short grain cooked brown rice

1. Preheat the oven to 400°F.

2. Season the chicken on all sides with salt. Sprinkle the cornmeal on a sheet of waxed paper. Toss the chicken in the cornmeal.

3. Heat the coconut oil over medium-high heat in a large ovenproof skillet (such as Xtrema); add the chicken and brown about 2 minutes on each side. Remove to a plate.

4. Add the olive oil to the skillet and heat over medium heat; add the onion, celery, and garlic and sauté until tender, 6 to 7 minutes. Season the vegetables with salt to taste. Return chicken to the skillet. Add tomatoes, broth, green chilies, and taco seasoning; bring to a boil and cook for 3 minutes. Stir in the black beans, olives, and rice.

5. Cover skillet with foil and bake for 35 minutes.

379

Slow Cooker African Peanut, Red Lentil, & Turkey Stew

SERVES 4 TO 6

Here, we give turkey stew a bit of an exotic African twist. The flavors are complex enough to keep things interesting, but not so outlandish that the kids won't eat it. It's a family food for sure.

2 teaspoons cold-pressed extra-virgin olive oil

1 Spanish onion, finely chopped

1 tablespoon minced gingerroot

5 garlic cloves, crushed

½ pound ground pastured turkey

Unrefined sea salt, to taste

3 cups peeled and cubed sweet potatoes

1½ teaspoon curry powder

½ teaspoon garam masala

1 can (14 ounces) BPA-free chopped tomatoes

1 can (14 ounces) organic coconut milk

2 cups organic vegetable broth

2 tablespoons all-natural smooth peanut butter

1½ cups red lentils

1. Heat the oil in a large heavy skillet over medium heat. Add the onion, garlic, and ginger and sauté until the onion softens, 6 or 7 minutes. Add the ground turkey, season with salt, and sauté until meat is cooked through, about 4 minutes. Transfer the mixture to a 5- or 6-quart slow cooker.

2. To the slow cooker, add the sweet potatoes, curry powder, garam masala, tomatoes, coconut milk, broth, peanut butter, and lentils. Mix to blend ingredients well. Cover and cook on high for 30 minutes. Reduce heat to low and cook for 3 hours. Serve warm.

Slow-Cooked Black Beans with Chipotle, Pumpkin Seeds, & Whole Grain Cornbread Topping

SERVES 6

The chipotles give this slow-cooked one-dish dinner a subtle smoky-spicy kick, while the cornbread topping contributes an incredible comfy-cozy food quality. Ivy adapted the black bean recipe from a favorite childhood dish that called for sausage; after several attempts she was able to mimic the richness of the sausage by incorporating pumpkin seeds. Processing pumpkin seeds with liquid makes a nice thick cream that stands in for extra oil and meat; it sounds a little strange, but it works.

Black Beans

1 tablespoon cold-pressed extra-virgin olive oil

6 garlic cloves, crushed

1 onion, finely chopped

Unrefined sea salt, to taste

2 celery ribs, finely chopped

1 red bell pepper, finely chopped

1 ear of organic corn, corn kernels removed with a knife

2 chipotle peppers, seeds removed

1 cup organic vegetable broth

1 tablespoon organic Worcestershire sauce (such as Annie's Naturals)

¼ cup raw pumpkin seeds

2 tablespoons julienned sun-dried tomatoes packed in extra-virgin olive oil, rinsed and patted dry

2 cans (15 ounces each) BPA-free organic black beans, rinsed and drained

1 can (14.5 ounces) organic diced tomatoes, with juices

Whole Grain Cornbread Topping (recipe follows)

1. Heat the oil in a large heavy skillet over medium heat. Add the garlic and onion; sauté 3 or 4 minutes. Season with salt to taste. Add the celery and cook 2 to 3 minutes. Add the bell peppers and corn and cook until

vegetables are very tender, 2 to 3 minutes. Transfer the vegetables to a 5- or 6-quart slow cooker.

2. In a high-speed blender or food processor, add the chipotle peppers, broth, Worcestershire sauce, and pumpkin seeds. Blend or process until smooth and creamy. Transfer the mixture to the slow cooker.

3. Add the black beans and diced tomatoes to the slow cooker and gently stir all the ingredients together. Cook on high for 2½ hours. Spoon the Whole Grain Cornbread Topping on top of black bean mixture, spreading the mixture out with the back of a spoon, and cook on high for 1 hour. Let sit 30 minutes before serving. Serve warm.

Whole Grain Cornbread Topping

⅓ cup stone-ground cornmeal (medium grind)

½ cup white whole wheat flour

1 teaspoon baking powder

¼ teaspoon unrefined sea salt

1 teaspoon raw honey

⅓ cup plain hemp milk

2 teaspoons cold-pressed extra-virgin olive oil

1 organic pastured egg

½ banana

1. In a small mixing bowl, whisk together the cornmeal, flour, baking powder, and salt. Set aside.

2. In a blender, add the honey, hemp milk, oil, egg, and banana; process until smooth and creamy.

3. Add the wet ingredients to the dry. Mix gently just to incorporate. Spoon on top of the beans as directed.

MEAT-FREE MONDAY MEALS

Veggies, Pasta, & White Beans with Lemony Cream Sauce

SERVES 4

This stick-to-your-ribs one-pot dinner is so divine you could easily serve it to guests. And here easy *is a double-entendre because it really is easy to prepare too. Nobody will believe the cream is dairy free!*

½ cup, plus 2 tablespoons pine nuts

2 tablespoons freshly squeezed lemon juice

¼ cup, plus 2 tablespoons water

½ teaspoon raw honey

¾ teaspoon fresh thyme

⅛ teaspoon unrefined sea salt, plus more to taste

1 pound asparagus, ends trimmed, cut on the diagonal into 2-inch segments

2 cups dry sprouted whole grain penne (such as Food for Life brand) or other whole grain penne

1 cup frozen petite peas

1 tablespoon cold-pressed extra-virgin olive oil

2 shallots, finely chopped

5 garlic cloves, minced

1 can (14.5 ounces) BPA-free organic cannellini beans

1. Place the pine nuts, lemon juice, water, honey, thyme and ⅛ teaspoon salt in a high-speed blender (such as a Vitamix); process for 1 full minute, or until smooth and creamy. Set aside.

2. Bring a large pot of salted water to a boil over medium-high heat. Add the asparagus to the boiling water and cook for 3 to 4 minutes. Add the sprouted whole grain pasta and cook for 4 minutes (if using regular whole grain penne, add it at the same time you add the asparagus and cook both for 7 to 8 minutes). Remove from heat and add the peas. Let the peas sit in the hot water for about 1 minute. Drain the asparagus, pasta and peas. Do not rinse pasta with water; you want to retain the pasta's natural starches so that the sauce will stick. Set pasta and vegetables aside.

3. Heat the oil in a large heavy saucepan over medium heat; add the shallots and garlic and sauté until the shallots are soft, 3 to 4 minutes. Stir in the beans and season with salt to taste.

4. Add the asparagus, pasta, and peas to the saucepan and gently toss to coat with the shallots, garlic, and beans. Stir in the prepared cream sauce. Season with salt to taste. Remove from heat and let sit 5 minutes before serving. Serve warm.

Thai Veggie Curry Stir–Fry

SERVES 4

This is one of our favorite family dinners. It is beyond delicious. One of the secrets to making a sensational stir-fry is to try to cut all of the vegetables into the same shape and size. Using a large wok is also a tremendous help. For a complete meal, serve over steamed short-grain brown rice or soba noodles. It's also wonderful with pan-seared cornmeal crusted tofu-bites scattered on top of the veggies just before serving. When we add tofu to this dish we like to marinate it for about 10 minutes in 2 tablespoons lime juice, 2 teaspoons raw honey, 1 teaspoon sesame oil, and 1 teaspoon red curry paste.

1 tablespoon organic extra-virgin coconut oil (such as Barlean's)

6 garlic cloves, crushed

3 tablespoons freshly grated gingerroot

1 shallot, finely chopped

2 teaspoons red curry paste (such as Thai Kitchen brand)

1 large eggplant, sliced into thin 1-inch-long strips

1 pound haricot vert, trimmed and cut into 1-inch pieces

Unrefined sea salt, to taste

¼ cup organic coconut milk

2 cups shiitake mushrooms, cut into bite-size pieces

1 red bell pepper, sliced into thin 1-inch-long strips

1 can (8 ounces) bamboo shoots, rinsed and drained

1 can (8 ounces) water chestnuts, rinsed and drained

1 cup chopped fresh basil

1 cup chopped fresh mint

1. Heat the oil in a large wok over medium heat. Add the garlic and ginger and sauté briefly, about 30 seconds. Add the shallots and sauté until just soft, about 2 minutes. Add the curry paste and sauté 30 seconds.

2. Add the eggplant and haricot vert. Stir-fry until the vegetables start to soften, 3 to 4 minutes. Season with salt to taste. Add the coconut milk and continue stir-frying about 2 minutes. Add the mushrooms and cook until they begin to soften, 2 to 3 minutes.

3. Add the red bell pepper and cook for about 2 minutes. Add the bamboo shoots and water chestnuts. Stir-fry until all the vegetables are of desired doneness, 2 to 3 minutes. Stir in the basil and mint and cook until just wilted. Remove from the heat and adjust the seasoning. (If you want a richer curry flavor dissolve a little bit of curry paste in about 2 tablespoons of coconut milk and pour on top of the vegetables.) Set the veggies aside to cool for a few minutes before serving. Serve warm.

Sprouted Whole Wheat Fettuccini (or Soba Noodles) with Cremini Mushrooms, Roasted Asparagus, & Pine Nut Crumble

SERVES 4

Here's an elegant spin on pasta primavera. If you aren't serving it on meat-free Monday you might also want to consider adding a few stone-ground corn flour–crusted and seared diver scallops on top of the pasta. To make it gluten free use 100% buckwheat soba noodles.

6 ounces uncooked sprouted whole grain fettuccini (or soba noodles)

4 cups asparagus, cut into 2-inch lengths

6 teaspoons cold-pressed extra-virgin olive oil

Unrefined sea salt, to taste

8 garlic cloves, crushed

¼ cup minced shallots

3 cups thinly sliced cremini mushrooms, brushed clean

¼ cup buttery white wine (we like Kendall Jackson Chardonnay)

¾ cup shredded parsley (see step 5)

½ cup pine nut crumbs (see step 5)

White pepper, to taste

1. Preheat the oven to 400°F. Lightly oil the bottom of a large cookie sheet.
2. Bring a large pot of salted water to a boil over high heat. Cook the fettuccini according to package directions. When the pasta is done, drain and set aside.
3. While the pasta is cooking, place the asparagus in the prepared pan and drizzle with 1 teaspoon of the oil. Season lightly with salt. Roast the asparagus for 15 minutes, or until desired doneness. Remove from the oven and set aside.
4. Heat the remaining 5 teaspoons of oil in a very large skillet over medium heat. Add the garlic and shallots; sauté until the shallots soften, 2 to 3 minutes. Add the mushrooms and cook until soft, 3 to 4 minutes. Add the wine and cook until liquid is reduced and the skillet is almost dry. Stir in the cooked fettuccini and asparagus tips. Remove from the heat.

5. Place parsley in a food processor and pulse until parsley is shredded. Add the shredded parsley to the skillet. Add the pine nuts to the food processor and process into fine crumbs. Add the crumbs to the skillet and toss to combine ingredients. Season with white pepper and additional salt to taste. Stir to combine. Serve warm.

Spring Barley & Quinoa Risotto with Asparagus & Shiitake Mushrooms

SERVES 4

The word risotto means "little rice" in Italian and as much as we love creamy, traditional risotto made with Arborio rice (a refined, not healthy white rice) our Clean Cuisine version is every bit as good, and can be enjoyed 100 percent guilt-free. Dairy-free, loaded with antioxidants, spiked with healing shiitake mushrooms, and filled to the brim with fiber, this is a risotto you will feel good about eating, and feel good after too. It won't weigh you down, and makes for a delicious light and lively dinner served with a side of arugula or watercress salad. To make it dairy free use the pine nut crumbs instead of the Parmesan cheese.

1 tablespoon cold-pressed extra-virgin olive oil

6 garlic cloves, crushed

1 leek, finely chopped

½ pound shiitake mushrooms, trimmed, wiped clean and thinly sliced

Unrefined sea salt, to taste

White pepper, to taste

½ cup pearl barley

½ cup quinoa

½ cup buttery white wine (we like Kendall Jackson Chardonnay)

3 cups liquid (organic vegetable broth *or* ½ cup miso diluted in 3 cups water)

1 pound asparagus, tough ends trimmed, cut on the diagonal into 2-inch segments

Parmesan cheese or pine nut crumbs (optional; see step 4)

1. Heat the oil in a large heavy-bottomed saucepan over medium-low heat. Add the garlic, leek, and mushrooms and cook, stirring occasionally,

until the leeks and mushrooms begin to soften, 5 to 7 minutes. Season lightly with salt and pepper to taste.

2. Add the barley and quinoa and toast 2 to 3 minutes, stirring occasionally. Add the wine and cook, stirring, until evaporated, about 5 minutes.

3. Add 1 cup of the liquid and cook, stirring occasionally, for 10 minutes. Add the asparagus segments and 1½ cups more liquid and cook, stirring occasionally, for 15 minutes. Add the remaining ½ cup of the liquid and cook for an additional 5 to 10 minutes, or until liquid has been absorbed. Remove from the heat and cover to keep warm.

4. Optional: Sprinkle a small amount of freshly grated Parmesan cheese on top and cover with a lid to let the cheese melt *or* sprinkle pine nut crumbs on top. To make the crumbs, process in a food processor.

Mexican-Style Seared Tempeh with Salsa Verde

SERVES 4

In our house this dish pretty much serves one: Andy! He loves it so much that Ivy always has to double the recipe. Salsa verde is a classic vibrant green Mexican condiment that is really more like a sauce than a salsa. It is always made with tomatillos, but this version is not. (Ivy got the idea to make it on a day when she didn't want to schlep to the store for tomatillos.) Serve the tempeh, peppers, onions, and salsa verde over black rice or quinoa. Even better, try it with grilled or roasted corn on the cob. If you are still taking baby steps toward eating less meat, feel free to use chicken strips in place of the tempeh.

Salsa Verde

⅓ cup pine nuts

2 garlic cloves

½ jalapeño pepper, seeds removed, chopped

1 cup parsley leaves (or cilantro)

2 tablespoons capers

¼ teaspoon cumin

Unrefined sea salt, to taste

2 tablespoons freshly squeezed lime juice

3 tablespoons cold-pressed extra-virgin olive oil

¼ cup plus 2 tablespoons water

Place all ingredients in a food processor and process until smooth and creamy. Set aside. (Salsa verde can be made up to 3 days in advance and stored in a covered container in the refrigerator.)

Tempeh

2 teaspoons cold-pressed extra-virgin olive oil

8 ounces tempeh, sliced in half lengthwise and then sliced into thin strips

Unrefined sea salt, to taste

1 large onion, thinly sliced

1 tablespoon freshly squeezed lime juice

1 red bell pepper, thinly sliced

1. Pour the oil in a large heavy skillet and tilt the pan to coat the entire bottom surface in a thin layer of oil. Heat the oil over medium heat. When the pan is hot add the tempeh, making sure the bottom of each tempeh strip is touching the pan. Season the tempeh with salt to taste and cook until it starts to turn golden brown, 2 to 3 minutes. Gently flip and cook for 2 to 3 minutes on the other side.
2. Add the onions and lime juice, and sauté until the onions soften, 5 minutes. Add the bell pepper, and sauté for 2 to 3 more minutes.
3. Pour the salsa verde into the pan, increase the heat to high, and bring to a boil. Lower the heat to simmer, cover, and cook for 5 minutes. Remove from heat and let sit for 5 minutes. Serve warm.

Szechuan Lettuce Wraps with Dipping Sauce

SERVES 4

Who doesn't love lettuce wraps? Not only are they tasty but they're also loads of fun to eat! We've noticed lettuce wraps becoming increasingly popular as menu items at restaurants, and our son just loves them. (Hey, who could blame the little guy? We love them too.) Unfortunately, time and time again we've found restaurant-style lettuce wraps to be greasy and unpleasantly heavy. Our Clean Cuisine vegan version uses crumbled tempeh but is still hearty and filling and loaded with flavor. It will fill you up and it's not the least bit greasy. And our dipping sauce is much lower in refined sugar (thanks to the puréed mango) than the sauces you'd get at a restaurant. The mango contributes sweetness but doesn't add a mango flavor. To make it gluten free use San J gluten-free soy sauce.

Dipping Sauce

⅓ cup mango pieces

3 garlic cloves

1-inch piece gingerroot, peeled and coarsely chopped

3 tablespoons plum sauce (such as Wok Mei)

3 tablespoons high-quality soy sauce (or nama shoyu or San J gluten-free soy sauce)

¼ cup rice wine vinegar

1 teaspoon sesame oil

Place all of the ingredients in a food processor or blender and blend or process until smooth and creamy. Set aside.

Lettuce Wraps

3 tablespoons freshly squeezed lime juice

2 tablespoons plum sauce (such as Wok Mei)

1 tablespoon high-quality soy sauce (or nama shoyu or San J gluten-free soy sauce)

2 tablespoons raw cashews

1 tablespoon sesame oil

1 tablespoon minced gingerroot

1 tablespoon crushed garlic

2 carrots, shredded

2 scallions, shredded

1 package (8 ounces) tempeh, shredded

12 large romaine lettuce leaves, rinsed and patted dry

1. In a food processor, add the lime juice, plum sauce, soy sauce, and cashews; process until smooth and creamy. Set aside.
2. Heat the oil in a large heavy skillet or wok over medium heat; add the ginger and garlic and sauté 30 seconds. Add the carrots and stir-fry for 2 to 3 minutes. Add the scallions and stir-fry for 2 to 3 minutes. Add the tempeh and stir-fry 2 to 3 minutes.
3. Drizzle the lime-soy sauce over the tempeh mixture and stir-fry 2 to 3 minutes. Serve the tempeh mixture in a large bowl with lettuce leaves and dipping sauce on the side.

FISH ON FRIDAY DINNERS

Cod Masala Stew

SERVES 4

This rich and creamy curry and turmeric-charged Indian-inspired stew has become one of our favorite cod dishes. And talk about easy to make! Fragrant and ever-so-slightly sweet, this stew makes a light meal on its own, but for heartier appetites serve over steamed black rice or millet.

2 teaspoons cold-pressed extra-virgin olive oil

1 tablespoon freshly grated gingerroot

5 garlic cloves, crushed

1 shallot, finely chopped

1 teaspoon ground turmeric

1 tablespoon curry powder

2 tomatoes, cored and chopped

1 mango, chopped

Unrefined sea salt, to taste

Juice from 1 whole lime

½ cup organic vegetable broth

1½ pounds cod, cut into bite-size pieces and lightly salted

1 cup frozen organic petite peas, thawed

1. Heat the oil in a large heavy skillet over medium heat; add the ginger, garlic, and shallot and sauté until shallot soften, 3 to 4 minutes. Add the turmeric and curry and cook 1 minute. Stir in the tomatoes and mango and cook for 3 minutes. Season with salt to taste.
2. Add the lime juice and vegetable broth and bring to a boil. Reduce the heat and simmer, covered, 8 to 10 minutes. Add the fish and peas. Cook until fish is cooked through, about 3 minutes. Remove from the heat and set aside to cool for 10 minutes. Serve warm.

Summer Panzanella with Pan-Seared Salmon & Corn

SERVES 4 TO 6

There are oodles of variations of this Tuscan tomato-bread salad but ours is particularly summery with the addition of the corn. Perfect for a summer supper. The trick is to let the flavors blend without allowing the bread to disintegrate into mush (using sprouted whole grain bread and toasting it to crispy crouton perfection from the start is a big help).

Croutons & Corn

2 ears of organic corn, husks on

Unrefined sea salt, to taste

4 slices sprouted whole grain bread, crusts removed, cut into bite-size squares

Cold-pressed extra-virgin olive oil (in a spritzer bottle)

1. Preheat oven to 375°F.
2. Place the corn directly on the oven rack. Arrange the bread on a large baking sheet and spritz lightly with the oil. Season with salt to taste. Bake the bread 8 to 9 minutes, until crisp and lightly colored on the outside but still soft on the inside. Set croutons aside and let cool.
3. Continue cooking the corn for another 15 minutes, or until desired doneness. Remove from the oven and peel back the husks. Use a knife to remove the corn kernels. Set aside.

Salmon

Organic extra-virgin coconut oil (such as Barlean's)

2 (8 ounces each) center-cut wild Alaskan salmon fillets

Unrefined sea salt, to taste

Freshly ground black pepper, to taste

Lemon juice, to taste

Lightly oil the bottom of a large heavy skillet and heat over medium-high. Season the salmon with salt and pepper on both sides and add to the hot skillet. Sear salmon for 3 minutes on one side. Flip the salmon and squeeze some lemon juice on top. Sear on the other side until it flakes easily, about 3 minutes (be careful not to overcook). Remove from the skillet and break into bite-size pieces. Set aside.

The Salad

2 pounds ripe heirloom tomatoes, peeled, seeded, and chopped

1 tablespoon cold-pressed extra-virgin olive oil

2 garlic cloves

1 teaspoon anchovy paste

2 tablespoons hemp seeds

2 tablespoons freshly squeezed lemon juice

¼ red onion, finely chopped

1 cucumber, peeled, seeded, and chopped

¼ cup chopped basil leaves

2 cups arugula, trimmed

Unrefined sea salt, to taste

Freshly ground black pepper, to taste

1. Drain the tomatoes in a sieve to remove excess liquid while you prepare the rest of the ingredients.
2. Place the olive oil, garlic, anchovy paste, hemp seeds, and lemon juice in a high speed blender or food processor; blend or process until smooth and creamy.
3. In a bowl, combine the tomatoes, corn, onion, cucumber, basil, arugula, salt, and pepper. Drizzle the vinaigrette on top and toss to coat. Add the croutons and toss again. Arrange the salmon on top of the salad. Let sit at room temperature for 10 to 15 minutes for flavors to fully develop. Serve at room temperature.

New Orleans–Style Shrimp in BBQ Sauce

SERVES 4

We got the idea for this recipe from Ruth's Chris Steak House, but ours is totally butter free and the barbecue sauce contains zero added sugar. It's sensational served over steamed black rice or on top of a bed of mashed caulitatoes (cauliflower mashed potatoes). P.S. The barbecue sauce can be prepared 3 days in advance and stored in a covered container in the fridge.

BBQ Sauce

1 teaspoon cold-pressed extra-virgin olive oil

1 jalapeño, finely chopped

2 garlic cloves

1 cup fresh or frozen mango pieces

4 pitted dates

¼ teaspoon cayenne pepper

¼ teaspoon unrefined sea salt

1 teaspoon paprika

2 tablespoons apple cider vinegar

1 teaspoon organic Worcestershire sauce (such as Annie's Naturals)

1 teaspoon liquid smoke

2 tablespoons water

Heat the oil in a small skillet over medium heat; add the jalapeño and sauté until softened, 3 or 4 minutes. Transfer to a blender or food processor. Add the remaining ingredients; blend or process until smooth and creamy. Set the sauce aside. The sauce will taste very spicy at first, but it will mellow out considerably when it's cooked with the shrimp.

Shrimp

1½ pounds (21 to 25 count) shrimp, peeled and patted very dry

Unrefined sea salt, to taste

4 teaspoons cold-pressed extra-virgin olive oil, divided

6 garlic cloves, crushed

1 onion, sliced

1 cup beer, divided

½ cup finely chopped parsley

1. Season the shrimp with salt. Add 2 teaspoons of the oil to a large heavy skillet and heat over medium; add the garlic and sauté 30 seconds. Add shrimp, making sure each piece is flat on the skillet, and cook for about 1½ minutes per side. (Do not to overcook the shrimp or they will end up tasting like erasers!) Remove the shrimp from the skillet and set aside.

2. Add the remaining 2 teaspoons of oil and the onion to the skillet. Season with salt to taste and sauté until very soft, 5 or 6 minutes. Add ½ cup of the beer and cook until reduced by half. Add the BBQ Sauce and remaining ½ cup of beer and simmer for 5 to 6 minutes. Stir in the shrimp and cook until warmed through, 1 more minute. Add the parsley. Remove from the heat and serve at once.

Company-Is-Coming Filet of Sole with Mustard Horseradish Sauce

SERVES 4

This is one of our go-to fish dinners for entertaining. It gets rave reviews every time. Filet of sole has a wonderfully delicate texture that stands up well to stronger seasonings, such as the mustard and horseradish here. Although sole is often one of the easiest fish to find on the market, if you can't find it or you want to use another fish feel free to try another mild white fish, such as sea bass, halibut, tilapia, or red snapper. Note: Look for prepared horseradish in the refrigerated section of the supermarket.

Mustard Horseradish Sauce

⅓ cup plus 2 tablespoons pine nuts

1 tablespoon prepared horseradish

2 teaspoons Dijon mustard

1 teaspoon brown sugar

¼ cup plus 3 tablespoons water

2 teaspoons organic Worcestershire sauce (such as Annie's Naturals)

1 tablespoon freshly squeezed lemon juice

Place all ingredients in a high-speed blender and blend until smooth and creamy. Set aside.

Sole

2 slices toasted sprouted whole grain bread, crusts removed

3 teaspoons cold-pressed extra-virgin olive oil, divided

1 large shallot, finely chopped

½ pound small button mushrooms, brushed clean, sliced thin

Unrefined sea salt, to taste

Freshly ground black pepper, to taste

4 filets (5 or 6 ounces each) sole, rinsed and patted dry with paper towels

½ cup finely chopped parsley

1. Position a rack in the lower part of the oven. Preheat the oven to 425°F. Lightly oil a 9- by 12-inch baking dish.

2. Place the bread in a food processor and pulse several times to make coarse crumbs. Add 1 teaspoon of the oil and pulse a few more times. Set aside.

3. Heat the remaining 2 teaspoons of the oil in a large skillet over medium heat; add the shallot and sauté, stirring, for 1 minute. Add the mushrooms and cook, stirring and tossing, until just wilted, 2 to 3 minutes. Season with salt and pepper to taste. Add the Mustard Horseradish Sauce and bring just to a simmer. Remove from heat.

4. Place the sole in the prepared baking dish in a single layer and spoon the sauce over the filets. Sprinkle the bread crumbs evenly over the top. Bake 10 to 15 minutes, until the fish is opaque throughout when pierced with a sharp knife (the timing depends on the thickness of the fish). Remove from oven.

5. Preheat the broiler. Slip the baking dish under the broiler and broil to brown the top, 1 minute. Carefully remove the fish with a spatula and plate. Sprinkle parsley on top. Serve at once.

Blake's Seafood Thai Chowder

SERVES 4 TO 6

We just had to name this recipe after our son because making it was his idea. Blake actually helped Ivy make the dish every step of the way, including shopping for the ingredients, chopping the vegetables, and peeling the shrimp. We go to Thai restaurants a lot, and Blake loves the exotic flavors of Southeast Asia. He was very enthused with how this dish turned out (not surprising because most kids think the food they prepare is delicious!). But this dish really is divine. We promise. Adjust the amount of coconut milk to get the broth consistency you prefer.

1 tablespoon organic extra-virgin coconut oil (such as Barlean's)

2 tablespoons minced gingerroot

1 green chile pepper, seeds removed, diced

1 red onion, finely chopped

Unrefined sea salt, to taste

3 carrots, finely chopped

2 red bell peppers, finely chopped

2 teaspoons red curry paste

1 cup water

3 cups organic vegetable broth

¼ to ½ cup organic coconut milk

3 tablespoons freshly squeezed lime juice

1 tablespoon brown sugar

1 teaspoon curry powder

1 pound assorted white fish (such as sea bass, halibut, red snapper, and cod)

¾ pound shrimp, peeled (leave tail fin attached) and deveined

15 to 20 mussels in the shell, well-scrubbed

½ cup very finely chopped cilantro

1. Heat the oil in a large heavy saucepan over medium heat; add the ginger, green chile, and onion. Season with salt to taste and sauté until the onion softens, 4 to 5 minutes. Add the carrots and bell peppers and sauté until the carrots are soft, 5 to 6 minutes. Season with more salt to taste.

2. Stir in the red curry paste and cook for 1 minute. Add the water, vegetable broth, coconut milk, lime juice, sugar, and curry powder. Cover partially and cook over low heat for 15 minutes.

3. Add the fish pieces and cook over low heat for 7 minutes. Add the shrimp and mussels and continue to barely simmer until the fish is opaque throughout when pierced with a sharp knife, the shrimp are pink, and the mussels have opened, 5 to 6 minutes. Discard any mussels that do not open. Taste and adjust the seasoning. Remove from the heat. Sprinkle the cilantro on top and give a quick stir. Serve at once.

River House–Style Baked Grouper with Brandied Bread Crumbs in Parchment

SERVES 4

Baked grouper in parchment is one of our favorite entrées at the River House, a restaurant in North Palm Beach that we love and visit frequently. (In her younger days Ivy was a hostess there; actress Susan Lucci would often eat there when in town.) At the River House they prepare their grouper on a bed of greens topped with brandied bread crumbs and then bake the whole thing in parchment. The combination is just to-die-for delicious. This is not the River House's official recipe, but it is absolutely wonderful! If you can't find grouper you can use just about any thick white fish (halibut, haddock, sea bass, snapper).

4 filets (5 ounces each) grouper, rinsed and patted dry

2 teaspoons cold-pressed extra-virgin olive oil

4 tablespoons brandy

2 slices sprouted whole grain bread, crusts removed

4 garlic cloves, chopped

¼ cup plus 2 tablespoons pine nuts

2 tablespoons chopped parsley

½ teaspoon unrefined sea salt

2 teaspoons organic extra-virgin coconut oil (such as Barlean's)

6 cups baby spinach leaves

1. Preheat the oven to 425 °F. Cut 4 pieces of parchment (or aluminum foil) that will enclose each fish filet completely.

2. Place the fish filets in a large self-sealing plastic bag and add the olive oil and 2 tablespoons of the brandy. Transfer the fish to the refrigerator and let marinate for at least 10 minutes.

3. Place the bread and garlic cloves in a food processor and pulse several times until you have coarse bread crumbs; remove and set aside. Place the pine nuts, parsley, and salt in the food processor and pulse several times until you have coarse pine nut crumbs; remove and set aside.

4. Heat the coconut oil in a medium-size skillet over medium heat; add the garlicky bread crumbs and cook until toasty, 4 to 5 minutes. Drizzle the remaining 2 tablespoons of brandy on top and cook until it evaporates, about 2 minutes. Add the pine nut mixture and cook for 1 more minute. Set aside.

5. Lay the sheets of parchment on a flat surface. Lightly brush an area in the center, about the size of the fish, with olive oil. Divide the spinach among the four sheets. Remove the fish from the marinade, season with salt on all sides, and lay on top of the spinach. Divide the bread crumb mixture and spoon on top of the fish, using your fingers to lightly press the mixture into the fish.

6. Fold the parchment to form a packet around each piece of fish. All edges of the packet should be folded to create a seal, but there should be an empty space, like a small tent, above the filet. Place the packets on a rimmed baking sheet and bake. The timing depends on the thickness of the filets: a 1½- to 2-inch-thick filet will take 18 to 20 minutes; smaller filets may be ready in 15 minutes. To check, remove the baking sheet from the oven and open one of the packets, taking care to avoid the hot steam that escapes. The cooked filet will look white and flake easily. If the fish is undercooked, refold the packet, and continue cooking.

Mom's Cleaned-Up Clean Cuisine Tuna Casserole

SERVES 6

Ivy's mom, Gail (our photographer at www.CleanCuisine.com), worked hard to clean up one of Ivy's favorite childhood dishes. Ivy actually loves the cleaned-up tuna casserole better than her mom's original version. This was also one of the recipes Ivy served at the official Clean Cuisine taste-testing party to her friends, Cherie, Carla, Claudia, Paula, and Susan, and the ladies loved it.

6 ounces (dry weight) quinoa spaghetti (such as Ancient Harvest)

⅓ cup raw macadamia nuts, chopped

½ cup Uncle Sam cereal

2 tablespoons plus 1 teaspoon cold-pressed extra-virgin olive oil

1 cup raw whole cashews

1 organic pastured egg

1 cup water

1 cup chopped onion

2 celery ribs, finely chopped

2 carrots, finely chopped

Unrefined sea salt, to taste

2 red bell peppers (or 1 red and 1 green), finely chopped

2 tablespoons finely chopped parsley

1 tablespoon chopped thyme (optional)

2 cans (5 ounces each) BPA-free and pole-caught canned water-packed tuna (such as Planet Wild), drained

¼ cup grated pastured Cheddar or pecorino Romana cheese

1. Preheat the oven to 350°F. Lightly oil the bottom and sides of a 8- by 13-inch casserole dish.

2. Cook the spaghetti according to package directions. Drain and set aside.

3. While the pasta is cooking, place the macadamia nuts in a food processor and pulse until crumbly, 6 to 7 times. Add the cereal and 1 teaspoon of the oil; pulse until the cereal is well blended with the nuts, 4 to 5 times. Set mixture aside.

4. Add the cashews, egg, and water to a high-speed blender; blend until smooth and creamy. Set cashew cream aside.

5. Heat the remaining 2 tablespoons of oil in a large heavy skillet over medium heat; add the onion and sauté until soft, 7 to 8 minutes. Add the celery and carrots and sauté 2 minutes. Season with salt to taste. Add the bell peppers and sauté for 2 minutes. Add the parsley, thyme, and tuna; mix well to combine. Season with salt to taste.

6. Add the cooked spaghetti, cheese, and cashew cream; mix ingredients well. Transfer the mixture to the casserole dish. Sprinkle the cereal-nut mixture over top. Bake for 20 minutes, or until casserole is firm. Remove from the oven and allow the casserole to cool at least 15 minutes before serving.

GREAT GREEN SIDES

Sautéed Collards & Cherries

SERVES 4

Mild-tasting collards and sweet, tangy cherries complement each other perfectly. And the spicy ginger adds both flavor and anti-inflammatory benefits.

¾ pound collard greens

1 tablespoon organic extra-virgin coconut oil (such as Barlean's)

3 shallots, thinly sliced

4 garlic cloves, crushed

1 tablespoon minced gingerroot

1 tablespoon balsamic vinegar

Unrefined sea salt, to taste

1 cup fresh cherries, pitted and quartered

¼ cup pine nuts (optional)

1. Wash the collard greens thoroughly. Remove the stems that run down the center by holding the leaf in your left hand and stripping the leaf

down with your right hand. (The tender young leaves in the heart of the collards don't need to be stripped.) Stack 6 to 8 leaves on top of one another, roll up, and slice into ½- to 1-inch-thick slices. Set aside.

2. Heat the oil in a large saucepan over medium heat. Add the shallots, garlic, and ginger; sauté until the shallots are tender, 4 to 5 minutes. Add the collards and vinegar and sauté until collards begin to wilt, about 4 minutes. Season with salt to taste and stir in the cherries. Cover and cook for a few more minutes, until the collards are nicely wilted. Serve warm. If desired, place the pine nuts in a mini food processor and process into crumbs; sprinkle pine nuts on top of the collards.

Braised Escarole with Sun-Dried Tomatoes

SERVES 4

Escarole is a type of endive considered to be the least bitter of that leafy veggie family and when cooked it not only mellows considerably but also takes on a delicate buttery-like quality that is absolutely delicious. If you want to get a little fancy with this dish, try adding an extra teaspoon of olive oil in step 1 and 3 ounces of cut shiitake mushrooms along with the garlic, shallots, and sun-dried tomatoes; sauté until mushrooms are soft and then add the escarole in step 2.

1 tablespoon cold-pressed extra-virgin olive oil

4 garlic cloves, minced

1 shallot, finely chopped

⅓ cup julienned sun-dried tomatoes packed in extra-virgin olive oil, rinsed with water and patted dry with paper towels

2 bunches escarole, washed and chopped (about 8 cups)

Unrefined sea salt, to taste

¼ cup organic vegetable broth

1 tablespoon balsamic vinegar

1. Heat the oil in a large heavy saucepan over medium heat; add the garlic, shallots, and sun-dried tomatoes and sauté until the shallots are soft, 3 to 4 minutes.
2. Add the escarole, toss to coat in the oil and cook, stirring constantly, for 2 to 3 minutes. Season with salt to taste. Add the vegetable broth and vinegar, and cook, stirring occasionally, until the escarole is very, very wilted, for 5 to 6 minutes.

Curried Kale Chips

SERVES 4

Everybody loves a side of chips. Why not health things up a bit and serve kale chips instead of potato chips? And yes, kids will eat these.

> 2 big handfuls kale, stems removed and leaves torn into roughly 1½-inch pieces
>
> 2 teaspoons cold-pressed extra-virgin olive oil
>
> 2 teaspoons tahini
>
> 1 tablespoon nutritional yeast
>
> 2 teaspoons curry powder
>
> Unrefined sea salt, to taste

1. Preheat oven to 325°F. Position the rack on the bottom of the oven.
2. Line a large baking sheet with parchment paper.
3. Toss the kale with the olive oil, tahini, and nutritional yeast. Spread the kale out on the parchment paper and sprinkle with curry powder and salt. Bake until just crispy, 15 to 18 minutes.

Asian Stir-Fried Spinach with Sesame Seeds & Garlic

SERVES 4

Sometimes a simple, classic greens side dish is all it takes to round off a meal. This one goes particularly well with Japanese, Asian, and Thai entrées.

> 1 tablespoon sesame seeds
>
> 2 teaspoons sesame oil
>
> 8 garlic cloves, crushed
>
> 8 cups organic baby leaf spinach
>
> Unrefined sea salt, to taste

1. Heat a wok over medium heat; add the sesame seeds and dry-fry, stirring constantly, until golden brown, 1 to 2 minutes. Transfer to a small bowl and set aside.

2. Heat the oil in the wok over medium heat; when hot, add the oil, garlic, spinach, and salt. Stir-fry until the spinach wilts and is coated in oil, about 2 minutes.

3. Sprinkle the dry-fried sesame seeds on top and toss well. Serve warm.

Super-Easy Smoked Turnip Greens with Diced Tomatoes

SERVES 4

These greens are super easy because you don't have to chop or wash them. For this recipe we use frozen chopped turnips because they not only cut down on chopping but they also taste really, really good. You can use the time you saved to make another Clean Cuisine recipe. Smile.

> 1 tablespoon plus 1 teaspoon cold-pressed extra-virgin olive oil
>
> 6 garlic cloves, chopped
>
> 1 shallot, finely chopped
>
> Unrefined sea salt, to taste
>
> 1 can (14.5 ounces) BPA-free organic diced tomatoes
>
> 1 tablespoon liquid smoke
>
> 1 pound frozen chopped turnips

1. Heat the oil in a large saucepan over medium heat; add the garlic and shallots and sauté until the shallots are soft, 4 to 5 minutes. Season with salt to taste.

2. Add the tomatoes and liquid smoke, increase the heat to high and cook until juices start to evaporate, 4 to 5 minutes. Add the turnips and use a spoon to break the frozen pieces apart. Cook until the turnips are tender and most of the liquid has evaporated, 7 to 8 minutes. Season with salt to taste. Serve warm.

Broccoli Rabe with Golden Raisins, Garlic, & Capers

SERVES 4

We're always up for a dose of different. This deliciously different savory greens dish is perfect eaten alone but it can be a complete meal tossed with sprouted whole grain bread and sprinkled with some pine nut crumbs. If you want to stretch this dish, you can add chopped frozen spinach and a little more olive oil at the very end and cook until spinach wilts.

1 large bunch broccoli rabe

1 tablespoon plus 1 teaspoon cold-pressed extra-virgin olive oil

1 teaspoon anchovy paste

8 garlic cloves, finely chopped

¼ cup capers

¼ cup golden raisins

Unrefined sea salt, to taste

1 tablespoon balsamic vinegar

1. Trim the thick tough stems from the broccoli rabe just below where the stems branch or the leaves start. Rinse the broccoli rabe and pat dry.

2. Heat the oil and anchovy paste in a large heavy cast-iron skillet over medium heat; add the garlic, capers, and raisins and sauté for about 1 minute. Add the broccoli rabe, toss to coat in the oil and garlic, and reduce the heat to low. Cook, stirring occasionally, until the broccoli rabe starts to wilt. As it is cooking, season several times with salt. Add the balsamic vinegar and continue cooking until the balsamic vinegar evaporates and the broccoli rabe is very, very tender, 15 to 20 minutes total.

VEGILICIOUS SIDES

Leeks à la Grecque with Grape Tomatoes

SERVES 4

The term Leeks à la Grecque *translates to "Greek-Style Leeks," but the recipe hails from France. À* la Grecque *simply refers to a sauce that generally consists of olive oil, lemon juice, and seasonings. You can serve this dish warm or cold, and it makes a great topping for whole grains such as brown rice or quinoa.*

> 1 tablespoon plus 1 teaspoon cold-pressed extra-virgin olive oil
>
> 3 medium leeks, sliced into thin rounds and washed very well then patted dry
>
> Unrefined sea salt, to taste
>
> Freshly ground black pepper, to taste
>
> 8 ounces grape tomatoes, sliced in half lengthwise
>
> 2 tablespoons freshly squeezed lemon juice
>
> 2 tablespoons finely chopped thyme
>
> 2 tablespoons finely chopped kalamata olives (optional)

1. Heat 1 tablespoon of the oil in a large heavy saucepan over medium heat; add the leeks, cover and cook, stirring occasionally, until they are quite soft, 6 to 7 minutes. Season with salt and pepper to taste.

2. Add the remaining 1 teaspoon of oil, the tomatoes, lemon juice, thyme, and olives (if using) and sauté until the tomatoes soften and just begin to burst, 4 to 5 minutes. Remove from the heat and season with more salt and pepper. Set aside and let sit for at least 10 minutes before serving. Can be served warm or cold.

Mashed Cauliflower

SERVES 6

It seems as though everybody has a recipe for mashed cauliflower these days. But a lot of the recipes we have seen call for too much oil, butter, cheese, or cream. Ours has just a teeny bit of oil (especially considering we use two heads of cauliflower) and no butter or dairy. But it does have taste.

¼ **cup hemp seeds**

2 tablespoons nutritional yeast

⅓ **cup water**

1 garlic clove

1 teaspoon cold-pressed extra-virgin olive oil

2 small heads cauliflower, cut into florets

Unrefined sea salt, to taste

Paprika and finely chopped scallions (optional)

1. Place the hemp seeds, nutritional yeast, water, garlic, and oil in a high-speed blender; blend until smooth and creamy. Set hemp cream aside.
2. Cut off the cauliflower florets and discard the core.
3. Put about 1 inch of water in the bottom of a pot. Add a steamer basket, cover, and bring the water to a boil. Place the cauliflower in the hot steamer, cover, and steam for 8 to 10 minutes.
4. Remove cauliflower, discard the water in the pot, and remove the steamer basket. Return the cauliflower to the pot. Pour in the hemp cream and use an immersion blender to process the cauliflower until smooth and creamy (you can process cauliflower and hemp cream in a food processor). Season with salt to taste. Transfer the mashed cauliflower to a serving bowl, and dust with paprika and sprinkle with scallions, if desired. Serve warm.

Party-Favorite Stuffed Peppers

SERVES 6

With their stuffed jewel-like presence these peppers make the perfect party entrance! This is actually the go-to side Ivy often brings to potlucks and dinner parties because they have such a festive appearance. They taste delicious too, making them truly ideal for entertaining. Best of all, they take only a few minutes to prepare, then you pop them in the oven for 35 minutes, and they're done. They actually taste best at room temperature, so you can absolutely make them in advance if you are bringing them to a party.

3 large sweet yellow peppers, sliced in half, seeds removed and stems cut off

2 tablespoons cold-pressed extra-virgin olive oil

1 cup very finely chopped fresh basil

¼ teaspoon dried oregano

¼ teaspoon dried thyme

5 garlic cloves, minced

1 tablespoon freshly squeezed lemon juice

2 teaspoons anchovy paste

8 ounces baby bella mushrooms, wiped clean and very finely chopped

½ pint cherry tomatoes, cut in quarters

Unrefined sea salt, to taste

1. Preheat the oven to 400°F.
2. Place the peppers on a large, lightly oiled baking sheet. Set aside.
3. Place the oil, basil, oregano, thyme, garlic, lemon juice, and anchovy paste in a mini food processor and process until smooth and creamy. Set aside.
4. In a large mixing bowl, add the mushrooms, tomatoes, and herb mixture. Season with salt to taste. Stir to combine.
5. Spoon the mushroom-tomato mixture into the pepper halves (stuff them generously). Place the stuffed peppers in the oven, and bake for 35 minutes, or until the peppers are soft and the outer edges are slightly brown. Serve warm or at room temperature.

Thanksgiving Day Green Bean Casserole with Pumpkin Seed Crumble

SERVES 6

Ivy has been tweaking her green bean casserole recipe for the entire decade that we have been married—every year it gets a little more healthful and tastier too. Back in 2009 Ivy was asked to do a Thanksgiving menu makeover feature for Natural Health magazine incorporating ten of Dr. Oz's superfoods, and a version of this recipe appeared in the magazine (pumpkin seeds were the superfood used in this dish), but Ivy has since tweaked the recipe even more. It's also a standby on our Thanksgiving table.

⅓ cup raw cashews

¾ cup water

Unrefined sea salt, to taste

1½ pounds green beans, ends snapped and broken into bite-size pieces

5 ounces baby portabella mushrooms, brushed clean and stems discarded

2 tablespoons plus 2 teaspoons cold-pressed extra-virgin olive oil

1 tablespoon minced garlic

7 ounces shiitake and oyster mushroom mix, cut into bite-size pieces

White pepper, to taste

2 tablespoons white whole wheat flour

½ cup raw pumpkin seeds, plus more for garnish

¼ cup whole wheat panko crumbs (such as Ian's Natural Foods)

1. Place the cashews and water in a high-speed blender or mini food processor and blend or process until smooth and creamy. Set cashew cream aside.
2. Preheat oven to 425°F. Lightly oil a 9- by 13-inch glass baking dish. Set aside. Prepare an ice bath.
3. Fill a large pot with water and add a generous amount of salt; bring the water to a boil. Add the beans and cook until fork-tender, 5 to 6 minutes. Drain the beans in a colander and immediately plunge them into an ice bath. Drain the beans again in a colander. Dry the beans with a kitchen towel or paper towels (don't skip this part!). Set aside.
4. Break the portobello mushroom tops into pieces using your hands.

5. In a large skillet over medium heat, heat 1 tablespoon of the oil; add the garlic and sauté for 1 minute. Add all of the mushrooms and sauté until soft, about 5 minutes. Season with salt and white pepper to taste. Remove from the heat. Add the cooked green beans to the skillet with the mushrooms and gently toss to mix. Transfer the green bean–mushroom mixture to the prepared baking dish. Season with salt to taste.

6. To the same skillet, add 1 tablespoon of the oil and the flour; cook over low heat, whisking constantly, for 1 minute. Add the cashew cream very, very slowly and continue whisking until all of the cream is used and the mixture is creamy and smooth, about 2 minutes. Season with salt and white pepper to taste. Add this roux to the green bean–mushroom mixture and gently toss to coat.

7. Add the pumpkin seeds, panko crumbs, and remaining 2 teaspoons of olive oil to a food processor; process by pulsing about 10 times. Season with salt and pulse again. Top the casserole with the pulsed pumpkin seed mixture. Bake, uncovered, for 10 minutes or until lightly golden. Garnish with whole pumpkin seeds before serving.

Roasted Harvest Vegetable Salad with Roasted Cranberry Vinaigrette

SERVES 6

Seasonal food doesn't get much more seasonal than during the holidays. But holiday food absolutely has to be special, this is nonnegotiable. Our roasted harvest vegetable salad is so special you could certainly serve it for Christmas or Thanksgiving dinner. Ivy brought it to Andy's parents' house for Thanksgiving one year and it was a huge hit with our whole family. It marries the flavors of the holidays into a sensationally satisfying and exceptional salad. To make it dairy free omit the blue cheese.

Roasted Cranberry Vinaigrette

¼ cup fresh cranberries

¼ cup plus 1 tablespoon cold-pressed extra-virgin olive oil

2 tablespoons white raisins

1 tablespoon plus 2 teaspoons balsamic vinegar

2 teaspoons raw honey

2 garlic cloves

½ teaspoon Dijon mustard

Unrefined sea salt, to taste

1 tablespoon water

1. Preheat the oven to 400°F.
2. Place the cranberries, 1 tablespoon of the oil, the raisins and 2 teaspoons of the balsamic vinegar in a small ovenproof skillet. Roast the cranberries for 20 minutes. Remove and set aside to cool.
3. Transfer all of the contents from the roasted cranberries (including the liquid) to a high-speed blender. Add the remaining ¼ cup of oil, 1 tablespoon of balsamic vinegar, and the honey, garlic, mustard, salt, and water. Process until smooth and creamy. Set the vinaigrette aside.

Salad

24 red pearl onions, peeled

4 large carrots, peeled and halved lengthwise and cut into ⅓-inch-wide pieces

4 large parsnips, peeled and halved lengthwise and cut into ⅓-inch-wide pieces

2 teaspoons cold-pressed extra-virgin olive oil

Unrefined sea salt, to taste

Freshly ground black pepper, to taste

2 tablespoons chopped rosemary

8 ounces arugula

2 ripe pears, cut into thin strips

½ cup chopped raw pecans

6 tablespoons crumbled blue cheese (optional)

1. Preheat the oven to 400°F. Lightly oil a large baking sheet.
2. In a large bowl, combine the onions, carrots, and parsnips. Add the oil and season with salt and pepper to taste; toss to coat evenly. Scatter the vegetables in the prepared pan and roast for 20 minutes. Remove the vegetables from the oven and sprinkle with the rosemary. Toss to combine and return the vegetables to the oven. Roast for another 20 minutes, or until the vegetables are very tender and just begin to brown. Remove from the oven and set aside to cool.
3. In a large salad bowl, combine the arugula, pears, and roasted vegetables. Drizzle the vinaigrette on top (the cranberry vinaigrette is rather

thick and a little goes a long way). Season with salt and pepper to taste and gently toss the mixture together. Sprinkle the pecans and blue cheese, if using, on top. Serve at room temperature.

411

Moroccan Carrot Salad

SERVES 4

This salad is totally oil free, and yet it is still every bit as moist as traditional carrot salad. The cumin and cardamom add an exotic Moroccan twist.

1 orange, peeled and cut into segments

¼ cup slivered almonds

¼ teaspoon ground cumin

⅛ teaspoon ground cardamom

2 tablespoons freshly squeezed lime juice

Unrefined sea salt, to taste

10 ounces carrots, shredded

¾ cup chopped fresh mint

½ cup dark raisins

1. Place the orange segments, almonds, cumin, cardamom, lime juice, and salt to taste in a high-speed blender. Blend until smooth and creamy. Set the vinaigrette aside.
2. In a large serving bowl add the shredded carrots, mint, and raisins. Pour the vinaigrette on top of the carrot mixture, and toss gently to coat. Season with salt to taste. Let the salad sit for at least 20 minutes to allow the flavors to fully develop before serving. Serve at room temperature.

Italian Eggplant Caponata

SERVES 6

A caponata is a Sicilian relish-like dish made of chopped vegetables, usually eggplant, and it seems every serious Italian culinary enthusiast has his or her own interpretation. Some versions are stripped down, and others seem to have a ridiculously endless ingredient list. While our adaptation leans mostly

412

toward stripped down, it is no less tasty than any others, just way easier to make! And with a lot less oil too. You'll love the rustic mellow flavor it delivers. It's also extremely versatile and can be served as an appetizer (it is especially good on sprouted whole grain crostini). We also enjoy it as a topping for whole grains, including quinoa and brown rice, and on top of grilled or broiled fish. Oh! And it is just divine mixed with lentils.

1 package (9 ounces) frozen artichoke hearts

2 tablespoons plus 2 teaspoons cold-pressed extra-virgin olive oil

⅓ cup pine nuts

¼ cup yellow raisins

1 large Spanish onion, chopped in ½-inch pieces

6 garlic cloves, crushed

1 medium eggplant, cut into ½-inch cubes

1 red bell pepper, chopped

Unrefined sea salt, to taste

Freshly ground black pepper, to taste

⅓ cup chopped kalamata olives

1 can (14.5 ounces) roasted diced tomatoes

1 tablespoon balsamic vinegar

¼ cup finely chopped basil

1. Preheat the oven to 400°F.
2. Place the frozen artichokes on a baking sheet and drizzle with 1 teaspoon of the oil. Roast for 20 minutes. Remove from the oven and use kitchen shears to cut into bite-size pieces. Set aside.
3. Place the pine nuts and raisins in a mini food processor and process into crumbs. Set aside.
4. Heat the remaining 2 tablespoons plus 1 teaspoon oil in a large heavy saucepan over medium heat; add the onion, garlic, and pine nut–raisin crumble and sauté until the onion softens, 6 to 7 minutes. Add the eggplant, bell pepper, and chopped roasted artichokes and cook until the eggplant is soft, 6 to 7 minutes. Season with salt and pepper to taste.
5. Add the olives, tomatoes, and vinegar and simmer for 10 to 15 minutes. Remove from the heat and add the basil. Season with more salt and pepper to taste. Let sit and cool for at least 15 minutes before serving. Serve warm or at room temperature.

Slow Cooker Fennel Braised with Artichokes

SERVES 4

This melt-in-your-mouth medley of Mediterranean-flavored vegetables is delicious as a side dish and spectacular served over grilled or broiled fish. It also makes a surprisingly satisfying sandwich filler nestled between two slices of toasted sprouted whole grain bread.

1 package (9 ounces) frozen artichoke hearts

2 fennel bulbs, stems and leaves trimmed and bulbs cut lengthwise into ½-inch-thick slices

1 tablespoon plus 2 teaspoons cold-pressed extra-virgin olive oil

Unrefined sea salt, to taste

Freshly ground black pepper, to taste

1 medium onion, halved and cut into slices

6 garlic, cloves crushed

2 teaspoons chopped rosemary

½ teaspoon dried oregano

½ teaspoon dried thyme

1 tablespoon white whole wheat flour

¼ cup dry white wine

¾ cup organic vegetable broth

1 can (14.5 ounces) organic fire-roasted diced tomatoes

1. Preheat the oven to 400°F.

2. Place the frozen artichokes and fennel on a baking sheet and drizzle with 2 teaspoons of the oil. Season with salt and pepper to taste. Roast for 25 minutes, or until the fennel is soft. Remove from the oven and set aside.

3. Heat the remaining 1 tablespoon of oil in a large heavy skillet over medium heat; add the onion and garlic and sauté until the onion is soft, 7 to 8 minutes. Add the rosemary, oregano, and thyme and season with salt and pepper to taste. Stir in the flour until the onions are coated. Add the wine and heat to boiling. Add the broth and tomatoes and stir until boiling.

4. Layer half of the fennel slices in a 5- or 6-quart slow cooker; cover with half of the artichokes and then half of the sauce. Repeat the layers. Cover and cook for 2 hours on high or 4 hours on low, or until vegetables are very tender. Let vegetables sit for at least 15 minutes before serving. Serve warm or cold.

Gingered Brussels Sprout Hash with Golden Raisins

SERVES 4

Think you don't like Brussels sprouts? Then you haven't tried these! Andy is not particularly fond of Brussels sprouts but he always asks for seconds when Ivy serves them like this.

2 teaspoons cold-pressed extra-virgin olive oil

1 tablespoon freshly grated gingerroot

2 shallots, thinly sliced

Unrefined sea salt, to taste

Freshly ground black pepper, to taste

2 tablespoons unrefined apple cider vinegar

⅓ cup golden raisins

1 tablespoon organic extra-virgin coconut oil (such as Barlean's)

1 pound Brussels sprouts, trimmed, halved lengthwise and cut into ⅛-inch slices

¼ cup water

1½ tablespoons orange juice concentrate

1. Heat the olive oil in a medium-size skillet over medium heat; add the ginger and shallots, season with salt and pepper to taste, and cook until the shallots are soft, about 8 minutes. Add the vinegar and raisins and cook until the liquid evaporates and the raisins soften, 4 to 5 minutes. Remove the shallot mixture from the skillet and set aside.

2. Heat the coconut oil in the same skillet over medium heat; add the Brussels sprouts, season with salt and pepper to taste, and sauté for 7 to 8 minutes. Add the water and orange juice concentrate and cook until the liquid evaporates, 8 to 10 minutes. Add the shallot mixture and season with salt and pepper to taste. Cook for an additional minute. Remove from the heat. Serve warm or at room temperature.

Tomatoes à la Provençal

SERVES 4

Tomatoes stuffed with bread crumbs, herbs, and garlic is the perfect make-ahead vegetable dish for dinner. To make this in advance, prep the tomatoes up until step 4 and store them in the refrigerator for up to 6 hours before cooking. This dish goes wonderfully with chicken, fish, lamb, and tofu steaks. And they look so pretty too!

> **4 firm, ripe, red tomatoes about 3 inches in diameter**
>
> **Unrefined sea salt, to taste**
>
> **Freshly ground black pepper, to taste**
>
> **3 garlic cloves**
>
> **1 shallot, chopped**
>
> **½ cup chopped parsley**
>
> **¼ cup pine nuts**
>
> **1 slice sprouted whole grain bread, torn into bite-size pieces**
>
> **1 tablespoon chopped rosemary**
>
> **1 teaspoon cold-pressed extra-virgin olive oil**

1. Set an oven rack in the upper third of the oven. Preheat the oven to 400°F.
2. Remove the stems, and cut the tomatoes in half crosswise. Gently press out the juice and seeds. Sprinkle the halves lightly with salt and pepper.
3. Place the garlic, shallot, parsley, pine nuts, bread pieces, and rosemary in a food processor and pulse several times to chop finely. Add the oil and season with salt and pepper to taste; pulse several more times.
4. Fill each tomato half with a heaping spoonful of the bread-herb mixture. Drizzle with just a smidgen of olive oil. Arrange the tomatoes in a shallow roasting pan.
5. Shortly before you are ready to serve, bake the tomatoes for 10 to 15 minutes, or until they are tender but hold their shape and the bread crumb filling has lightly browned. Serve warm.

So Easy Eggplant Pizzas

SERVES 4

This recipe is so easy we almost feel silly calling it a recipe, but we shared it on our Clean Cuisine Facebook page, and it got so many "likes" and "shares" that we just had to share it here too. You'll love it. Oh, and leftovers make a great sandwich filler between two pieces of toasted sprouted whole grain bread.

> 1 whole eggplant, sliced into thin rounds about ¼ inch thick
>
> Unrefined sea salt, to taste
>
> ¾ cup Clean Cuisine marinara sauce (page 371) or prepared good-quality marinara (such as Rao's)
>
> ⅓ cup shredded organic pastured cheese (such as Cheddar)
>
> Dried oregano, to taste

1. Preheat oven to 400°F. Line a large baking sheet with parchment paper.
2. Place the eggplant rounds on the parchment paper and season with salt. Spoon a heaping tablespoon of marinara on top of each eggplant round. Sprinkle a smidgen of cheese on top of the marinara and a bit of oregano on top of the cheese.
3. Bake eggplant "pizzas" for about 20 minutes, or until cheese melts and eggplant is soft. Serve warm.

Pan Seared Radishes & Radish Greens

SERVES 4

For the longest time we both thought radishes were only good for being cut into delicate, diamond-faceted garnishes. The idea of eating a cooked radish never really crossed our minds. But these days we consider pan-seared peppery radishes and radish greens among our favorite vegetables. Try them and you too will be delighted.

Radish Greens

> ⅓ cup good-quality balsamic vinegar
>
> 1 tablespoon cold-pressed extra-virgin olive oil
>
> 5 garlic cloves, crushed
>
> 1 bunch radish greens, rinsed and chopped

Unrefined sea salt, to taste

Coarsely ground black pepper, to taste

1. Place the vinegar in a small saucepan and heat over low heat; cook until it is thick and syrupy, 10 to 15 minutes. Set aside.
2. Heat the oil and garlic in a large heavy skillet over medium-high heat; when the oil is hot, add the radish greens and sauté until wilted, 3 to 4 minutes. Season with salt and pepper to taste. Drizzle the balsamic reduction on top and set aside.

Radishes

2 teaspoons cold-pressed extra-virgin olive oil

1 tablespoon water

1 dozen medium radishes, thinly sliced

Unrefined sea salt, to taste

Heat the oil and water in a large heavy skillet over medium-high heat; add the radishes and cook until soft, 5 to 6 minutes. Season with salt to taste. Add the cooked radish greens to the skillet and toss to combine. Serve warm.

WHOLE GRAINS
& EARTHY SIDES

Gluten-Free Cranberry-Walnut Tabbouleh

SERVES 6 TO 8

While there's nothing wrong with the bulgur used in traditional tabbouleh recipes, gluten-free quinoa is a delicious alternative if you are gluten-sensitive or if you simply want a twist on the conventional. Eliminating the tomatoes and adding cranberries, walnuts, and mint adds an additional unusual spin and brings a fresh new flavor dimension to a classic favorite.

1 cup water

1 cup quinoa

3 tablespoons cold-pressed walnut oil or flax oil

⅓ cup freshly squeezed lemon juice

¼ cup red onion, minced

1 cup chopped parsley

¼ cup chopped mint

½ cup dried cranberries

1 cucumber, peeled, seeded, and chopped

½ cup raw walnuts, chopped

Unrefined sea salt, to taste

1. Bring the water to a boil in a large saucepan. Add the quinoa and cook until tender, about 15 minutes. Drain if necessary. Transfer quinoa to a large mixing bowl and set aside to cool.

2. To the bowl with the quinoa, add the the oil, lemon juice, onion, parsley, mint, cranberries, cucumber, and walnuts; toss to combine. Season to taste with salt. Cover and refrigerate for at least 1 hour before serving. Leftovers can be stored in a covered container in the fridge for up to 3 days.

Baked Quinoa Spinach Cakes

SERVES 4

These savory cakes are always such a hit with everyone. Ivy first created them for our sister-in-law, Kim Larson, because Kim is crazy for quinoa. Sophisticated but charming, they appeal to both grownups and kids. And, they can be made in a jiffy, especially if you precook your quinoa in a rice cooker. Quinoa can be cooked ahead and stored in the fridge up to 3 days.

1 organic pastured egg

2 tablespoons white whole wheat flour

2 tablespoons raw almond butter or tahini

1 tablespoon plus 1 teaspoon raw apple cider vinegar

1½ cups cooked quinoa

1 package (10 ounces) frozen chopped spinach, thawed and squeezed *very, very dry* with paper towels

¼ cup Spanish onion, diced

5 garlic cloves, crushed

½ teaspoon unrefined sea salt

1. Preheat the oven to 350°F. Lightly oil a large baking pan.
2. In a large bowl, combine the egg, flour, almond butter, and vinegar; mix well. Add the quinoa, spinach, onion, garlic, and salt. Stir until all ingredients are well combined.
3. Divide the mixture into ¼-cup portions and form into cakes, using your hands to gently shape and press the cakes together. Arrange the cakes in the prepared pan and bake 30 to 35 minutes, or until just golden and firm. Serve warm.

Kale & Olive Oil Mashed Potatoes

SERVES 4 TO 6

Ivy originally made this recipe for Thanksgiving dinner a few years back but it has since become a family dinner standby. The secret to this dish is to make sure the kale is chopped really, really well. If you want a heartier version simply double the amount of potatoes and pine nut cream. And whatever you do, please do not peel the potatoes, or you'll peel the fiber and a good dose of nutrients right off! Note: To chop the kale, pulse several times in a food processor.

> 1 pound golden potatoes, cut into chunks
> Unrefined sea salt, to taste
> ⅓ cup water
> ⅓ cup plus 1 tablespoon pine nuts
> 1 tablespoon cold-pressed extra-virgin olive oil
> 6 garlic cloves, crushed
> 6 cups finely chopped kale
> Freshly ground black pepper, to taste

1. Put the potatoes in a large pot and cover with water. Add salt and bring the water to a boil and continue boiling until they are tender, 15 to 20 minutes. Drain and set aside.

2. Place the water and pine nuts in a high-speed blender and process until smooth and creamy. Set aside.

3. Heat the oil in a large heavy saucepan over medium heat; add the garlic and kale and sauté until the kale begins to wilt, 4 to 5 minutes. Pour in the pine nut cream and continue cooking until the kale is very, very wilted. Remove from the heat and add the cooked potatoes. Use a potato masher to mash the potatoes into the creamy kale mixture. Season with salt and pepper to taste. Serve warm.

Wintery Roasted Root Vegetable Mash

SERVES 6 TO 8

This is a lively twist on mashed potatoes and absolutely perfect served as a wintery side dish. The tried-and-true method of open-pan roasting yields a much richer-tasting result than boiling the vegetables. Adding pear to the mix is a sweet and subtle touch. In the end, even though this is a considerably lighter dish than classic mashed potatoes, you won't feel gypped in the taste department.

2 sweet potatoes, peeled and chopped

1 pear, chopped, skins on

2 turnips, peeled and chopped

1 small rutabaga, peeled and chopped

2 teaspoons cold-pressed extra-virgin olive oil

Unrefined sea salt, to taste

⅓ cup pine nuts

3 tablespoons water

3 tablespoons freshly squeezed lemon juice

1 teaspoon lemon zest

¼ teaspoon ground cardamom, or to taste

1. Preheat the oven to 400°F.
2. Toss the sweet potatoes, pear, turnips, and rutabaga with the oil. Arrange the vegetables in 2 baking dishes. Season with salt to taste. Roast for 40 minutes, or until the vegetables are tender. Transfer the vegetables to a large mixing bowl.
3. Place the pine nuts, water, lemon juice, lemon zest, and cardamom in a food processor. Process until smooth and creamy. Pour the mixture into the bowl with the roasted vegetables.
4. Use an immersion blender to purée the vegetables; process until smooth and creamy. Season with additional salt and cardamom. Serve warm.

Fried Black or Brown Rice

SERVES 6 TO 8

In case you haven't heard, black rice is the new brown rice (see page 86). You can find black rice at natural foods stores across the country and at your local Asian market. You can also buy it online at Lotus Foods (LotusFoods.com). If you can't find black rice you can always substitute short-grain brown rice.

> 2 tablespoons organic extra-virgin coconut oil (such as Barlean's)
>
> 1 shallot, very finely chopped
>
> 1 tablespoon grated gingerroot
>
> 5 garlic cloves, crushed
>
> 1 or 2 red chile peppers, seeds removed, finely chopped
>
> 1 teaspoon ground cardamom, or to taste
>
> Unrefined sea salt, to taste
>
> 2 carrots, diced
>
> 1 red or orange bell pepper, very finely chopped
>
> 3 cups cooked black rice (page 423)
>
> Juice from 1 whole lime
>
> ½ cup shredded cilantro
>
> 1 tablespoon agave nectar

1. Heat the oil in a large heavy skillet over medium heat; add the shallot, ginger, garlic, and red chile pepper and sauté until the shallot is soft, 3 to 4 minutes. Season with cardamom and salt to taste.

2. Add the carrots and cook 2 to 3 minutes. Add the bell pepper and cook until all the vegetables are soft, 4 to 5 minutes.

3. Add the rice and toss to mix well with the vegetables. Add the lime juice. Stir-fry for 3 or 4 minutes. Add the cilantro and agave nectar and cook for 1 minute. Adjust the seasoning. Serve warm.

HOW TO COOK BLACK RICE

DRY RICE EXPANDS after cooking. Expect 1 cup of raw rice to yield 3 cups of cooked rice.

1¾ cups water

1 cup black rice

RICE COOKER METHOD

Place water and rice in a rice cooker and cook for approximately 45 minutes, or until the water is soaked up.

STOVETOP METHOD

Add water and rice to a pot and bring to a boil over high heat. Cover, reduce heat, and simmer 30 minutes.

Gluten-Free Soba Noodle Salad with Peanut Sauce

SERVES 6

Our photographer friend Lena Hyde gave Ivy the inspiration for this dish. Lena travels extensively and loves good, healthful food. Ivy didn't make too many changes to the original recipe other than adding the red cabbage, carrots, and scallions and reducing the oil a bit. We hope Lena likes it!

> NOTE: *The nama shoyu in this recipe is a special type of soy sauce that has not been pasteurized; it is made from cultured soybeans and is rich in enzymes and free of preservatives. You can buy it online or at any natural foods store. If you can't find it feel free to use regular soy sauce. Nama shoyu does contain some gluten so if you want a completely gluten-free soy sauce look for San J brand organic gluten-free soy sauce.*

8 ounces 100 percent buckwheat soba noodles

1 tablespoon plus 3 teaspoons toasted sesame oil

3 tablespoons all-natural creamy peanut butter

2 to 3 tablespoons nama shoyu soy sauce

2 tablespoons freshly squeezed lime juice

1 teaspoon crushed garlic

1 teaspoon red chili peppers

4 cups finely chopped red cabbage

2 cups finely chopped carrots

¾ cup finely chopped scallions

Unrefined sea salt, to taste

1. Bring a large pot of salted water to a boil; add the noodles and cook al dente according to the package directions. Drain the noodles.

2. While the noodles are cooking, in a small bowl, whisk together 2 teaspoons of the sesame oil, the peanut butter, soy sauce, lime juice, garlic, and red chili peppers. Set the sauce aside.

3. Heat the remaining 1 tablespoon plus 1 teaspoon sesame oil in a very large heavy skillet over medium heat; add the cabbage and carrots and sauté until the vegetables soften, 6 to 7 minutes. Add the scallions and sauté for 2 to 3 minutes. Season the vegetables with salt to taste. Pour the peanut sauce in with the vegetables and cook for 1 minute. Remove the skillet from the heat, add the cooked noodles, and toss well. Serve warm.

ALMOST GUILT-FREE
SWEET TREATS

Fresh Cinnamon Apple-Pecan Cake

SERVES 8 TO 10

Ivy has been making this cake for years, especially around the holidays (sure beats fruit cake). Although it tastes very sweet there is actually very little added sugar; most of the sweetness comes from the apples and raisins. It's very low in oil too. But not to worry, it still tastes decadent, as any good cake should. If you want to make this treat extra-special for the adults try drizzling a bit of brandy or amaretto on top just before serving. If you are an avid cake baker you will probably think we made a mistake with the recipe since the ingredients do not call for any added liquid or eggs; it's not a mistake, the recipe works because the apples provide a lot of moisture.

2 cups raw pecans

3 apples, cored and chopped (leave the skins on); keep the apples separate

½ cup packed brown sugar

1½ teaspoons ground cinnamon

1¾ teaspoons baking soda

½ teaspoon unrefined sea salt

1 cup yellow or black raisins

3 tablespoons plus 1 teaspoon organic extra-virgin coconut oil (such as Barlean's), melted

1½ cups white whole wheat flour

1. Preheat the oven to 350°F. Oil a 9-inch round cake pan.
2. Add 1½ cups of the pecans to the bowl of a food processor and pulse several times to finely chop. Add 1 of the chopped apples along with the sugar, cinnamon, baking soda, and salt. Pulse several more times so that some chunks remain. Add another chopped apple, and pulse again until the apples are chopped but not mushy. Add the raisins and 2 tablespoons of the melted oil and pulse again until the ingredients are well blended. Add the flour and process until moist (batter will be heavy and rather lumpy). Transfer the batter to the cake pan and set aside.
3. To the food processor add the remaining ½ cup pecans, chopped apple, and 1 teaspoon oil; pulse several times until ingredients are finely chopped. Scatter the mixture on top of the cake batter.
4. Bake for 30 to 40 minutes (checking after 30 minutes), or until a toothpick inserted in the center comes out clean. Set aside on a wire rack to cool for 10 minutes before slicing.

Blueberry Upside-Down Cake

SERVES 8

This self-decorating cake is always such a hit at dinner parties. The perfect sweet ending! Don't worry about the olive oil affecting the flavor of the cake; it contributes a savory flavor that is absolutely delicious. Please don't try a substitute oil!

1 cup packed brown sugar, divided in half

4 tablespoons organic extra-virgin coconut oil, divided in half and melted

2½ cups frozen organic blueberries, semithawed

Juice from 1 whole lemon

1¼ cups white whole wheat flour

1 teaspoon baking powder

½ teaspoon baking soda

¼ teaspoon unrefined sea salt

2 organic pastured eggs

2 tablespoons cold-pressed extra-virgin olive oil

½ cup plain, unsweetened hemp milk

1 banana, mashed

1 teaspoon pure lemon extract

1. Preheat the oven to 350°F. Lightly oil a 9-inch springform pan.
2. In a small mixing bowl, mix together ½ cup of the sugar with 2 table-spoons of the coconut oil and spread evenly over the bottom of the pan. Toss the blueberries lightly with the lemon juice; spread them out evenly over the bottom of the pan.
3. In a medium bowl, mix together the remaining ½ cup sugar and the flour, baking powder, baking soda, and salt.
4. In a high-speed blender, add the eggs and blend for 1 full minute, until frothy. Add the remaining 2 tablespoons of coconut oil, the olive oil, hemp milk, banana, and lemon extract. Process until smooth and creamy. Add the wet ingredients to the dry and mix well. Carefully spread the batter (it will be thick!) over the blueberries.
5. Place the pan on a large baking sheet to catch any drips and bake the cake for 45 minutes, or until a toothpick inserted in the middle of the cake comes out clean. Let the cake cool for 15 minutes on a rack.
6. Transfer the cake to the refrigerator and cool for 2 to 3 hours so the blueberries can set.
7. Flip the cake. Release the latches on the springform pan. Run a paring knife around the edges of the cake to loosen it. Carefully press the bottom up to the top rim of the pan. When you get the bottom of the pan up to the top rim place a serving platter over the cake and invert it, carefully pressing the bottom of the loosened springform pan toward the platter. Carefully remove the bottom of the springform pan. Cut cake into wedges and serve.

Spirited Chocolate Sauce

Chocolate connoisseurs will be on cloud nine after trying this decadent choc-olate sauce that gets a "spirited" lift from amaretto, an Italian sweet almond-flavored liqueur. Adding unsweetened cocoa powder gives the sauce an antioxidant boost and an added richness that is to-die-for delish. Once re-frigerated, the sauce is almost fudge-like (if you'd like a thinner sauce, dilute

with 1 tablespoon of water at a time). Drizzle over any fruit you like; we par-
ticularly love it over grilled pineapples and fresh raspberries. Leftovers can be

stored in the refrigerator in a covered container for up to 4 days.

1 small bar (1.2 ounces) Beyond Organic brand fine Italian dark chocolate (see below) or ⅓ cup plus 2 tablespoons dark vegan chocolate chips

1 tablespoon organic extra-virgin coconut oil (such as Barlean's)

2 tablespoons amaretto

2 tablespoons water

2 tablespoons good quality unsweetened cocoa powder

1. Place the chocolate and oil in a small saucepan; heat over low heat until the chocolate begins to melt. Add the amaretto and water; use a fork to whisk ingredients together. Continue heating over low heat until the chocolate melts. Add the cocoa powder and stir to combine. Remove from the heat. Drizzle over fresh or grilled fruit.

A CHOCOLATE IN A CLASS OF ITS OWN: BEYOND ORGANIC FINE ITALIAN DARK CHOCOLATE

BY NOW ANY health-conscious chocolate lover on the face of the earth has certainly heard a tidbit or two about the benefits associated with eating a little dark, high-quality chocolate now and then. The fact that the plant-based saturated fat in chocolate is stearic acid and does not raise cholesterol is undoubtedly comforting, and who couldn't be just a little excited about the connection moderate chocolate consumption has with reduced blood pressure, improved blood vessel health, and the lowering of bad LDL cholesterol and elevation of good HDL cholesterol? Such sweet news is often attributed to a class of antioxidant phytonutrients in chocolate called flavonoids. Because Ivy is a lover of all things chocolate, she is constantly on the lookout for new scientific studies about chocolate (maybe one that says eating chocolate is the secret to making fine hair grow thick?). Although we can't attribute any health or beauty benefits to chocolate other than the ones bona fide health-conscious chocolate lovers are already aware of, we can introduce you to the best-tasting and healthiest chocolate we have yet to find. Beyond Organic Chocolate is crafted in Italy by fifth-generation chocolatiers, so it tastes absolutely nothing like the mass-market chocolate candy bars you have surely tried in the past. But beyond that, Beyond Organic is dairy-free and created from certified organic artisanal dark chocolate infused with flaxseeds. Yes, chocolate that tastes decadent but is also a source (even if small) of omega-3s and fiber too! Beyond that, Beyond Organic Chocolate is GMO-free and contains antioxidants as well as probiotics. Chocolate honestly never tasted so sweet (and nearly guilt free!). Learn More at GoBeyondFoods.com.

Broiled Bananas with Rum-Raisin Sauce

SERVES 4

A version of this dessert has been in Ivy's recipe repertoire for almost a decade. As the years have gone by she has tweaked it here and there. This version, although it's the most healthful one by far with very little oil and zero added sugar, is actually the tastiest. We serve it, with rave reviews, to guests all the time. It is over-the-top delicious with a small scoop of coconut ice cream (such as Coconut Bliss).

Sauce

2 whole oranges, peeled and cut into segments

5 tablespoons rum

4 tablespoons water

6 pitted dates

1 teaspoon organic extra-virgin coconut oil (such as Barlean's)

½ cup golden or dark organic raisins

Dash of nutmeg

1. Place oranges, rum, water, and dates in a high-speed blender and process until smooth and creamy.

2. Pour the orange-rum mixture into a medium-size skillet and add the oil and raisins. Place the skillet over medium heat and gently stir until the oil melts. Cook, stirring constantly, until the sauce is thickened, about 2 minutes. Stir in the nutmeg, then taste and adjust the

seasoning. Remove from the heat and cover to keep warm. The sauce can be made a few days in advance.

Bananas

4 bananas

Organic extra-virgin coconut oil, for brushing onto bananas

1 tablespoon freshly squeezed lemon juice

½ cup raw pecan crumbs (see note below)

1. Position the oven broiler rack about 5 inches from the heat source. Preheat the broiler. Lightly coat a cookie sheet with coconut oil.
2. Peel the bananas and cut in half lengthwise and crosswise. Arrange the strips, uncut-side up, in the baking dish. Lightly brush the tops of the bananas with the oil and drizzle with lemon juice.
3. Broil the bananas for about 5 minutes, watching closely, until the bananas are lightly browned. When done, remove the bananas from the oven and *gently* peel them off the cookie sheet with a spatula.
4. For each serving, artfully arrange the banana sections on a dessert plate. Drizzle with the sauce and sprinkle with the pecan crumbs. Serve at once.

Note: To make pecan crumbs, place ½ cup raw pecans in a high-speed blender or mini–food processor and blend or process into crumbs. The pecan crumbs can be stored in the freezer in a self-sealing plastic bag for up to 2 months.

Stovetop Apple & Cherry Crumble
SERVES 8 TO 10

We drastically reduced the sugar in this recipe compared to typical fruit crumble desserts. Ivy was even able to sneak some chia seeds into the crumbly topping! We especially love this treat served with a small scoop of ice cream made from coconuts (such as Coconut Bliss). The secret to getting the crumbly topping just right is to make sure the coconut oil is very cold and hard.

Crumbly Topping

¾ cup white whole wheat flour

6 tablespoons sugar

¾ teaspoon baking soda

½ teaspoon baking powder

¼ teaspoon ground cinnamon

Pinch of unrefined sea salt

3 tablespoons plain hemp milk

1 tablespoon plus 1 teaspoon *very cold* organic extra-virgin coconut oil

3 tablespoons chia seeds (such as Barlean's)

Whisk together the flour, sugar, baking soda, baking powder, cinnamon, and salt. Pour the hemp milk in and use a fork to wet the flour. Add the coconut oil and use your hands to crumble the ingredients together. Add chia seeds and continue crumbling the ingredients together. Set the crumb mixture aside.

Fruit Filling

2 Granny Smith apples, chopped (keep the skins on!)

2 bags (10 ounces each) frozen cherries

½ cup white raisins

¼ cup date sugar or brown sugar

Pinch unrefined sea salt

2 tablespoons amaretto

2 tablespoons freshly squeezed lemon juice

¼ cup water

1. Add all of the ingredients to a medium heavy skillet. Bring the liquid to a boil and cook, stirring occasionally, until the cherries are thawed and the fruit is very soft, about 4 minutes.
2. Use your fingers to scatter the crumbly topping over the fruit. Cover with a lid and cook for 8 or 10 minutes. Remove lid and remove from the heat. Let sit for at least 20 minutes so the fruit can set. Spoon out into dessert bowls and serve with a small scoop of coconut ice cream, if desired. Adults can add a little extra splash of amaretto.

Pumpkin Custard

SERVES 4

This pretty much tastes exactly like pumpkin pie but without the crust, yet it maintains the perfect sweetness with only a fraction of the sugar used in traditional pumpkin pie. It is made with unconventional ingredients (including-hemp seeds, dates, and coconut milk) but we assure you it tastes just like the real deal pumpkin pie! And it's much easier to make too.

3 tablespoons hemp seeds

½ cup water

5 pitted dates

¾ cup canned pumpkin (or fresh roasted pumpkin, mashed)

¼ cup packed plus 2 tablespoons brown sugar or date sugar

½ cup organic coconut milk

1 teaspoon freshly grated gingerroot

2 organic pastured eggs

1 teaspoon ground cinnamon

¼ teaspoon ground allspice

⅛ teaspoon ground cloves

1. Preheat the oven to 350°F. Lightly grease four 4-ounce ramekins with extra-virgin coconut oil.
2. Put the hemp seeds, water, and dates in a high-speed blender and blend until smooth and creamy. Add the pumpkin, brown sugar, coconut milk, ginger, eggs, cinnamon, allspice, and cloves; process for at least 1 full minute, or until all ingredients are smooth and silky. Pour mixture into prepared ramekins.
3. Place ramekins in a large baking pan. Add hot water around ramekins to a depth of 1 inch. Place the baking pan on middle oven rack and bake for 50 to 55 minutes, or until custard is firm and no longer jiggly. Remove from the oven and set aside on a wire rack to cool and set. Serve at room temperature or chilled.

Clean Cuisine Chia & Chocolate Cookies

Ivy's dad, Norman, loves these cookies so much that when we asked him what
*he wanted for his eighty-sixth birthday the first thing he said was, "How
about those chia cookie things?" They are just beyond delicious. And you
can't just eat one. Also, for what it is worth, although they are not totally gluten free, because they are made with barley flour they contain considerably
less gluten than cookies made with wheat flour.*

YIELDS 24 COOKIES

- 1½ cups raw almonds
- 8 pitted dates
- 2 cups barley flour
- ¼ cup chia seeds (such as Barlean's)
- ½ cup organic extra-virgin coconut oil, softened
- ½ cup pure maple syrup
- ½ teaspoon unrefined sea salt
- ½ cup vegan mini chocolate chips

1. Preheat the oven to 350°F.
2. Put the almonds in a food processor and process into crumbs. Transfer the almond crumbs to a large mixing bowl. Put the dates in the food processor and pulse 6 to 7 times, or until well ground. Add the dates to the almonds.
3. To the mixing bowl, add the flour, chia seeds, coconut oil, maple syrup, and salt. Combine all ingredients with a wooden spoon. Form the mixture into tablespoonful balls and space them evenly on a large cookie sheet. Using your index finger, make an indent in each cookie. Fill the indent in each cookie with 4 or 5 mini chocolate chips.
4. Bake for 18 minutes. The cookies should be done but the chocolate will not totally be melted. As soon as you remove the cookies from the oven, take the back of a spoon and gently press down on the chocolate so that it melts. Set the cookies aside to cool and harden for at least 15 minutes before eating.

Key Lime, Blueberry, & Coconut Cloud Custards

SERVES 4

Ivy created these key lime custards as a special treat for Andy as a Clean Cuisine alternative to his favorite dessert in the whole world, key lime pie. Andy loves key lime pie so much that we had to include it in our wedding menu in 2000. And believe it or not, he loves these key lime custards every bit as much as pie. They are just that good!

> 1½ cups frozen organic wild blueberries
>
> 3½ teaspoons arrowroot
>
> ⅓ cup plus 2 tablespoons sugar
>
> 2 tablespoons real key lime juice (such as Nellie of Joe's)
>
> 2 organic pastured eggs
>
> 5 raw macadamia nuts
>
> 1 cup organic coconut milk

1. Preheat the oven to 350°F.
2. Mix the blueberries with 1½ teaspoons of the arrowroot and 2 tablespoons of the sugar. Set aside.
3. Fill a large casserole dish one fourth of the way up with water. Arrange four 6-ounce ramekins in the water. Divide the blueberry mixture among the ramekins.
4. In a high-speed blender (such as a Vitamix), add the remaining 2 teaspoons arrowroot and ⅓ cup sugar and the key lime juice, eggs, macadamia nuts, and coconut milk. Process until smooth and creamy. Pour the key lime–coconut mixture over the blueberries.
5. Bake for 35 to 40 minutes, or until the custards are set. Remove from the oven and set aside to cool for at least 15 minutes. Transfer to the refrigerator and cool for 1 hour before serving. Serve chilled.

THANK YOU!

Doing business with friends and family is something most people advise against, but we find it works perfectly well for us. Ivy's mom, Gail Ingram, has been working with us for years proofreading, doing recipe development, recipe testing, and serving as our food stylist. When we started CleanCuisine.com she soon became our official website food photographer; she also presents the exercise photos in Chapter 8. Thanks to Gail, our recipes on CleanCuisine.com look so enticing that even people who don't care about eating clean get inspired! Gail has infinite talent, boundless energy, and more generosity than just about anyone. Not only does she help us with our work, she has been a tremendous help over the years pitching in whenever needed with our son, Blake. There is no way Ivy could have managed the lengthy recovery from her surgery while writing this book without Gail's help. We just don't know how we could ever manage without her. XOXOX

Our friend and business partner, Samantha Gardner . . . we don't even know where to start thanking you. Clean Cuisine would not be what it is—and might not even exist—without her. Samantha wears more hats than we can count. She juggles all of the online marketing, web development, graphics, and behind-the-scenes nuisances and "techy stuff" that go into running an online business and she picks up the slack whenever Ivy gets overwhelmed, which can happen at any given moment! She keeps Ivy focused and organized, again, not an easy job. Ivy went with a hunch when she first met Samantha that she would make the perfect business partner, and she was right. We couldn't ask for a better partner, or friend.

Linda Konner, our hardworking, determined, and always supportive agent, thank you so very much for your candid direction, enthusiasm, and commitment to us and to this project. We know we can always count on

435

Linda to guide us in the right direction. Her wisdom and advice throughout the years have been invaluable.

To our dear friend Cherie Fromson, no matter what we need—whether it is business or personal, we can always ask Cherie. She's trekked with Ivy to New York City to be her food stylist for national TV appearances, she's turned her kitchen upside down and into Clean Cuisine recipe testing headquarters weekend after weekend, she's done hundreds of pushups and squats rehearsing for the Clean Cuisine workout DVD, she made the Clean Cuisine Salad Booster a reality, and she saved the day over and over during Ivy's lengthy recovery from surgery. Most important . . . she is a true friend.

To the team at Penguin: a very special thank-you to our publisher, Leslie Gelbman, for her wholehearted commitment to Clean Cuisine and unwavering support. To our wonderful editor, Denise Silvestro, for her instrumental role in getting this project off the ground, for keeping the ball rolling, and for supporting our Clean Cuisine message so enthusiastically. Meredith Giordan, thank you for always being so quick to respond, so easy to work with, and so very organized. To our managing editor, Pamela Barricklow, and editorial director, Susan Allison, thank you both for your hard work and attention to detail. Judith Murello Lagerman, thank you for the sensationally "clean" cover and the new look of "Clean Cuisine"—we love the mint leaves! And a big shout-out to the sales, marketing, and PR team, we are so lucky to have such a hardworking group in our corner. Thank you all!

Our fitness expert pals and consultants: husband and wife team, Marissa and Gary Lavin, thank you both for your input on the workouts and for the catchy "Sizzle, Sculpt, Slim, Stretch & Strengthen" concept. You not only contributed function but added a sprinkling of fun too (a key component of any good workout!). And to our dear friend Mike Gibbs, your fitness knowledge is incredible and your help rehabbing Ivy while she recovered from surgery was so invaluable and so deeply appreciated. You came into our lives at a critical time and we will always, always be grateful for your help.

Our biggest thank-you to our online Clean Cuisine community! This book would not exist if it weren't for you. Thank you all!!! To Allison Janse, Peter Vegso, and Kim Weiss, we will forever be thankful to all of you for opening the doors to the exciting world of book publishing. And, Natalie Morales, we don't know what else to say other than a very big and most sincere thank-you. Jack Nicklaus, we will always be grateful for your early support when we needed it most. To one of Ivy's oldest friends, Susan Malt Josephson, for being such a trouper going through with the Clean Cuisine workout DVD while pregnant, and for always being a true friend. And to Rana Burr, her continuous tech support and wonderful marketing ideas are much appreciated.

437

To Ivy's dad, Norman Ingram, for instilling in Ivy an entrepreneurial spirit, for encouraging her to think for herself, and for teaching the importance of persistence. Clean Cuisine would not exist if it weren't for the tremendous influence Ivy's dad has had on her. We are also both most appreciative of the time Norm spends with our son, as we know the life lessons he is passing on are invaluable and will help him so much.

To Andy's parents, Elaine and Ken Larson, we thank you for always being ready to help us as we navigate our busy professional schedules and we thank you for your help and dedication when it comes to turning our son into a man and for helping him learn to appreciate life, nature, and the simpler joys in life.

And to our dear son, Blake, thank you for bringing us such joy and happiness. Your sunny disposition, great sense of humor, kind heart, energy, and fun spirit bring us such delight every day. We love you so very much and we look forward to sharing in the great things we know you are going to do.

The products and brands listed here are some of our favorite staple pantry items. When appropriate, we have also included a link to the brand's website so you can do your own searches in your local area or to learn more details. By no means is this a complete list because new products appear on the market every day! Also, don't forget when possible to connect with local farms and vendors.

CULINARY OILS

Organic extra-virgin coconut oil: Barlean's Organic Oils (barleans .com/clean)

Cold-pressed extra virgin olive oil: Costco's Kirkland (costco.com), McEvoy Ranch (mcevoyranch.com), Trader Joes' California Estate (traderjoes.com), Whole Food's 365 Everyday Value 100% California Unfiltered (wholefoodsmarket.com), Lucini Premuium (lucini.com)

Macadamia nut oil: NOW Foods (nowfoods.com)

Cold-pressed organic flax oil: Barlean's Organic Oils (barleans.com/ clean)

Walnut oil: Roland (rolandfood.com) or Flora (florahealth.com)

Hemp oil: Nutiva (nutiva.com) or Tempt (livingharvest.com)

Truffle oil: Roland (rolandfood.elsstore.com)

SPICES, HERBS, CONDIMENTS, SEEDS, & NUTS

Clean Cuisine Superfood Salad Booster: (CleanCuisineSaladBooster .com)

Unrefined sea salt: Real Salt (realsalt.com)

White pepper: Simply Organic (simplyorganic.com)

Red pepper flakes: Simply Organic (simplyorganic.com)
Garam masala: Simply Organic (simplyorganic.com)
Taco seasoning: Simply Organic (simplyorganic.com)   439
Miso: Miso Master brand Sweet White Miso (great-eastern-sun.com)
Red curry paste: Thai Kitchen (thaikitchen.com)
Raw apple cider vinegar: Bragg (bragg.com)
Soy sauce, unpasteurized: Ohsawa namu shoyu (goldminenatural
    foods.com) or gluten-free: San-J (san-j.com)
Organic Worcestershire sauce: Annie's Naturals (annies.com) or 365
    Organic (wholefoodsmarkets.com)
Liquid smoke: Colgin (colgin.com)
Organic chia seeds: Barlean's (barleans.com/clean)
Organic hemp seeds: Nutiva (www.Nutiva.com)
Ground flax seeds: Barlean's Forti Flax (barleans.com/clean)
Organic dried fruits and raw nuts: Diamond Organics (OrganicFruits
    andNuts.com)

BEANS, BROTH, SAUCES, ETC.
Raw almond butter (no sugar, no salt, no oils): MaraNatha (maranatha
    foods.com)
Organic BPA-free beans (any type of beans): Eden Organic (edenfoods
    .com)
Organic vegetable broth: Pacific Naturals (pacificnaturals.com), Imag-
    ine (imaginefoods.com), or read the labels on in-store brands
BPA-free boxed tomatoes (no sugar, no salt, no oils): Pomì (pomi.it)
Prepared marinara: Rao's (raos.com) or Amy's (amys.com)

BREAKFAST CEREALS
Uncle Sam cereal with flax seeds (attunefoods.com)
Post Shredded Wheat'n Bran (postfoods.com)
Ezekiel 4:9 sprouted whole grain cereal (almond, cinnamon raisin,
    golden flax, or original) (foodforlife.com)

BREADS, FLOURS, AND BAKING
Sprouted whole grain bread, wraps, and English muffins: Food for Life
    (foodforlife.com)
Manna bread: Manna Organic Bakery (mannaorganicbakery.com)

White whole wheat flour: King Arthur Flour (kingarthurflour.com)

Stone-ground cornmeal: Bob's Red Mill (bobsredmill.com)

Unsweetened cocoa powder: Green & Black's (greenandblacks.com) or Ghirardelli (ghirardelli.com)

Dark chocolate chips, dairy free: Sunspire organic chocolate chips (sunspire.com)

PASTAS AND RICE

Sprouted whole grain pasta: Food for Life (foodforlife.com)

Whole grain quinoa pasta: Ancient Harvest (quinoa.net) or Eden Foods (edenfoods.com)

Black rice: Lotus Foods (lotusfoods.com)

Black Rice Pad Thai: Annie Chun (anniechun.com)

MEATS, SEAFOOD, TOFU (AND A TINY BIT OF CHEESE)

Organic sprouted tofu: Nasoya (nasoya.com) or Trader Joe's (traderjoes.com)

Tempeh: Lightlife (lightlife.com)

Ground beef, grass-fed and organic: US Wellness Meats (grasslandbeef.com) or Beyond Organic (gobeyondfoods.com)

BPA-free sustainable line-caught wild tuna: Wild Planet (wildplanetfoods.com)

Organic pastured eggs: Vital Farms (vitalfarms.com)

Grass-fed lamb and poultry: US Wellness Meats (grasslandbeef.com)

Organic grass-fed cheese: Natural by Nature (natural-by-nature.com) or Beyond Organic (gobeyondfoods.com)

Nut cheese: Dr-Cow (Dr-cow.com)

DRINKS

Sparkling water: San Pellegrino (sanpellegrino.com) or Perrier (perrier.com)

Green tea: Kirkland Signature Green Tea (costco.com) or Ito En teas (www.itoen.com)

Unsweetened plain hemp milk: Tempt (livingharvest.com)

Unsweetened plain almond milk: Silk (silkpurealmond.com) or Pacific (pacificfoods.com)

Matcha Japanese Green Tea powder: Teavana (teavana.com)

Coconut water: O.N.E. Coconut Water (onedrinks.com)
Kombucha Probiotic Beverage: GT's Organic Raw Kombucha (www
.synergydrinks.com)

FRUITS, DESSERTS, AND SNACKS ON THE GO
Frozen organic berries: Cascadian Farm (cascadianfarm.com)
Organic chocolate bars: Beyond Organic with flax seeds (gobeyond
foods.com)
Coconut ice cream: Coconut Bliss (coconutbliss.com)
Snack bars: Good Greens (goodgreens.com) or Lärabar (larabar.com)

NUTRITIONAL ENHANCEMENTS AND SUPPLEMENTS
Barlean's (barleans.com/clean)
- Barlean's Greens
- Barlean's Ultra High Potency Omega Swirl Fish Oil and Total
  Omega Vegan Swirl
- Barlean's Ultra EPA-DHA capsules
- Barlean's evening primrose oil
Juice Plus+ caspules (juiceplus.com)
Green Vibrance (vibranthealth.us)
New Chapter Berry Green (newchapter.com)
Clean Cuisine Essentials (CleanCuisineandMore.com/supplements)
Clean Cuisine Probiotic Blend (CleanCuisineandMore.com/supple
ments). Use the code GIFT to receive a 20 percent discount off your
first order.
Dr. Ohhira's Probiotics (drohhiraprobiotics.com)
Kyolic Aged Garlic Extract (kyolic.com)

IN THE KITCHEN
High Speed Blender: Vitamix® (vitamix.com) Use code 06-006758 for
free shipping.
Non-Toxic Ceramic Cookware: Xtrema™ (ceramcor.com/clean) Use
code ccx10 for 10% off.
All-Natural, Non-Toxic Food Storage Containers: FridgeX Silicon
(ceramcor.com/clean) Use code ccx10 for 10% off.
Aprons: Flirty Aprons (flirtyaprons.com)
Recipe Holder: Recipe Rock (cleancuisineandmore.com/recipe-rock)

FITNESS

Full Fitness Fusion DVDs (cleancuisineandmore.com/fullfitness fusion)

Fitness Equipment (CleanCuisineandMore.com/equipment)

> **KEEP IN TOUCH** with Ivy and Andy to get the latest on additional healthy products, Clean Cuisine recipes, workouts, and more by signing up for their weekly e-newsletter at CleanCuisine.com.

NOTES

CHAPTER ONE

1 Centers for Disease Control and Prevention, "Obesity and Overweight," last updated August 28, 2012, www.cdc.gov/obesity/childhood/data.html.
2 Angel Gil-Izquierdo, Maria I. Gil, and Federico Ferreres, "Effect of Processing Techniques at Industrial Scale on Orange Juice Antioxidant and Beneficial Health Compounds," *Journal of Agricultural and Food Chemistry* 50, no. 18 (2002): 5107–14, available at http://pubs.acs.org/doi/abs/10.1021/jf020162%2B.
3 S. Endres, T. Eisenhut, and B. Sinha, "n-3 Polyunsaturated Fatty Acids in the Regulation of Human Cytokine Synthesis," *Biochemical Society Transactions* 23, no. 2 (1995); 277–81.
4 U. A. Ajani, E. S. Ford, and A. H. Mokdad, "Dietary Fiber and C-Reactive Protein: Findings from National Health and Nutrition Examination Survey Data," *Journal of Nutrition* 134, no. 5 (2004): 1181–85.

CHAPTER TWO

1 D. Mozaffarian, T Hao, E. B. Rimm, et al., "Changes in Diet and Lifestyle and Long-Term Weight Gain in Women and Men," *New England Journal of Medicine* 364, no. 25 (2011): 2392–404.
2 W. C. Willett, M. J. Stampfer, J. E. Manson, et al., "Intake of Trans Fatty Acids and Risk of Coronary Heart Disease among Women," *Lancet* 341, no. 8845 (1993): 581–85.
3 J. Brody, "Huge Study of Diet Indicts Fat and Meat," *New York Times*, May 8, 1990.
4 T. Colin Campbell and Thomas M. Campbell, *The China Study* (BenBella Books, Dallas, 2006).
5 E. T. Poehlman, P. J. Arciero, C. L. Melby, and S. F. Badylak, "Resting Metabolic Rate and Postprandial Thermogenesis in Vegetarians and Nonvegetarians," *American Journal of Clinical Nutrition* 48, no. 2 (1988): 209–13.
6 P. K. Newby, K. L. Tucker, and A. Wolk, "Risk of Overweight and Obesity among Semivegetarian, Lactovegetarian, and Vegan Women," *American Journal of Clinical Nutrition* 81, no. 6 (2005): 1267–74.
7 S. Tonstad, T. Butler, R. Yan, and G. E. Fraser, "Type of Vegetarian Diet, Body Weight, and Prevalence of Type 2 Diabetes," *Diabetes Care* 32, no. 5 (2009): 791–96.
8 C. Pelletier, P. Imbeault, and A. Tremblay, "Energy Balance and Pollution by Organochlorines and Polychlorinated Biphenyls," *Obesity Reviews* 4, no. 1 (2003): 17–24.
9 A. Tremblay, C. Pelletier, E. Doucet, and P. Imbeault, "Thermogenesis and Weight Loss in Obese Individuals: A Primary Association with Organochlorine Pollution," *International Journal of Obesity and Related Metabolic Disorders* 28, no. 7 (2004): 936–39.

CHAPTER THREE

1   S. E. McCann, J. L. Fredenheim, J. R. Marshall, and S. Graham, "Risk of Human Ovarian Cancer Is Related to Dietary Intake of Selected Nutrients, Phytochemicals and Food Groups," *Journal of Nutrition* 133, no. 6 (2003): 1937–42.

2   K. A. Steinmetz and J. D. Potter, "Vegetables, Fruit and Cancer Prevention: A Review," *Journal of the American Dietetic Association* 96, no. 10 (1996): 1027–39.

3   J. A. Satia, A. Littman, C. G. Slatore, et al., "Long-Term Use of Beta-Carotene, Retinol, Lycopene, and Lutein Supplements and Lung Cancer Risk: Results from the VITamins And Lifestyle (VITAL) Study," *American Journal of Epidemiology* 169, no. 7 (2009): 815–28. J. Virtamo, P. Pietinen, J. K. Huttunen, et al., "Incidence of Cancer and Mortality Following Alpha-Tocopherol and Beta-Carotene Supplementation: A Postintervention Follow-Up," *Journal of the American Medical Association* 290, no. 4 (2003): 476–85.

4   A. G. Dulloo, C. Duret, D. Rohrer, et al., "Efficacy of a Green Tea Extract Rich in Catechin Polyphenols and Caffeine in Increasing 24-h Energy Expenditure and Fat Oxidation in Humans," *American Journal of Clinical Nutrition* 70, no. 6 (1999): 1040–45.

5   C. S. Mizuno, G. Ma, S. Khan, et al., "Design, Synthesis, Biological Evaluation and Docking Studies of Pterostilbene Analogs inside PPARalpha," *Bioorganic & Medicinal Chemistry* 16, no. 7 (2008): 3800–08.

6   A. Khan, M. Safdar, M. M. Ali Khan, et al., "Cinnamon Improves Glucose and Lipids of People with Type 2 Diabetes," *Diabetes Care* 26, no. 12 (2003): 3215–18.

CHAPTER FOUR

1   F. B. Hu and W. C. Willet, "Optimal Diets for Prevention of Coronary Heart Disease," *Journal of the American Medical Association* 288, no. 20 (2002): 2569–78.

2   A. T. Merchant, H. Vatanparast, S. Barlas, et al., "Carbohydrate Intake and Overweight and Obesity among Healthy Adults," *Journal of the American Dietetic Association* 109, no. 7 (2009): 1165–72.

3   U. A. Ajani, E. S. Ford, and A. H. Mokdad, "Dietary Fiber and C-Reactive Protein: Findings from the National Health and Nutrition Examination Survey Data," *Journal of Nutrition* 134, no. 5 (2004): 1181–85.

4   L. A. Bazzano, "Effects of Soluble Dietary Fiber on Low-Density Lipoprotein Cholesterol and Coronary Heart Disease Risk," *Current Atherosclerosis Reports* 10, no. 6 (2008): 473–77.

5   G. R. Howe, E. Benito, R. Castelleto, et al., "Dietary Intake of Fiber and Decreased Risk of Cancers of the Colon and Rectum: Evidence from the Combined Analysis of 13 Case-Control Studies," *Journal of the National Cancer Institute* 84, no. 24 (1992): 1887–96.

6   www.gallup.com/poll/151181/Weight-Quarterly.aspx accessed 9/24/12.

7   C. L. Bodinham, G. S. Frost, and M. D. Robertson, "Acute Ingestion of Resistant Starch Reduces Food Intake in Healthy Adults," *British Journal of Nutrition* 103, no. 6 (2010): 917–22.

8   T. Colin Campbell and Thomas M. Campbell, *The China Study* (BenBella Books, Dallas, 2006).

9   R. M. van Dam, A. W. Visscher, E. J. Feskens, et al., "Dietary Glycemic Index in Relation to Metabolic Risk Factors and Incidence of Coronary Heart Disease: The Zutphen Elderly Study," *European Journal of Clinical Nutrition* 54, no. 9 (2000): 726–31.

10   R. J. Barnard, E. J. Ugianskis, D. A. Martin, and S. B. Inkeles, "Role of Diet and Exercise in the Management of Hyperinsulinemia and Associated Atherosclerotic Risk Factors," *American Journal of Cardiology* 69, no. 5 (1992): 440–444.

11   S. H. Holt, J. C. Miller, P. Petocz, and E. Farmakalidis, "A Satiety Index of Common Foods," *European Journal of Clinical Nutrition* 49, no. 9 (1995): 675–90.

12   F. J. He, C. A. Nowson, and G. A. MacGregor, "Fruit and Vegetable Consumption and Stroke: Meta-Analysis of Cohort Studies," *Lancet* 367, no. 9507 (2006): 320–26.
L. Dauchet, P. Amouyel, S. Hercberg, and J. Dallongeville, "Fruit and Vegetable Consumption and Risk of Coronary Heart Disease: A Meta-Analysis of Cohort Studies," *Journal of Nutrition* 136, no. 10 (2006): 2588–93.

13   J. M. Douglass, I. M. Rasgon, P. M. Fleiss, et al., "Effects of a Raw Food Diet on Hypertension and Obesity," *Southern Medical Journal* 78, no. 7 (1985): 841–44.

14   L. Kohlmeier, J. D. Kark, E. Gomez-Garcia, et al., "Lycopene and Myocardial Infarction Risk in the EURAMIC Study," *American Journal of Epidemiology* 146, no. 8 (1997): 618–26.

15   K. E. Schroder, "Effects of Fruit Consumption on Body Mass Index and Weight Loss in a Sample of Overweight and Obese Dieters enrolled in a Weight-Loss Intervention Trial," *Nutrition* 26, no. 7–8 (2010): 727–34.

16   Y. Papanikolaou and V. L. Fulgoni, "Bean Consumption Is Associated with Greater Nutrient Intake, Reduced Systolic Blood Pressure, Lower Body Weight, and a Smaller Waist Circumference in Adults: Results from the National Health and Nutrition Examination Survey 1999–2002," *Journal of the American College of Nutrition* 27, no. 5 (2008): 569–76.

17   N. M. McKeown, M. Yoshida, P. F. Jacques, et al., "Whole-Grain Intake and Cereal Fiber Are Associated with Lower Abdominal Adiposity in Older Adults," *Journal of Nutrition* 139, no. 10 (2009): 1950–55.

18   P. Koh-Banerjee, M. Franz, L. Sampson, et al., "Changes in Whole-Grain, Bran, and Cereal Fiber Consumption in Relation to 8-yr. Weight Gain among Men," *American Journal of Clinical Nutrition* 80, no. 5 (2004): 1237–45.

19   H. I. Katcher, R. S. Legro, A. R. Kunselman et al., "The Effects of a Whole Grain-Enriched Hypocaloric Diet on Cardiovascular Disease Risk Factors in Men and Women with Metabolic Syndrome," *American Journal of Clinical Nutrition* 87, no. 1 (2008): 79–90.

20   "Nutrition and Aging Skin: Sugar and Glycation." *Clinics in Dermatology.* 28, no. 4 (2010): 409-11.

CHAPTER FIVE

1   J. Sabate, "Nut Consumption and Body Weight," *American Journal of Clinical Nutrition* 73, supplement 3 (2003): 647S–50S.

2   R. Jiang, J. E. Manson, M. J. Stampfer, et al., "Nut and Peanut Butter Consumption and Risk of Type 2 Diabetes in Women," *Journal of the American Medical Association* 288, no. 20 (2002): 2254–60.

3   G. Buckland, A. Agudo, N. Travier, et al., "Adherence to the Mediterranean Diet Reduces Mortality in the Spanish Cohort of the European Prospective Investigation into Cancer and Nutrition (EPIC-Spain)," *British Journal of Nutrition* 106, no. 10 (2011): 1581–91.

4   F. B. Hu, J. E. Manson, and W. C. Willett, "Types of Dietary Fat and Risk of Coronary Heart Disease: A Critical Review," *Journal of the American College of Nutrition* 20, no. 1 (2001): 5–19.

5   Dietary Reference Intakes for Energy, Carbohydrate, Fiber, Fat, Fatty Acids, Cholesterol, Protein, and Amino Acids (Macronutrients), *The National Academies Press* 2005, p. 504.

6   N. M. de Roos, M. L. Bots, and M. B. Katan, "Replacement of Dietary Saturated Fatty Acids by Trans Fatty Acids Lowers Serum HDL Cholesterol and Impairs Endothelial Function in Healthy Men and Women," *Arteriosclerosis, Thrombosis, and Vascular Biology* 21, no. 7 (2001): 1233–37.

7   V. Chajès, A. C. Thiébaut, M. Rotival, et al., "Association between Serum Trans-Monounsaturated Fatty Acids and Breast Cancer Risk in the E3N-EPIC Study," *American Journal of Epidemiology* 167, no. 11 (2008): 1312–20.

445

8   J. E. Chavarro, J. W. Rich-Edwards, B. A. Rosner, and W. C. Willett, "Dietary Fatty Acid Intakes and the Risk of Ovulatory Infertility," *American Journal of Clinical Nutrition* 85, no. 1 (2007): 231–37.

9   G. Misciagna, S. Centonze, C. Leoci, et al., "Diet, Physical Activity, and Gallstones—A Population-Based, Case-Control Study in Southern Italy," *American Journal of Clinical Nutrition* 69, no. 10 (1999): 120–26.

10   A. Kennedy, K. Martinez, C. C. Chuang, et al., "Saturated Fatty Acid-Mediated Inflammation and Insulin Resistance in Adipose Tissue: Mechanism of Action and Implications," *Journal of Nutrition* 139, no. 1 (2009): 1–4.

11   A. P. Simopoulos, "The Importance of the Omega-6/Omega-3 Fatty Acid Ratio in Cardiovascular Disease and Other Chronic Diseases," *Experimental Biological Medicine* 233, no. 6 (2008): 674–88.

12   M. Studer, M. Briel, B. Leimenstoll, et al., "Effect of Different Antilipidemic Agents and Diets on Mortality: A Systematic Review," *Archives of Internal Medicine* 165, no. 7 (2005): 725–30.

13   D. Bates, N. E. Cartlidge, J. M. French, et al., "A Double-Blind Controlled Trial of Long Chain *n*-3 Polyunsaturated Fatty Acids in the Treatment of Multiple Sclerosis," *Journal of Neurology, Neurosurgery, and Psychiatry* 52, no. 1 (1989): 18–22.

14   M. Peet and D. F. Horrobin, "A Dose-Ranging Study of the Effects of Ethyl-Eicosapentaenoate in Patients with Ongoing Depression Despite Apparently Adequate Treatment with Standard Drugs," *Archives of General Psychiatry* 59, no. 10 (2002): 913–19.

15   M. M. McCusker and J. M. Grant-Kels, "Healing Fats of the Skin: The Structural and Immunologic Roles of the Omega-6 and Omega-3 Fatty Acids," *Clinical Dermatology* 28, no. 4 (2010): 440–51.

16   P. D. Tsitouras, F. Gucciardo, A. D. Salbe, et al., "High Omega-3 Fat Intake Improves Insulin Sensitivity and Reduces CRP and IL6, but Does Not Affect Other Endocrine Axes in Healthy Older Adults," *Hormone and Metabolic Research* 40, no. 3 (2008): 199–205.

17   O. A. Gani, "Are Fish Oil Omega-3 Long-Chain Fatty Acids and Their Derivatives Peroxisome Proliferator-Activated Receptor Agonists?," *Cardiovascular Diabetology* 7 (2008): 6.

18   C. R. Ritch, R. L. Wan, L. B. Stephens, et al., "Dietary Fatty Acids Correlate with Prostate Cancer Biopsy Grade and Volume in Jamaican Men," *Journal of Urology* 177, no. 1 (2007): 97–101.

19   P. Casas-Agustench, P. Lopez-Uriarte, M. Bullo, et. al. "Acute Effects of Three High-Fat Meals with Different Fat Saturations on Energy Expenditure, Substrate Oxidation and Satiety" *Clinical Nutrition* 28, no. 1 (2009): 39–45.

20   R. Segura, C. Javierre, M. A. Lizarraga, and E. Ros, "Other Relevant Components of Nuts: Phytosterols, Folate and Minerals," *British Journal of Nutrition* 96, suppl. 2 (2006): D36–44.

21   N. I. Lipoeto, Z. Agus, F. Oenzil, et al., "Dietary Intake and the Risk of Coronary Heart Disease among the Coconut-Consuming Minangkabua in West Sumatra, Indonesia," *Asia Pacific Journal of Clinical Nutrition* 13, no. 4 (2004): 377–84.

22   A. Prior, F. Davidson, C. E. Salmond, and Z. Czochanska, "Cholesterol, Coconuts, and Diet on Polynesian Atolls: A Natural Experiment: the Pukapuka and Tokelau Island Studies." *American Journal of Clinical Nutrition* 34, no. 8 (1981): 1552–61

23   A. B. Feranil, P. L. Duazo, C. W. Kuzawa, and L. S. Adair, "Coconut Oil Is Associated with a Beneficial Lipid Profile in Pre-Menopausal Women in the Philippines," *Asia Pacific Journal of Clinical Nutrition* 20, no. 2 (2011): 190–95.

24   H. Tsuji, M. Kasai, H. Takeuchi, et al., "Dietary Medium-Chain Triacylglycerols Suppress Accumulation of Body Fat in a Double-Blind, Controlled Trial in Healthy Men and Women," *Journal of Nutrition* 131, no. 11 (2001): 2853–59.

25   J. Sabate, "Nut Consumption, Vegetarian Diets, Ischemic Heart Disease Risk, and All-Cause Mortality: Evidence from Epidemiological Studies," *American Journal of Clinical Nutrition* 70, suppl. 3 (1999): 500S–03S.

notes

26 C. M. Albert, J. M. Gaziano, W. C. Wilett, and J. E. Manson, "Nut Consumption and Decreased Risk of Sudden Cardiac Death in the Physicians' Health Study," *Archives of Internal Medicine* 162, no. 12 (2002): 1382–87.

27 R. U. Almario, V. Vonghavaravat, R. Wong, and S. E. Kasim-Karakas, "Effects of Walnut Consumption on Plasma Fatty Acids and Lipoproteins in Combined Hyperlipidemia," *American Journal of Clinical Nutrition* 74, no. 1 (2001): 72–79.

28 J. D. Curb, G. Wergowske, J. C. Dobbs, et al., "Serum Lipid Effects of a High-Monounsaturated Fat Diet Based on Macadamia Nuts," *Archives of Internal Medicine* 160, no. 8 (2000): 1154–58. S. Rajaram, K. Burke, B. Connell, et al., "A Monounsaturated Fatty Acid-Rich Pecan-Enriched Diet Favorably Alters the Serum Lipid Profile of Healthy Men and Women," *Journal of Nutrition* 131, no. 9 (2001): 2275–79.

29 J. Sabate, "Nut Consumption and Body Weight," *American Journal of Clinical Nutrition* 78, suppl. 3 (2003): 647S–50S.

30 R. Jiang, J. E. Manson, M. J. Stampfer, et al., "Nut and Peanut Butter Consumption and Risk of Type 2 Diabetes in Women," *Journal of the American Medical Association* 288, no. 20 (2002): 2254–60.

CHAPTER SIX

1 Food and Nutrition Board, Institute of Medicine of the National Academies, "Dietary Reference Intakes for Energy, Carbohydrate, Fiber, Fat, Fatty Acids, Cholesterol, Protein, and Amino Acids," last updated September 2002, www.iom.edu/Reports/2002/Dietary-Reference-Intakes-for-Energy-Carbohydrate-Fiber-Fat-Fatty-Acids-Cholesterol-Protein-and-Amino-Acids.aspx.

2 Rip Esselstyn, *The Engine 2 Diet*, (Hachette Book Group, New York, 2009) and http://engine2diet.com/question/are-plant-proteins-complete-proteins.

3 C. N. Meredith, W. R. Frontera, K. P. O'Reilly, and W. J. Evans, "Body Composition in Elderly Men: Effect of Dietary Modification during Strength Training," *Journal of the American Geriatric Society* 40, no. 2 (1992): 155–62.

4 http://live.psu.edu/story/47514.

5 von Schacky, P. Angerer, W. Kothny, et al., The Effect of Dietary Omega-3 Fatty Acids on Coronary Atherosclerosis. A Randomized, Double-Blind, Placebo-Controlled Trial," *Annals of Internal Medicine* 130, no. 7 (1999): 544–62. K. He, E. B. Rimm, A. Merchant, et al., "Fish Consumption and Risk of Stroke in Men," *Journal of the American Medical Association* 288, no. 24 (2002): 3130–36. J. M. Geleijinse, E. J. Giltay, D. E. Grobbee, et al., "Blood Pressure Response to Fish Oil Supplementation: Metagregression Analysis of Randomized Trials," *Journal of Hypertension* 20, no. 8 (2002): 1491–99. C. M. Albert, H. Campos, M. J. Stampfer, et al., "Blood Levels of Long-Chain *n*-3 Fatty Acids and Risk of Sudden Death," *New England Journal of Medicine* 346, no. 15 (2002): 1113–18.

6 D. Mozaffarian, R. N. Lemaitre, L. H. Kuller, et al. "Cardiac Benefits of Fish Consumption May Depend on the Type of Fish Meal Consumed: The Cardiovascular Health Study," *Circulation* 107, no. 10 (2003): 1372–77.

7 A. Ramel, M. T. Jonsdottir, and I. Thorsdottir, "Consumption of Cod and Weight Loss in Young Overweight and Obese Adults on an Energy Reduced Diet for 8-Weeks," *Nutrition, Metabolism, and Cardiovascular Disease* 19, no. 1 (2009): 690–96.

8 P. Y. Lin and K. P. Su, "A Meta-analytic Review of Double-blind, Placebo-controlled Trials of Antidepressant Efficacy of Omega-3 Fatty Acids," *Journal of Clinical Psychiatry* 68, no. 7 (2007): 1056-61.

9 J. Zhang, S. Sasaki, K. Amano, and H. Kesteloot, "Fish Consumption and Mortality from all Causes, Ischemic Heart Disease and Stroke: An Ecological Study," *Preventative Medicine* 28, no. 5 (1999): 520–29.

10 P. W. Davidson, G. J. Myers, C. Cox, et al., "Effects of Prenatal and Postnatal Methylmercury Exposure from Fish Consumption on Neurodevelopment: Outcomes

at 66 Months of Age in the Seychelles Child Development Study," *Journal of the American Medical Association* 280, no. 8 (1998): 701–07. G. J. Myers, P. W. Davidson, C. Cox, et al., "Prenatal Methylmercury Exposure from Ocean Fish Consumption in the Seychelles Child Development Study," *Lancet* 361, no. 9370 (2003): 1686–92.

11 U. S. Barzel and L. K. Massey, "Excess Dietary Protein Can Adversely Affect Bone," *Journal of Nutrition* 128, no. 6 (1998): 1051–55.

12 D. E. Sellmeyer, K. L. Stone, A. Sebastian, and S. R. Cummings, "A High Ratio of Dietary Animal to Vegetable Protein Increases the Rate of Bone Loss and the Risk of Fracture in Postmenopausal Women. Study of Osteoporotic Fractures Research Group," *American Journal of Clinical Nutrition* 73, no. 1 (2001): 118–22.

13 D. Feskanich, W. C. Willett, M. J. Stampfer, and G. A. Colditz, "Milk, Dietary Calcium, and Bone Fractures in Women: A 12-Year Prospective Study," *American Journal of Public Health* 87, no. 6 (1997): 992–97.

14 D. Geskanich, P. Weber, W. C. Willett, et al., "Vitamin K Intake and Hip Fractures in Women: A Prospective Study," *American Journal of Clinical Nutrition* 69, no. 1 (1999): 74–79.

15 A. Host, "Frequency of Cow's Milk Allergy in Childhood," *Annals of Allergy, Asthma, and Immunology* 89, no. 6, suppl. 1 (2002): 33–37.

16 A. M. Collins, "Xenogeneic Antibodies and Atopic Disease," *Lancet* 1, no. 8588 (1988): 734–37.

17 M. Knip, S. M. Virtanen, K. Seppä, et al., "Dietary Intervention in Infancy and Later Signs of Beta-Cell Autoimmunity," *New England Journal of Medicine* 363, no. 20 (2010): 1900–08.

18 S. Raimondi, J. B. Mabrouk, B. Shatenstein, et al., "Diet and Prostate Cancer Risk with Specific Focus on Dairy Products and Dietary Calcium: A Case-Control Study," *Prostate* 70, no. 1 (2010): 1051–65.

19 D. Malosse, H. Perron, A. Sasco, and J. M. Seigneurin, "Correlation between Milk and Dairy Product Consumption and Multiple Sclerosis Prevalence: A Worldwide Study," *Neuroepidemiology* 11, nos. 4–6 (1992): 304–12.

CHAPTER SEVEN

1 R. C. Cabot, "The Relation of Alcohol to Atherosclerosis," *Journal of the American Medical Association* 43 (1904): 774–75.

2 P. Boffetta and L. Garfinkel, "Alcohol Drinking and Mortality among Men Enrolled in an American Cancer Society Prospective Study," *Epidemiology* 1, no. 5 (1990): 342–48. G. Maskarinec, L. Meng, and L. N. Kolonel, "Alcohol Intake, Body Weight, and Mortality in a Multiethnic Prospective Cohort," *Epidemiology* 9, no. 6 (1998): 654–61.

3 J. M. Gaziano, T. A. Gaziano, R. J. Glynn, et al., "Light-to-Moderate Alcohol Consumption and Mortality in the Physicians' Health Study Enrollment Cohort," *Journal of the American College of Cardiology* 35, no. 1 (2000): 96–105.

4 T. Truelsen, M. Gronbaek, P. Schnohr, and G. Boysen, "Intake of Beer, Wine, and Spirits and Risk of Stroke: The Copenhagen City Heart Study." *Stroke* 29, no. 12 (1998): 2467–72.

5 M. S. Elkind, F. Sciacca, B. Boden-Albala, et al., "Moderate Alcohol Consumption Reduces Risk of Ischemic Stroke: The Northern Manhattan Study," *Stroke* 37, no. 1 (2006): 13–19.

6 A. Tjønneland, J. Christensen, A. Olsen, et al., "Folate Intake, Alcohol and Risk of Breast Cancer among Postmenopausal Women in Denmark," *European Journal of Clincal Nutrition* 60, no. 2 (2006): 280–86.

7 C. G. Solomon, F. B. Hu, M. J. Stampfer, et al., "Moderate Alcohol Consumption and Risk of Coronary Heart Disease among Women with Type 2 Diabetes Mellitus," *Circulation* 102, no. 5 (2000): 494–99.

8 M. J. Stampfer, G. A. Colditz, W. C. Willet, et al., "A Prospective Study of Moderate

Alcohol Drinking and Risk of Diabetes in Women." *American Journal of Epidemiology* 128, no. 3 (1988): 549–58.

9   M. J. Davies, D. J. Baer, J. T. Judd, et al., "Effects of Moderate Alcohol Intake on Fasting Insulin and Glucose Concentrations and Insulin Sensitivity in Postmenopausal Women: A Randomized Controlled Trial," *Journal of the American Medical Association* 287, no. 19 (2002): 2559–62.

10   A. Larson and I. Larson *The Gold Coast Cure: The 5-Week Health & Body Makeover,*" Health Communications, Inc., Deerfield Beach, 2005.

11   L. Cordain, E. D. Bryan, C. L. Melby, and M. J. Smith, "Influence of Moderate Daily Wine Consumption on Body Weight Regulation and Metabolism in Healthy Free-Living Males," *Journal of the American College of Nurtition* 16, no. 2 (1997): 134–39.

12   http://www.cnn.com/2010/HEALTH/03/08/women.drink.weight/index.html.

13   L. Wang, I. M. Lee, J. E. Manson, et al., "Alcohol Consumption, Weight Gain, and Risk of Becoming Overweight in Middle-Aged and Older Women," *Archives of Internal Medicine* 170, no. 5 (2010): 453–61.

14   J. R. Greenfield, K. Samaras, A. B. Jenkins, et al., "Moderate Alcohol Consumption, Dietary Fat Composition, and Abdominal Obesity in Women: Evidence for Gene-Environment Interaction," *Journal of Clinical Endocrinology and Metabolism* 88, no. 11 (2003): 5381–86.

15   S. Liu, M. K. Derdula, D. F. Williamson, et al., "A Prospective Study of Alcohol Intake and Change in Body Weight among US Adults," *American Journal of Epidemiology* 140, no. 10 (1994): 912–20.

16   H. S. Kahn, L. M. Tatham, C. Rodriguez, et al., "Stable Behaviors Associated with Adults' 10-Year Change in Body Mass Index and Likelihood of Gain at the Waist," *American Journal of Public Health* 87, no. 5 (1997): 747–54.

CHAPTER EIGHT

1   T. M. Manini, J. E. Everhart, K. V. Patel, et al., "Daily Activity Energy Expenditure and Mortality Among Older Adults," *Journal of the American Medical Association* 296, no. 2 (2006): 171–79.

2   A. Chatzinikolaou, I. Fatouros, A. Petridou, et al., "Adipose Tissue Lipolysis Is Unregulated in Lean and Obese Men during Acute Resistance Exercise," *Diabetes Care* 31, no. 7 (2008): 1397–99.

3   J. L. Talanian, S. D. Galloway, G. J. Heigenhauser, et. al., "Two Weeks of High-Intensity Aerobic Interval Training Increases the Capacity for Fat Oxidation During Exercise in Women." *Journal of Applied Physiology* 102, no. 4 (2007): 1439-47.

4   D. S. Petitt, S. A. Arngímsson, and K. J. Cureton, "Effect of Resistance Exercise on Postprandial Lipemia," *Journal of Applied Physiology* 94, no. 2 (2003): 694–700.

5   E. G. Trapp, D. J. Chisholm, J. Freund, and S. H. Boutcher, "The Effects of High-Intensity Intermittent Exercise Training on Fat Loss and Fasting Insulin Levels of Young Women," *International Journal of Obesity* (London) 32, no. 4 (2008): 684–91.

6   A. McTiernan, B. Sorensen, M. L. Irwin, et al., "Exercise Effect on Weight and Body Fat in Men and Women," *Obesity* (Silver Spring) 15, no. 6 (2007): 1496–512.

CHAPTER NINE

1   R. H. Fletcher and K. M. Fairfield, "Vitamins for Chronic Disease Prevention in Adults: Clinical Applications," *Journal of the American Medical Association* 287, no. 23 (2002): 3127–29.

2   E. J. Gardner, C. H. Ruxton, A. R. Reeds, "Black Tea—Helpful or Harmful? A Review of the Evidence." *European Journal of Clinical Nutrition* 61, no. 1 (2007); 3–18.

3   S. Kuriyama, T. Shimazu, K Ohmori, et al., "Green Tea Consumption and Mortality Due to Cardiovascular Disease, Cancer, and All Causes in Japan: The Ohsaki Study," *Journal of the American Medical Association* 296, no. 10 (2006): 1255–65.

4   U. Heinrich, C. E. Moore, S. De Spirt, et. al., "Green Tea Polyphenols Provide Photoprotection, Increase Microcirculation, and Modulate Skin Properties of Women." *Journal of Nutrition* 141, no. 6 (2011); 1202–08.

5   A. G. Dulloo, C. Duret, D. Rohrer, et al., "Efficacy of a Green Tea Extract Rich in Catechin Polyphenols and Caffeine in Increasing 24-h Energy Expenditure and Fat Oxidation in Humans," *American Journal of Clinical Nutrition* 70, no. 6 (1999): 1040–05.

6   J. M. Geleijnse, C. Vermeer, D. E. Grobbee, et al., "Dietary Intake of Menaquinone Is Associated with a Reduced Risk of Coronary Heart Disease: The Rotterdam Study," *Journal of Nutrition* 134, no. 11 (2004): 3100–05.

7   G. C. Gast, N. M. de Roos, I. Sluijs, et al., "A High Menaquinone Intake Reduces the Incidence of Coronary Heart Disease," *Nutrition, Metabolism, and Cardiovascular Diseases* 19, no. 7 (2009): 504–10.

8   B. W. Hollis, "Circulating 25-Hydroxyvitamin D Levels Indicative of Vitamin D Sufficiency: Implications for Establishing a New Effective Dietary Intake Recommendation for Vitamin D," *Journal of Nutrition* 1235, no. 2 (2005): 317–22.

9   K. L. Munger, S. M. Zhang, E. O'Reilly, et al., "Vitamin D Intake and Incidence of Multiple Sclerosis," *Neurology* 62, no. 1 (2004): 60–65.

10   C. Stevinson, M. H. Pittler, and E. Ernst, "Garlic for Treating Hypercholesterolemia. A Meta-Analysis of Randomized Controlled Trials," *Annals of Internal Medicine* 133, no. 6 (2000): 420–29.

11   T. Ishikawa, Y. Fujiyama, O. Igarashi, et al., "Effects of Gammalinolenic Acid on Plasma Lipoproteins and Apolipoproteins," *Atherosclerosis* 75, nos. 2–3 (1989): 95–104.

INDEX

Page numbers in **bold** indicate charts and tables; those in *italic* indicate figures and photographs.

451